Poverty and Fertility in India

Poverty and Fertility in India

Demographic Field Theory Perspective

SHEKHAR MUKHERJI

RAWAT PUBLICATIONS
Jaipur • New Delhi • Bangalore • Mumbai • Hyderabad • Guwahati

ISBN 81-316-0085-8

Published by
Prem Rawat for **Rawat Publications**
Satyam Apts, Sector 3, Jawahar Nagar, Jaipur 302 004 (India)
Phone: 0141 265 1748 / 7006 Fax: 0141 265 1748
E-mail: info@rawatbooks.com
Website: www.rawatbooks.com

New Delhi Office
4858/24, Ansari Road, Daryaganj, New Delhi 110 002
Phone: 011 2326 3290

Also at Bangalore, Mumbai, Hyderabad and Guwahati

Typeset by Rawat Computers, Jaipur
Printed at Chaman Enterprises, New Delhi

Dedicated to

Professor Rudolf J. Rummel

Emeritus Professor of Political Science,
University of Hawaii at Manoa, Honolulu, Hawaii, USA

to whom I am very grateful for his proposed links between demographic, socio-economic and population policies – a concept which formed main idea of Demographic Field Theory here.

Contents

List of Illustrations

List of Tables

Preface

The study of causal linkages between abject poverty, on the one hand, and high fertility and high infant mortality, on the other, has not been yet adequately and satisfactorily investigated in India, nor elsewhere. Though this crucial issue should have been the most pertinent concern of greatest national importance, but, most unfortunately, this was never given its due and proper attention by scholars and planners in India. Consequently, although India was the first country in the world to initiate family planning programme (since 1951), but her achievement in controlling population explosion was not at all spectacular. One of the most important reasons for such failure was tunnel vision of the policy makers and scholars and their persistent refusal to face and resolve the most basic causal relationships between poverty and high fertility in India. Unless the most basic problem of India is tackled, the so-called super structure of family welfare and public health services falls as house of cards! In the meantime, six decades of most precious time have vanished. The main objective of this book, thus, is to draw the attention of politicians, planners, policy makers and scholars to this vital issue of supreme national importance.

Not only there is a lack of sound and mathematically verifiable theoretical and analytical design to unfold the nexus between poverty and fertility, but there is also a dearth of detailed data on income poverty and other indices of deprivation at the individual level, on the one hand, and also of fine-grained demographic, socio-economic and population policy/programme data at the same unit of observations, on the other. Such lacuna hampered unfolding of the crucial nexus between poverty and fertility.

Recently, however, National Family and Health Surveys (NFHS) and reports have provided very good data and excellent description of levels of fertility, mortality, family planning and MCH in various Indian states. But, so far, adequate and threadbare analytic and synthetic investigations have not yet been made to unfold the crucial aspect: why fertility and mortality remain very high in many poverty-stricken states (like Uttar Pradesh, Madhya Pradesh, Bihar, Rajasthan), or what are the crucial determinants of fertility and mortality in Indian situation? What are the basic causal relations between poverty and fertility in India? How could we reduce abject poverty and high fertility in the country?

Unfortunately, NFHS surveys were never concerned with such basic and most crucial issues, and so never collected 'poverty' data, nor attempted to unravel causal linkages between poverty and fertility in India. Sadly, the conventional demographers or population scientists are not concerned with unfolding such crucial nexus. These are most unfortunate trends, specially in highly populous and poverty-stricken country, like India.

Answer to such crucial population questions needs a comprehensive and holistic approach of analysis, which would encompass demographic, socio-economic, and policy-programme variables, treating them simultaneously, not in isolation.

The Demographic Field Theory approach, as developed and successfully tested by the present author during 1975-83, and associated canonical models, provide answers to such basic questions, and thereby highlights the most fundamental changes that are required in present policies and society in Indian context. This study provides some very crucial findings that emerged out of application of the Demographic Field Theory to analyze demographic, socio-economic, and policy-programme data of Indian states, using recent NFHS-I survey data (1992-93), and also of NFHS-II survey of 1998-99.

In so doing, whatever data from NFHS surveys could be utilized for proxy measurements of poverty (and fertility), were made in this study, and hence the relations between indirect indices of poverty and fertility were found by performing various Demographic Field Theory models and canonical analyses.

Attempts have been thus made, and it was rewarding, as the findings mathematically confirmed the dismal truth, which conventional researchers have ignored since last six decades.

Even after sixty years of India's independence, it is very disheartening that India's fertility and infant mortality rates remain at very high level, and, as the findings have shown time and again, these are primarily caused due to abject poverty and widespread illiteracy among the people, specially females.

The main purpose of this study is to draw urgent attention of the scholars, planners and the policy makers of India to such dismal situation, specially to the basic cause-and-effect relationship between poverty and high fertility in India and her numerous neglected and backward states. Multitudes of very highly powerful canonical linkages have repeatedly confirmed the basic truth that it is the widespread illiteracy and concomitant abject poverty among the masses, specially females, which is the root cause of persistently high fertility and very high infant mortality. Unless and until such oppressive situations are not relieved, no improvement in demographic and socio-economic condition would happen in India.

Findings have conclusively demonstrated that nothing is going to change in India, unless we set our priorities right and provide the barest essentials of food and functional education to the poor masses and the downtrodden. This calls for soulful efforts for providing (a) massive poverty eradication programmes and universal female literacy programmes, all over India, specially in the neglected, remote and inaccessible regions, and (b) concerted efforts for improving health services and family planning services therein. Alleviation of people's basic living condition and poverty eradication must precede all other efforts for the improvement of their reproductive health and general health. Without the fulfilment of the first condition, as the findings repeatedly shown, the motivation for adopting the small family norm is very difficult to emerge. This is the basic lesson from this investigation. I do sincerely hope that all stake holders will take notice of these hard realities, before it is too late for India and her people.

This study was undertaken in 1995, and the research monograph completed in 1997. But, due to my manifold research activities over successive period and my perfectionist attitude, I always wanted to add more, update and revise again. As such, it got delayed. Meantime, NFHS-II data were also collected (during 1998-99). So, I have also briefly analyzed these data, and presented in Chapter 10, and found that almost similar patterns of results persisted that emanated from canonically analyzing earlier NHFS-I sets. So, all major findings remained the same, albeit in modified form; and this tremendously testified the strength of my central theoretical and analytical design, as well as the most important policy implications of main findings. Nothing changes in India overnight. Even data of Census 2001 or Sample Registration Survey (SRS, 2003) have not revealed any drastic changes in fertility, nor in precarious socio-economic condition of common people.

In this book, most recent demographic situation in India is also examined with the help of Census 2001 and SRS data (2003). Socio-economic situation is investigated with various Census 2001 data on social and cultural tables, educational tables, and housing tables. Most recent health situation in various states is explored with two Reproductive and Child Health (RCH) survey data of 1998-99 and 2002-04. Hence, the crucial causal relationship between poverty and fertility is examined, time and again, with most recent data, and the findings are found to be very relevant.

In short, this study deals with one of the most crucial issues – abject poverty and high fertility in India. These are the most glaring problems, which demand our immediate attention and permanent solution. Unless these are solved, unfortunately, India would remain a poor Third World country, in spite of her recent so-called 'software super-power' fame. Unless the life of the poorest of the poor in India is improved, we cannot afford any complacency! And, we cannot claim that we have performed our basic and most sacred duty to our fellow human beings!

The book is very respectfully dedicated to Professor Rudolf J. Rummel, Emeritus Professor in Political Science, University of

Hawaii at Manoa, Honolulu, Hawaii, USA to whom I am very much indebted for learning his Social Field Theory and canonical analyses in early 1970s during my PhD study. I am also very much indebted to him for his proposed concept of making a cross-country field-theoretic linkages between demographic, socio-economic-political-cultural, and population policy systems – the concept which was later expanded, structured and mathematically and empirically tested by me in the form of Demographic Field Theory formulations (during 1975-83), its constant refinements and its manifold verifications (1983-2001). Indeed, I am very grateful to him for his innovative ideas of 1975-76.

A study such as this needs help from many. I am grateful to Prof. K.B. Pathak and Prof. T.K. Roy, former Directors, International Institute for Population Sciences (IIPS), Mumbai, for project funding. I also sincerely thank Prof. G Rama Rao, Research Coordinator, for kindly distributing old draft, first, as xeroxed research monograph of IIPS.

My thanks also go to all concerned persons in NFHS survey and data processing team, who have provided excellent basic data. Without such good data, it was difficult to make inroads into current demographic, socio-economic and policy programme situation in India. Regarding analysis of data, a specific kind of field theoretic models and multivariate techniques were developed by me and employed in this study. In this respect, I am very sincerely grateful to Shri Robert Marshal, Assistant Research Officer (ARO) of the project for major computer programming help. Without this, numerous technical analyses would have been very difficult. I am also very much indebted to Shri M. Dharmar, Institute's former Programmer, who helped in some canonical analyses.

My sincere thanks also go to Shri Madhu Ratnam, and also Shri Dinesh Pon Dhas, other AROs, for setting tables from computer outputs. I am also sincerely grateful to Ms Sai Thakur, new ARO, who meticulously transferred former entire computer files into new MS-Word format. My thanks are also due to late Gopal Padmashali, Institute's Artist, for his expert cartographic help for inking and finalizing my all draft maps and figures. Shri Motital Mohare also helped in finalizing some maps of 1998-99. I am also very thankful to Shri R.B.

Lakhan for many cartographic and photographic assistance. I am also grateful to all others, not specifically mentioned here, but who have helped me in various ways.

Last, but not the least, my very special thanks and gratitude go to Shri Pranit Rawat and all in Rawat Publications for their professional excellence and utmost care for very nice and timely publication of the book.

As stated at the outset, this study was completed by July 1997. Although numerous research papers were already published, highlighting the main findings about causal relationships between poverty and fertility in India, but unfortunately, its publication as a book was much delayed due to some unavoidable circumstances.

However, nothing changes in India overnight, and the basic causal relationships of abject poverty and high fertility remain very much the same in India, even today (2005-06). Attempts are however made, as far as possible, to examine and highlight recent demographic and socio-economic situation, as well as health condition of the people in various states, and also to update the references and issues. Besides, the great utility and elegance of the Demographic Field Theory, as a novel and innovative analytic and theoretic tool to unfold the most complex causal relations between demographic system, socio-economic system and population system of any country and of the world, will remain very much relevant for a long time. Like a general analytic strategy, this theoretic tool can be effectively utilized for untangling the complex nexus of demographic-socio-economic-policy systems and for generating socio-economic development policies and population policies for any nation of the world.

Shekhar Mukherji

Message of Swami Vivekananda

"Feel, my children, feel; feel for the poor, the ignorant, the downtrodden; feel till the heart stops and brain reels and you think you will go mad – then pour the soul out at the feet of the Lord, and then will come the power, help, and indomitable energy."

Swami Vivekananda (1893)
(Complete Work, Centenary Volume IV, 1963, p. 367)

1

Introduction

"Say, the ignorant Indian, the poor and destitute Indian, the Brahmin Indian, the Pariah Indian is my brother" (Swami Vivekananda, 1896, Complete Work, Centenary Volume IV, 1963, p. 480).

"Arise, awake, for your country needs this tremendous sacrifice" (Swami Vivekananda, 1893, Complete Work, Centenary Volume III, 1963, p. 318).

Complex Economic-Demographic Linkages

The greatest human problem of this Planet Earth now has been its very rapidly growing population explosion and concomitant issues of maintaining sustainable development, without deteriorating the humanity's cradle, the earth's environment. As International Conference on Population and Development (UNFPA, ICPD, Cairo, 1994) had emphasized, the world's the then population of 5.8 billion will cross 12 billion by the year 2050, unless its birth rate is drastically reduced now by vigorously adopting fertility reduction measures. If fertility in the developing countries can be drastically reduced from now on, then chances may arise that the world's population may be stabilized at 8.5 billion by year 2025, and the war on hunger, famine, destruction, and environmental catastrophe can be averted. Given this global context, very high fertility in South Asia, specially in India, is all the more alarming!

Complex interrelationships between economic factors and fertility behaviour are not yet well understood and specially so in low-income country like India. Most demographers and economists argue that high level of fertility of household actually deteriorates its well-being, and its income, household consumption, savings, and investment, and consequently, generates poverty (Coale and Hoover, 1958, pp. 11-31; Demeny, 1972, pp. 1-12; Srinivasan, 1988, pp. 94-101; Gilispie, 1998, pp. 34-38). According to them, high fertility at household level causes poverty. While their arguments are quite strong that per capita foodgrains intake or size of landholdings decreases as size of family increases, and that very little is left for savings, investment, or raising level of living; but such arguments often fail to answer to crucial questions: Why, at the first place, is level of fertility high only among the poor families? Why, is it low among urbanized, educated and affluent families?

Thus, very few demographers ever question the above hypothesis and ever ask themselves: of the two factors, poverty and fertility, which one is the cause, and which one is the effect? Is it not true that poverty-stricken condition of households is conducive to give births to excessive number of children? Is it not true that poverty and illiteracy make it imperative to give births to a large number of children as a means of more hands of labour and old age security? Such crucial issues urgently need very intensive and extensive research.

This book, thus, deals with crucial causal linkages between poverty and high fertility in India, from a theoretical perspective, called the *Demographic Field Theory*. Crucial issue of poverty, widespread female illiteracy and high fertility in India should be given their due and tremendous focus in population research and action plans, which is very sadly missing. Most Indian demographers, geographers and social scientists forgot this very crucial issue, and also forgot Mother India. It is strongly urged in this study that we must emphasize upon this crucial issue and do meaningful research on this interface. Intensive analysis of these crucial aspects is done here by canonically analyzing recent National Family and Health Survey (NFHS-I) (1992-93) data, and later NFHS-II (1998-99) data. Unfortunately, NFHS did not collect economic or poverty data, so female illiteracy data is taken as 'proxy' indicator of poverty. Results show that widespread poverty, or very high female illiteracy is the main *cause,* and high fertility and high infant mortality are the *effects.* This crucial cause-and-effect relationship has repeatedly emerged through many very high powered canonical analyses, and this relationship must be highlighted in policies and action programmes.

It is very sad that most Indian population specialists/social scientists forgot their sacred duty to unfold this 'truth' and to help the poor and downtrodden through committed research, and by planning for the poor. Evidence of such great lacuna can be easily seen, e.g., even the word 'poverty' cannot be easily found in 26 reports of NFHS-I 1992-93 survey (NFHS, 1994a, 1994b, 1995), nor in another 26 reports of NFHS-II 1998-99 survey (NFHS, 2000). Neither nexus between poverty and population was highlighted in National Population Policy, 1994 (Ministry of Health, Government of India, 1995), nor in National Population Policy, 2000 (Ministry of Health, Government of India, 2000). Nor in the recent National Rural Health Mission Document (NRHM, 2005). These are eye-openers. So, the main purpose of the book is to unfold such crucial relationship, and consequently draw the attention of scholars and planners, policy makers and the administrators, before it reaches a catastrophe.

The basic issue is to find answers to some such questions: Why fertility and mortality remain very high in many states (UP, MP, Bihar, Rajasthan)? Or, what are the crucial determinants of fertility and mortality in India? Answer to such crucial questions need a holistic approach, which would encompass demographic, socio-economic, and policy-programme variables, treating simultaneously, not in exclusion of each other.

The Demographic Field Theoretic approach, as developed and successfully tested by the present author (Mukherji, 1977b, pp. 250-266; 1983a, pp. 161-177; 1983b, pp. 1-141), and associated canonical models, provide answers to such basic questions; and highlights most fundamental changes required in Indian policies and society. This study provides some very crucial findings that emerged out of the application of the Demographic Field Theory to analyze demographic, socio-economic, and policy-programme data of Indian states, using recent NFHS survey data of 1992-93 (NFHS, 1995, various tables) and also 1998-99 sets (NFHS, 2000). Attempts have been thus made, and it was rewarding that the findings mathematically and empirically confirmed the dismal reality, which conventional researchers and policy makers are trying to ignore since last six decades.

Unfortunately, the NFHS team and its various reports have not attempted such thread-bare and highly powerful mathematical canonical analyses. The results of are presented throughout the book, which are confirmed mathematically by performing very high powered canonical models and their manifold findings.

Crucial Demographic and Socio-Economic Problems in India

Demographic and socio-economic situation of India is very precarious. Even after 60 years of India's independence, it is very disheartening that India's fertility and infant mortality rates have remained very high, and these are primarily caused due to abject poverty and widespread illiteracy among people, specially among the females. Total fertility rate (TFR), or the average number of children per mother, is still at 3.4 level (in 1992-93), which is far higher than the replacement level, or 2.1 children. Rural TFR is still 3.7 children per mother (1992-93), which is 36 per cent higher than urban TFR of 2.7 children. Considerable variations also occur in this all-India TFR, for instance, TFR is as high as 4.82 children in Uttar Pradesh, 4 in Bihar, 4.25 in Arunachal Pradesh, and 3.90 in Madhya Pradesh. Rural TFR is still much higher, e.g., in Uttar Pradesh it is as high as is 5.19 children, followed by 4.15 in Bihar and 4.11 in Madhya Pradesh. Thus, in spite of considerable family planning campaign and practices in India since 1951, not much dent upon fertility level is yet made.

Situation of infant mortality is no better either. According to NFHS-I (1992-93), infant mortality rate (IMR) is still very high: 78.5 deaths of infants per 1,000 live born children within the first year; and under-five mortality is 109.3 deaths per 1,000 children born during five years preceding survey. Unfortunately, IMR sometimes exceeds 100 per 1,000 live births (112 in Orissa, 100 in Uttar Pradesh). In rural India, sometimes, it exceeds even 116.9 in Orissa and 108 in Uttar Pradesh. In 1992-93, under-five child mortality (CMR) in rural India exceeds 130 per 1,000 live births in many states (152 in Uttar Pradesh, 146 in Bihar, 145 in Madhya Pradesh, and 135 in Orissa). Indeed, tremendous dent upon infant mortality and child mortality is very urgently needed. In India, IMR and TFR are intimately connected, so we need to reduce IMR much before TFR can be expected to decline.

The socio-economic situation of India is not very heartening either. Recent figures of the Planning Commission have estimated that population below poverty level is about 360 million in 1997, about 37 per cent of total population. Chronic problems of abject rural poverty, swelling of urban poverty, widespread adult and female illiteracy, pronounced regional disparity, acute unemployment, and a sluggish economic growth have plagued India since last three decades. All such conditions need vast systems transformations immediately.

Set within this context, interactions of demographic-geographic-socio-economic-cultural variables and population policies are very complex and not yet well understood. Analytical research is still very much required to ascertain those linkages in highly populous but developing countries like India, and similarly placed countries, which are still characterized by high TFR and IMR, low level of agricultural and industrial development, and respective governments still attempting (or not attempting) to reduce high fertility by adopting some population policies (Mukherji, 1982d, pp. 1-30). Many UN and World Bank reports have reiterated upon the great need for further research for better understanding of the complex links between demographic behaviour, socio-economic-cultural systems of societies, and population and development policies enacted to onset fertility decline (UN, 1992, pp. 51-83; 1993, pp. 3-9; World Bank, 1990, pp. 56-89; 1993, pp. 25-60).

Although the need for such kinds of research is long felt (UN, 1973, pp. 4-9), but suitable methodologies to determine such linkages are yet lacking. Set within this context of the research need and conceptual-methodological gap, it becomes very necessary to unentangle the complex web of interrelationships between the demographic behaviour (i.e., fertility/mortality/migration behaviour), geographic-socio-economic-cultural systems of the society, and various population policies enacted to affect demographic behaviour. Only with a proper understanding of such complex policy-demographic linkages, within socio-economic context, alternative population and development policies may be generated which would be more effective to quicken fertility transition in developing countries (Berelson, 1969, pp. 533-543; Coale and Hoover, 1958, pp. 43-44; Demeny, 1972, pp. 1-12; Rummel and Mukherji, 1981, pp. 1-81; Srinivasan, 1988, pp. 94-101). Thus, the overall objective of this study is to achieve better comprehension of this complex demographic-socio-economic-policy nexus, and to identify those socio-economic factors and policies which will quicken fertility-mortality decline in developing countries.

We need to know how a population policy works, whether it acts in alignment with the existing socio-economic milieu, or operates contrary to the social nexus, and therefore has little chance of success. We also need to know how the prevailing structure and forces of the socio-economic system of society affect the demographic behaviour of its population.

The Need for Comprehensive Approach

The Demographic Field Theoretic Approach, as developed and successfully tested by the present author during 1976-83 (Mukherji, 1983b, pp. 1-141), and associated canonical models (Mukherji, 1985d, pp. 1-20; 1985e, pp. 1-12), provide answers to above-mentioned basic questions; and thereby highlights the most fundamental changes required in the present policies and society in Indian context. This study provides some very crucial findings that emerged out of application of the Demographic Field Theory to analyze demographic, socio-economic, and policy-programmes data of Indian states, using recent NFHS-I survey data (1992-93) (NFHS, India, 1994).

The Demographic Field Theory attempts, by using canonical model, to ascertain causal relations between:

(a) demographic behaviour of different regions, or states, or individuals;
(b) geo-social-economic-cultural systems of those regions, or states, or individuals; and
(c) various population policies or programmes followed by those regions, or states, or individuals.

Specific Objectives

Following are the specific objectives of the study:

(a) to evolve a new theory, called the *Demographic Field Theory*, as a theoretical and analytical methodology of ascertaining the causal linkages between (i) geo-social-economic system of different states-cum-population policies adopted/followed by those states, on the one hand, and (ii) resulting demographic behaviour (fertility and mortality behaviour) of respective states on the other;

(b) to identify what socio-economic factors determine demographic behaviour;

(c) to ascertain what population policies or programmes are in alignment to the existing socio-economic nexus, and thus have more chance of success; and conversely, what population policies are contrary to the existing social milieu and thus stand little chance of success to onset fertility/mortality decline; and

(d) finally, based on the findings, to generate alternative population and development policies for India.

Relation between Poverty and Fertility Unraveled in Most Studies

NFHS did not collect poverty data, nor studied poverty situation, rather made a crude proxy index, termed Standard of Living Index (SLI), based on binary (yes-no type) information on items of possessions of the households. Items considered were: if the household have land, cattle, shelter, radio, cycle, watch, TV, utensils, etc.! As if, mostly poor Indian households can have such costly consumer goods! Some may even wonder, why were such items like car, scooter, micro oven, home theatre, liquor cabinet, or women's fashion magazine not included?

Problems with such a gross SLI measure is that it cannot capture the degree, intensity and the extent of poverty among the chronically poor and the very poor people, nor among the completely dispossessed people – who unfortunately live in the bottom pit of poverty, and who do not possess none of those items. Neither land, nor cattle, shelter, radio, cycle, or watch; nor even a water pitcher, and who perpetually live in perilous, damned, and most hapless poverty situation! Indeed, they constitute a very large segment of the rural population, mostly poor peasants, landless agricultural labourers, village operatives, masons, weavers, and an ocean of unemployed and underemployed rural workers. They constitute completely deprived people.

Very seldom the conventional demographers, bereft from such stark reality, have ever met them. Nor did their survey workers. As a result, this ocean of dispossessed masses are ticked and lumped together as one large undefined category in the survey, under that unscientific SLI measure. Thus, this SLI measure cannot decipher the poor, from the very poor, chronically poor, and those who sadly live in the bottom pit of poverty! Consequently, no causal relations between *'poverty'* and *'fertility'* do emerge in such research design, nor are reflected in such survey reports!

During the severe drought in Gujarat and Rajasthan in 1997-99 – exactly during the same period when NFHS-II survey were conducted – tens of millions of completely dispossessed and wretchedly poor people were forced to leave their villages and out-migrate in search of water, and they had only one small earthen pitcher with them, nothing else! No bicycle, no watch, no radio, no another cloth, and not even another earthen pitcher! Their photos also appeared in some newspapers. That was the stark and cruel reality! The basic truth which stares us in our face. But, unfortunately, the elitist Indian demographers, population scientists, geographers and social scientists still refuse to open their eyes and hearts, and look at the truth. Had they ever really seen and felt the stark reality of extreme poverty in Indian villages, then, they would have automatically motivated to measure and unravel the extent and character of poverty among hundreds of millions of the rural dispossessed, and had found the causal relations between high poverty and high fertility. Could have found long ago.

In 1998, before NFHS-II survey began, this author suggested to the NFHS organizers to include just minimum 1-2 page questionnaire, in their total package of questions, for direct measurement of income poverty (like various consumption expenditure data, or data of intake of basic food items, cereals, pulses, etc., or direct measurement of agricultural income), instead of gross SLI. But, that suggestion was summarily rejected. I was terribly amazed. As if, in India, population studies can ever scientifically be made, without directly referring to 'poverty' situation among the three hundred millions people! Wished, better sense would prevail soon among the Indian academia!

And, consequent to all such lacunae, no clear relationship between *'poverty and fertility'* and *'poverty and mortality'* can ever be found in such conventional demographic research. As a result, persistent problems of poverty and high fertility continued unresolved in India. Such crucial research remained always ignored and ridiculed. Thence, population research remained limited, and policy prescriptions, misdirected.

Organization of the Book

This study has following nine specific objectives:

- To present a brief outline of the Demographic Field Theory which was evolved as a conceptual and analytical means of determining multivariate linkages between the geo-social-economic systems of a society or a region and population policies on the one hand, and the demographic behaviour of that region, on the other.
- To demonstrate the use of a methodology consisting of principal components analysis and canonical models to assess the effects of population policies upon demographic behaviour, in the context of the socio-economic system of a region/society.
- To discuss the results of empirical tests of the theory, by taking different Indian states as units of observations, and by performing various canonical models.
- To repeat canonical analysis for each of major Indian states, by taking individual level data of the women respondents. It is surmised that such micro-level investigations may unravel some intriguing results that cannot be found from macro-level analysis.
- To devise 'Poverty Index' measurement using the individuals level data and causally relate them to fertility and infant mortality rates, for each major states, by performing a series of 25 canonical tests.
- To unravel changes that happened during 1992-93 to 1998-99 period in India's demographic, socio-economic and population programmes sets by performing a series of canonical analyses with NFHS-II data.

- To thoroughly examine recent-most data of Census 2001, Sample Registration Survey data of 2003, and Reproductive and Child Health data of 2002-04, and evaluate the changes, if any, in demographic, socio-economic, and health services in India.
- To highlight the policy implications of main findings for demographic development and welfare planning of Indian states.
- To recommend specific useful socio-economic development policies for poverty alleviation and illiteracy reduction, and health policies for demographic transition in India.

All the above nine objectives are interrelated, each issuing from the previous one.

Both NFHS-I survey data (1992-93) (Chapters IV to VIII) and NFHS-II survey data (1998-99) (Chapter X) are utilized, and many crucial findings are generated, based on author's unique Demographic Field Theoretic model. Various canonical findings have great policy import (Chapters IX, X, and XI). In Chapter XI, Reproductive and Child Health Survey data (Round I, 1998-99 and Round II, 2002-04) are also examined, as well as Census 2001 (available only in 2005) and Sample Registration Survey (SRS data of 2003) (available only in 2006). Hence, the study provides recent-most pictures, as far as possible.

It must be specifically mentioned, right at the outset, that NFHS surveys and their reports do not deal with people's poverty, nor with its crucial relations with fertility, and infant mortality. Nor these surveys ever collected data on poverty measures of the respondents, or the states. These are great lacunae of these surveys and studies.

On the other hand, this book has specifically dealt with this crucial relationship between poverty and fertility (by using female illiteracy as a proxy indicator of poverty). Besides, it has also evolved and developed indirect measures of poverty levels of the women respondents (by using indices of female illiteracy, lack of water and toilet facilities in the households, lack of health services to the female respondents, and the like), and have ascertained the causal relations between poverty and fertility. In this respect, this research is novel and unique and makes very valuable contribution to demographic and population studies, as well as to geographical and population policy research. Besides, these findings on poverty and fertility have great national importance for India, and similar countries.

2

The Demographic Field Theory

"You must have an iron will if you would cross the ocean. You must be strong enough to pierce mountains" (Swami Vivekananda, 1893, Complete Work, Centenary Volume VI, 1963, p. 297).

"Test everything, try everything, and then believe it, and if you find it for the good of many, give it to all" (Swami Vivekananda, 1894, Complete Work, Centenary Volume III, 1963, p. 528).

The Field Concept in Social Sciences and Previous Studies

In geography, although there has been a lot of studies made on spatial organization (Abler, Adams, and Gould, 1971, pp. 12-51) and spatial behaviour (Wolpert, 1965, pp. 158-180), but so far very little research is done to link and integrate the spatial behaviour to spatial structure. Essentially, such linkages and integration between the structure of attributes (of places, or people, or individuals) and the patterns of spatial behaviour between them required a field theoretic approach – an approach which could causally link the behaviour of the objects towards each other to the attributes of the objects themselves and their differences, all seen in an integrative manner. Evidently, for a long time, there has been a gap between the research need felt and the theoretical-cum-methodological ways and means of achieving such integrative design.

It was the classic work of German psychologist Kurt Lewin (1951, pp. 1-250), which showed the pathway towards such an integrative approach. For the first time in social sciences, Lewin presented a *Psychological Field Theory* in which he attempted to explain the behaviour of the juvenile delinquents in German prisons by integrating their behaviour with their social attributes and couching both behaviour and attributes in the context of the specific environment in which the delinquents were placed in.

However, Lewin's field theory was descriptive, loosely fashioned, and not structurally organized; nor was it presented in a form that could be mathematically verifiable or testable. According to his own statements, his field theory was not a theory, rather a method, and a philosophy to view behaviour and attributes in their causal relations. However, Lewin's basic research interest was to unfold juvenile delinquency (not population and demography).

The credit for formulating and successfully testing a theoretically organized and mathematically testable field theory in social sciences goes to Rudolf J. Rummel (1965, pp. 183-97) who contributed a new *Field Theory of Social Action* in order to explain the conflict behaviour within nations and between nations. Rummel, in his life-long contributions to field theories, also provided new formulations, titled as *Dynamic Psychological Field* (1975, pp. 1-150) in which he dealt with the dynamics of conflict and war between the individuals and the peoples, as well as between the nations. In 1979, Rummel published his classic book, *Field Theory Evolving* (1979, pp. 1-152), which summed up his life-long research on social-psychological field theories in an evolving fashion, along with a socio-philosophical context, where he explored into the roots of violence and war in the minds of man! Thus, his basic research interests are political science and international relations, not demography.

It must be mentioned that in geography and the studies of spatial behaviour, the credit goes to Brian Berry (1966, 1969) who for the first time gave a spatial translation of the above-mentioned attempts of field theory formulation of psychology (of Lewin) and of political science (of Rummel). Berry, in his pioneering study of commodity flows and the spatial structure of the Indian economy (1966, pp. 6-151), has made a very laudable contribution by providing a spatial transformation of field theories of other sciences by referring it specifically to the spatial interactions between the places. In this study, he investigated the relationship between spatial economic structure and the commodity flows amongst the states of India, and postulated and tested that spatial patterns of attributes of places and of interactions between them are interdependent and isomorphic. That study, however, dealt with 'commodity flows' between various regions (states of India), it did not deal with human behaviour, nor migration.

However, later in another pioneering study, Berry (1969, pp. 21-31) extended his earlier work, postulated about the interdependency of spatial structure and spatial behaviour, and formulated a *General Field Theory of Spatial Behaviour*, in which he referred to migration. In the former study, he successfully tested his model by applying canonical analysis to data on commodity flows, whereas his second study was a general formulation of the theory, which referred to all spatial interactions, including migration between places, but, which he did not test in that study with real migration data. The present author is not aware of Berry's later papers in which he has tested his above-mentioned field theory model employing migration data. Nevertheless, it must be said that all the building blocks of the field theory model, linking spatial behaviour between regions (especially migration) to spatial structure, were there.

The third major attempt of field theory construction in geography and social sciences was that of the *Mobility Field Theory* of Mukherji (1975, pp. 10-383) in which he provided a full spatial rendering of Lewin's psychological field theory to spatial behaviour or mobility/migration behaviour of the individuals, along with philosophical perspective, theoretical text, and mathematical model, and also tested and verified with fine-grained field survey data.

In this connection, it must be indicated that although Berry's attempt was pioneering and very commendable, but it essentially referred to passive interactions between the regions; it did not refer to migration behaviour of the individual movers themselves who actually suffer locational stresses, who struggle to fulfil their basic needs, who evaluate various place utilities, who are the decision-makers themselves, and who actually perform the act of migration. All such crucial and complex aspects were not considered in Berry's both models (Mukherji, 1975, pp. 1-278; 1979a, pp. 1-81). These were done by the present author in a series of refining and redesigning attempts throughout 1970-75 (Mukherji, 1971, pp. 1-40; 1972a, pp.

1-25; 1972b, pp. 1-35; 1974, pp. 325-346; 1976a, pp. 1-25, and 1976b, pp. 21-32).

In the Mobility Field Theory, attempts were made by the present author to provide answers to all these crucial issues, by indicating causal relationships between the individuals' basic needs, as filtered through their place utility considerations of places of origins and destinations, and the resultant migration-mobility behaviour of the individuals that arises from attempting to satisfy those needs (Mukherji, 1975, pp. 25-121; 1979, pp. 1-80). The theory was tested with survey data and was found very successful and useful to explain migration behaviour of the individuals (people) (Mukherji, 1979b, pp. 18-32; 1979c, pp. 234-249). It was also found capable of generating concrete policy prescriptions to alleviate the problems associated with migration under duress (Mukherji, 1980, pp. 254-284; 1982a, pp. 1-248).

However, the above theoretical model referred to the individual mobility behaviour. If, on the other hand, we want to explain migration behaviour or flows between places or regions, we will need to re-design the entire structure of above Mobility Field Theory. This is the concern of another unique model, evolved and discussed in Mukherji (1993, pp. 183-202). This was termed *Spatial Field Theory.* In doing so, Berry's second model (1969), which postulated about spatial behaviour and spatial structure, provided considerable guidelines. However, it must be noted that Berry did not deal with demographic behaviour (like fertility/mortality), nor with Demographic Field Theory.

Related Previous Studies and Concepts in Demography

In 1974-75, Rudolf J. Rummel, a very renowned Professor of Political Science and International Relations, University of Hawaii (USA), had propounded and designed the concept of cross-country field-theoretic linkages between demographic set of variables, social-economic-political-cultural systems, and population policy systems therein (Rummel, 1974, pp. 1-18). He also proposed the use of canonical analysis for testing such linkages, across all major countries of the world, and also over time. This was first written and presented by him as a research proposal for National Science Foundation (NSF, USA) (Rummel, 1975, pp. 1-46). Rummel, mainly being a political scientist and keenly concerned with study of international relations between nations, was also very much concerned with unraveling causal linkages between some population growth variables and various socio-economic development indices of nations and their respective political and social policies. This research proposal was further expanded and some demographic components were further crystallized and elaborated during 1975-76 (with some demographic contributions from present author) and the entire work was subsequently published as a book in 1981 (Rummel and Mukherji, 1981, pp. 1-81). However, that proposed analysis of over-time, cross-country design of policy-demographic linkages, within the social field, could not be mathematically verified, nor empirically tested with data, due to lack of research funding. So, the entire idea got dropped, because of no funding available for his proposal. At that stage, the proposal was then mainly an analytical design, neither a Field Theoretic Study, nor a Demographic Field Theory.

Rummel's seed concept (of 1974-76) of linking three systems was not thrown into barren mind. The present author started seriously thinking about it throughout 1976-77, and later expanded, structured and given it a Demographic Field Theoretic perspective (Mukherji, 1977, pp. 250-66). Thus, began the present author's three decades old (1975-2006) persistent research interest and continuous effort to explore, innovate, crystallize, improve and persistently and empirically testify causal linkages between demographic systems, socio-economic systems, and population policy systems of India and the world (Mukherji, 1982b, pp. 12-16; 1982c, p. 4; 1983a, pp. 161-177; 1989b, pp. 343-373; and 1992, pp. 1-92). Due to such continuous effort, the Demographic Field Theory was first formulated by the present author and mathematically verified and empirically testified with Indian data in 1977 (Mukherji, 1977, pp. 250-66), and further structured and manifold verifications made which was published in 1983 (Mukherji, 1983, pp. 1-141). Rummel's innovative ideas provided the main seeds of thoughts for the Demographic Field Theory formulations, for which I am immensely indebted and grateful to my Professor in University of Hawaii (USA). The book is solemnly dedicated to my most revered Professor! He did not even know that I was religiously pursuing this idea since last 30 years!

However, at the same time, it must also be clearly stated that all major concepts of the Demographic Field Theory, its central notions, general statements, axioms, various formulations, matrix forms, numerous analytic designs, its ten-fold canonical models, empirical verifications and findings, its specific focus on poverty and high fertility, and all policy implications for wiping out poverty from the surface of India and the world – all these, as presented and testified in this book, are the results of 30 years of continuous effort of the present author (1975-2005).

The Demographic Field Theory was further testified with 1971-81 data of India (Mukherji, 1983, pp. 1-141) and subsequently with 1981-88 data (Mukherji, 1989, pp. 343-73). A global test of the Demographic Field Theory was made with demographic, socio-economic and population policy data (1990) sets of all major nations (numbering 130 excluding 50 small countries and colonies) of the world (Mukherji, 1992, pp. 1-91). Syndrome of poverty and fertility in India and the world was further explored and testified by Demographic Field Theory in Mukherji (1995, pp. 1-36; 1997a, pp. 1-6; 1997c, pp. 1-45; 1997e, pp. 1-12). The causal relations between Poverty Index and High Fertility among women in various states of India was unraveled in another study (Mukherji, 2000, pp. 1-25). Recently, in another major study the causal linkages between demographic behaviour, socio-economic systems and population policies of various states and of 91,000 women respondents were made, using NFHS-I survey data (Mukherji, 2000d, pp. 1-141).

The Demographic Field Theory, as evolved and presented here, is a very powerful, most useful, a novel and innovative analytic and theoretic tool – which is immensely capable of generating most pragmatic and most beneficial policy prescriptions for uplifting the common people of the Third World. It should be more widely utilized in demographic, geographic, and social research.

The Concept of Demographic Field

The demographic field is a system which consists of the following three parts (Mukherji, 1977, pp. 250-266):

(a) the individual family's socio-economic-cultural attributes and needs, including specific stresses in particular geographic setting;

(b) the family's knowingly or unknowingly-pursued population policy considerations regarding the family; and
(c) the different patterns of fertility, mortality, and migration behaviour of the family, and the complex inter-relationships between these three sub-systems.

All these are interdependent parts of the family's demographic field. A particular kind of demographic behaviour, e.g., a particular kind of fertility, mortality or migration behaviour of the family, is a resultant manifestation of changing constellations of all these co-existing facts of the life space of the family at a given time. Such behaviour is a change in the state of the *'field'* due to a change in the geo-socio-economic-cultural conditions of the family and its policy decisions.

The geo-socio-economic systems of the family form the nucleus of the demographic field (Mukherji, 1983b, pp. 1-141). The socio-economic needs and stresses in specific geographic setting are the sources of psychological tensions which generate motive forces for the family to mentally locomote – to think or to behave in a particular way – within the *demographic field* for a specific need gratification. For example, a decision is made that a child may be born in a family, or a migration should take place. Often, a conscious decision may not be taken, but some conscious/unconscious mental locomotion is involved. Although this is a mental locomotion – reaching out for a specific goal fulfilment – but it also has a physical manifestation, e.g., a migration is actually made, or a child is born, or a doctor/medicines brought to avert an infant death.

Studies have shown that a marked difference in fertility levels exists between urbanized educated families and semi-literate/illiterate rural peasant families. Caldwell (1982; 1988, pp. 71-96) has developed very useful concepts of inter-generational flows of wealth and veneration between parents and children, and causally connected these to demographic behaviour. Among urbanized educated families, children are regarded as more costly since a larger expenditure is incurred for rearing them, and fertility is dampened. Situation is, however, just the reverse among rural peasants'/labourers' families, among whom children are considered assets for they contribute to family earnings right from a very early age. As a result, the level of fertility is very high.

Caldwell studied these in terms of inter-generational wealth and veneration flows between children and parents. But, in the present concept of the *demographic field*, the concepts of the needs, poverty, stresses, roles, aspirations, and conscious or unconscious population policy considerations of the family are considered in an integrated manner. These aspects may be visualized within the concept of the demographic field (Figures 1(a) and (b)). In Figure 1(a), a specific pattern of the social needs, roles, aspirations, poverty and stresses of a rural peasant family, and in relation to these, specific population policy considerations, consciously or unconsciously followed by that family, may induce a specific type of demographic behaviour, e.g., high fertility, high mortality and poverty-induced migration.

Conversely, as shown in Figure 1(b), different sets of social needs, roles and aspirations of an educated urbanized family, and in relation to these, a different kind of population policy alternatives, consciously or unconsciously followed by that family, may induce a completely different pattern of demographic behaviour, e.g., low fertility, low mortality and upward social mobility due to migration.

Geographic-socio-economic systems of the needs, attributes and stresses also sample out the content and extent of information on the population policy considerations that are known, which, in turn, delineate the family's subjective policy space, within which a search for alternative population policies may occur. The family's geographic-socio-economic systems, therefore, determine the configuration of population policy space and also generate the 'demographic field' and cause a particular kind of fertility, mortality and migration behaviour to arise within the field. This binds every aspect of the demographic process within a single concept of the demographic field, and facilitates the assessment of the causal relations between:

(a) the geo-socio-economic systems;
(b) population policies; and
(c) demographic behaviour of the families.

At a higher level, this concept may be extended to explain a 'society's behaviour (Mukherji, 1983b, pp. 1-141; 1989b, pp. 343-373). A

Figure 1(a)

Demographic Field of a Rural Peasant Family

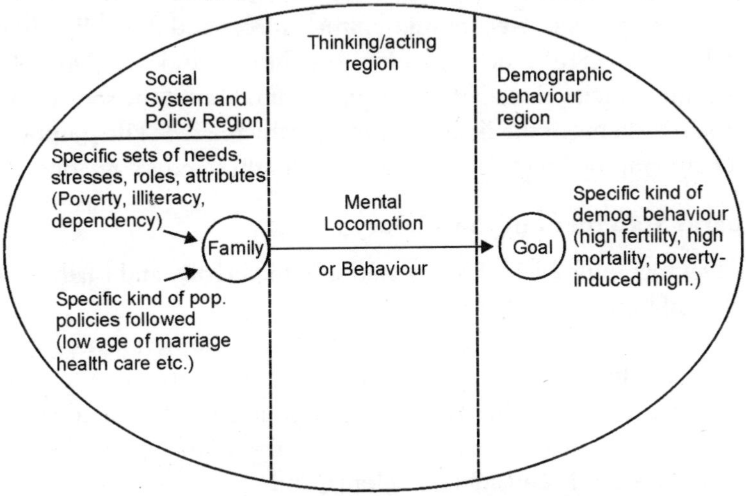

Specific patterns of social needs, aspirations, poverty and stresses of a rural peasant family and specific kind of population policy followed by the family, may induce it to show a specific kind of demographic behaviour.

Figure 1(b)

Demographic Field of Another Family (Urbanized-Educated-Affluent)

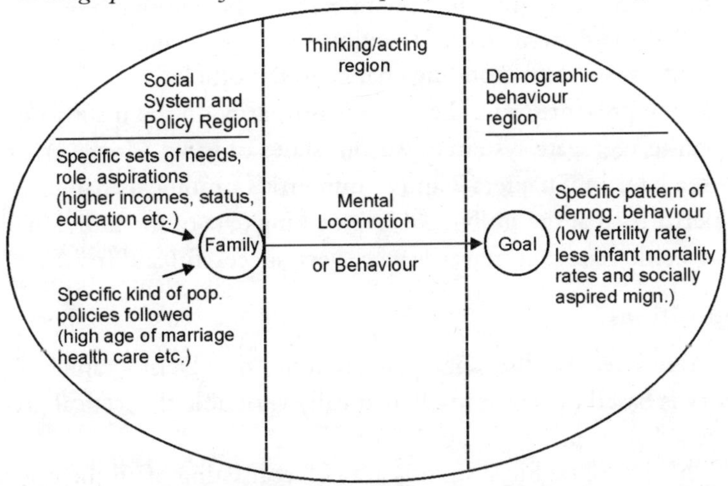

Different sets of social needs. roles, aspirations of an urbanised and educated affluent family and a different set of population policies adopted by that family, may induce to show on different kind of demographic behaviour pattern (mod./low fertility, less I.M.R.) and upward social mobility due to migration)

poverty-stricken society may feel it imperative to have high levels of fertility, and, consequently, suffer from high levels of infant mortality. In short, the geo-socio-economic-cultural forces and their alignments influence a society's demographic behaviour; and the prevailing population policies also operate through that nexus of the society. The three sub-systems of the field are thus causally related. The purpose of the Demographic Field Theory is to unravel these causal relations.

General Statement of the Theory

The Demographic Field Theory states, both verbally and mathematically (Mukherji, 1977; 1983b), that

(a) at the level of the family, the demographic behaviour of the family, located in a particular geographic setting, is a linear function of both that family socio-economic cultural attributes, needs and stresses, and in relation to those, the specific policies that the family considers or adopts; and

(b) at the level of the aggregate system, the structure of the geo-socio-economic-cultural attributes of the population, the structure of the population policies prevailing in those various states, and the resultant patterns of demographic behaviour of those states, are interdependent parts of the demographic system, called the *demographic field,* within which any change in one part generates a corresponding change in the other.

In the present study, the focus is primarily on the macro-model, i.e., on the aggregate system of various states of India. However, as we shall see later in Chapters 7 and 8, numerous canonical analyses were also performed at the individual level, taking data of the individuals in each specific state, and rewards were very successful and fruitful.

Propositions

With reference to the aggregate system, the Demographic Field Theory is based on seven mathematically verifiable theoretical propositions (Mukherji, 1983b, pp. 1-35):

(i) The demographic system is a 'field' consisting of all the relevant geo-socio-economic-cultural attributes of society, the population policies operating in that society, and all the different kinds of demographic behaviour in that society, and their complex interrelationships.

(ii) The demographic field may be analytically divided into a society's geo-socio-economic-cultural attributes (S), population policies (P), and demographic behaviour (D) spaces, into which the attributes, the policy variables, and the demographic behaviour are projected as vectors, with length and direction (Figures 3 to 5).

(iii) The socio-economic, population policy and demographic behaviour spaces are spanned by dimensions which generate the spaces and which are finite and empirically determinant (Figures 3 to 5).

(iv) Geographic units such as states (or settlements, regions, nations) are located as vectors in three spaces (S, P, and D), denoting, respectively, the geo-economic attributes of the units, their population policy considerations, and their demographic behaviour (Figures 3 to 5).

(v) Socio-economic vectors S_1, S_2, ... etc., in S space that describe the geo-socio-economic system of a society, and P_1, P_2, ... etc., that describe the population policies operating in that society, are the social 'field forces' determining the location of D_1, D_2, ... etc., of the vectors in D space according to the linear function:

$$\Sigma \beta_m D_m = \Sigma \alpha_q S_q + \Sigma \alpha_r{}^* P_r \qquad \text{..........(1)}$$

Here, betas, alphas, and alpha-stars are canonical weights. The basic proposition of the demographic field theory is that the demographic behaviour of a population, located in a particular geographical and social context, is a linear function of that population's specific geo-socio-economic-cultural attribute set, and in relation to that, of the specific kind of population policies that prevail in that particular society in a given space and time (Figure 6).

(vi) The direction and velocity of movement over time of a vector in the demographic behaviour space is along the resolution vectors of the forces, S and P, as a society's geo-socio-economic characteristics change, and as different population policies are enacted over time.

(vii) Demographic behaviour space D and combined S-P spaces are coincident such that the dimensions of one generate the other.

Figure 2 (a) and (b)

Socio-Economic Processes of Fertility Behaviour and Required Programmes

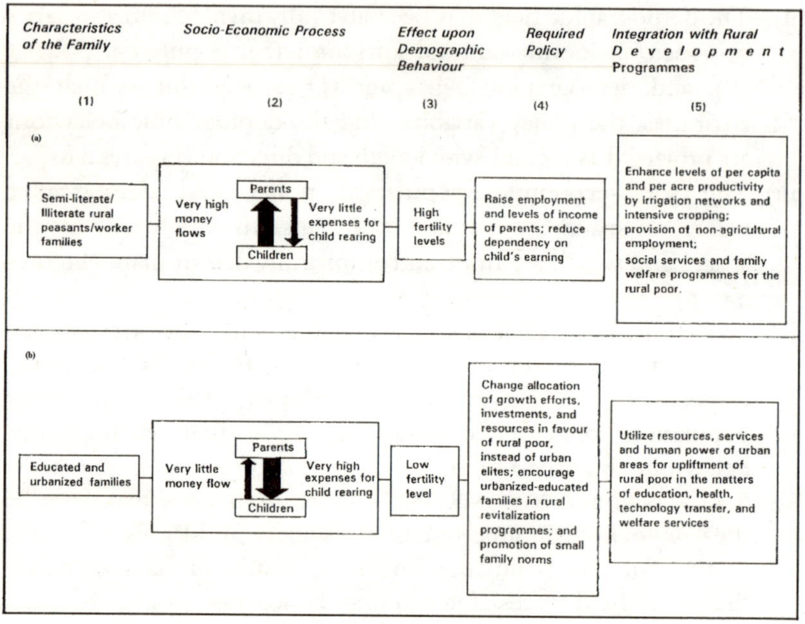

Figure 3

Demographic Space: Relative Location of Three State Vectors on Multi-dimensional Demographic Space

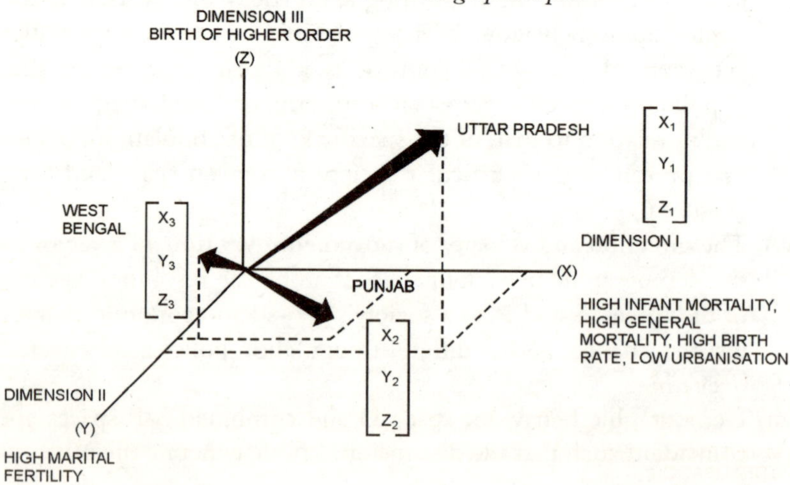

Figure 4

Socio-Economic Cultural Space: Relative Location of Three State Vectors on the Multi-dimensional Socio-Economic-Cultural Space

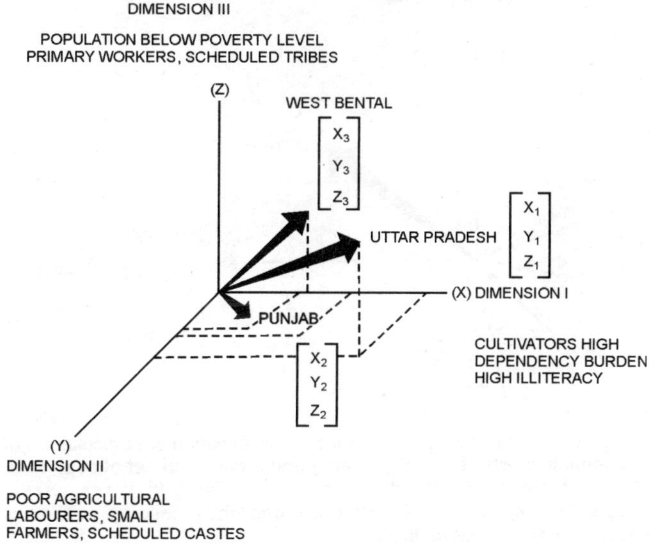

Figure 5

Population Policy Space: Relative Location of Three State Vectors on Multi-dimensional Population Policy Space

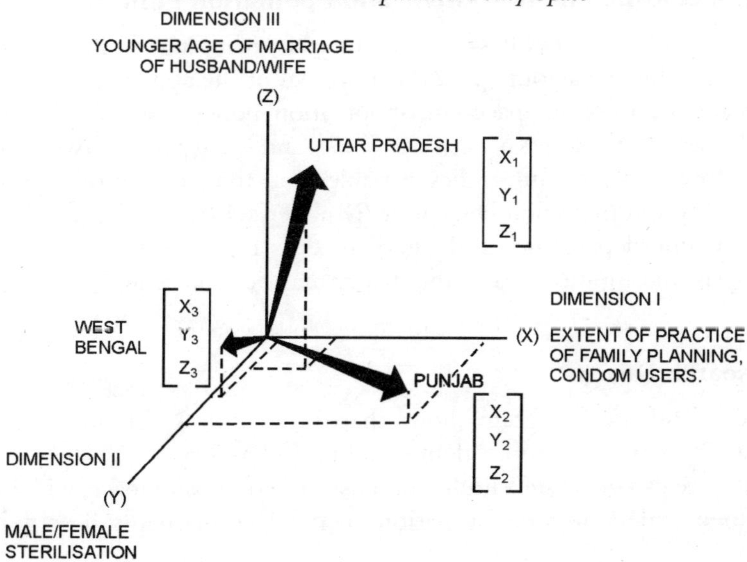

Figure 6

Demographic Behaviour Space: Demographic and Social-Policy Linkages

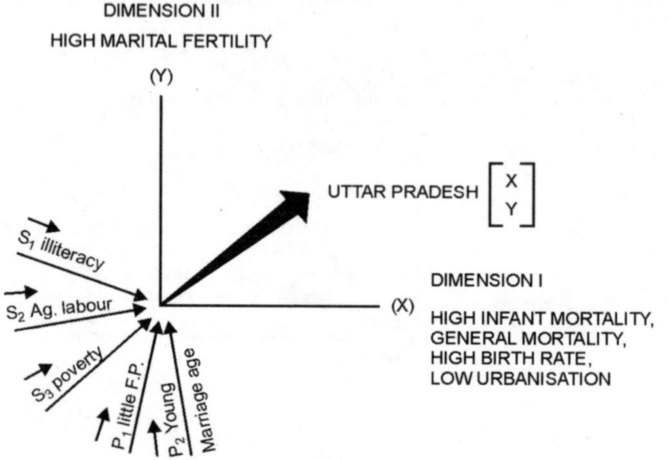

Demographic behaviour space: A specific combination of particular set of socio economic factors (S_1, S_2, S_3 etc.) and a particular set of population policy dimensions (P_1, P_2 etc.) acting as social field forces on the demographic vector of Uttar Pradesh and thus causing a specific demographic behaviour to occur.

Linkages between Demographic Behaviour, Geo-Socio-Economic System, and Population Policies

The crux of the theory lies in mathematically mapping out the bases of demographic behaviour space (D) into that of the combined space of geo-socio-economic space-cum-population policy space (S and P), and assessing the *degree of interdependencies* and *isomorphism* between the structure of social-cum-policy variables and the patterns of fertility, mortality and migration behaviour (Mukherji, 1983b, pp. 1-25). This test of interdependence and causal links is performed by canonical analysis. In canonical terms, the theory may be represented as:

$$D \sim (S + P)$$

Research Design

The hypothetical diagram shows that from innumerable number of data on socio-economic, demographic and policy variables across states, we can generate a multi-dimensional composite space, which is defined and delineated by various general components describing multivariate interrelationships between the socio-economic variables, demographic variables and population policy variables (Figure 3 to 6) (Mukherji, 1977, 1983b). In this space, each state can be projected as a vector (with length and direction) to represent a state's specification, relative to all others, on this space. Thus, both the general characteristics of the societies and of individual states can be untangled in this manner. These hypothetical dimensions can be found empirically also, as will be shown later (Figures 3 to 6).

Delineation of Separate Dimensions for Demographic, Socio-Economic and Policy Variables

These separate sets of dimensions and the isolation of their indicators would then enable one to define and measure the empirical interrelationships and major lines of forces within socio-economic processes, in population dynamics, and in policy inputs. For example, in Figures 3, 4 and 5, hypothetical indicators of demographic, social and population policy dimensions are shown, respectively. On each space, three states (Uttar Pradesh, West Bengal and Punjab) are shown to have their specific locations, relative to all others. Each of them share a specific combination of the common dimensions which spans the space. Thus, these figures represent both general dimensions and also state-specific, demographic, social and policy characteristics. Considerable effort is now going into indicator research, and yet little of this research has been making use of the power the methodological and computer developments have given us. Through the suggested research the indicators would be isolated – indicators which will define statistically independent trends in demographic behaviour, in socio-economic systems, and in population policies. These will not only measure major differences among the states, but will also span the economic, socio-cultural and demographic range of regions, and will be fully operational.

Assessment of Demographic-Policy Linkages, within Socio-Economic Field

Such linkages will be established by performing a canonical (regression) analysis on the three matrices of indicators, in which demographic variables will consist the dependent set and socio-economic variables-cum-population policy (or programme) variables will form the independent, or explanatory set. Such assessment of social, demographic and policy interrelationships across states (1992-93) would bear directly on population policy making and demographic research. These would shed light on many important questions and issues, such as on economic implications of rapid population growth; on interactions between social and economic development and fertility behaviour; on effects of spread of female education, or lack of it, on fertility control; and relative effectiveness of various population policies/programmes upon fertility and mortality reduction, within the context of socio-economic system (or field), and so forth.

Consider Uttar Pradesh, for example, having high infant mortality and high general mortality rates, high birth rates, and low urbanization, on demographic space (Figure 3). On socio-economic space (Figure 4), Uttar Pradesh shows more proportion of cultivators and high dependency burden and high illiteracy burden, as also quite high proportion of small farmers and landless agricultural labourers. Besides, on policy space (Figure 5), this state manifests more proportion of people in younger age of marriage, and considerably less family planning practices and use of contraceptives. So, the policy-demographic linkages within the socio-economic system may show that, for Uttar Pradesh, such characteristics like illiteracy, dependency, poverty, little family planning, and more younger people getting married at younger age – all are leading to very high fertility, high infant mortality and low urbanization (resultant Figure 6). The alternative policy will be raising the age of marriage, poverty alleviation, more spread of contraceptives, and above all, much greater provision of universal female literacy. Similar analysis can also be made for West Bengal, or Punjab or else. And, similar socio-economic-cum-policy-and-demographic linkages can also be extracted.

The policy relevance of this research design becomes at once very apparent from the canonical relationships between the demographic behaviour matrix, social matrix and policy matrix. For example, for some developed states, the findings may show that in a state, given only partial emphasis on family planning and more welfare-medical support, and in the absence of legalized abortion laws, the fertility rate cannot be reduced further. This would be more true for population growth in Uttar Pradesh or Bihar, especially under declining mortality conditions and the state's virtual pro-natal policy. For many Indian states, due to lack of old age security and little population control, such factors as low age of female marriage, low family income, low female education, and higher proportion of poor agricultural workers may cause high levels of fertility and mortality. Consequently, high rate of population growth will prevail. Hence, policy alternatives would be raising the legal age of marriage for the Indian women, more emphasis on effective measures of fertility control, simultaneously with mortality control and subsequent change in the present population policies and socio-economic policies.

Moreover, the linkages between demographic behaviour and population policies, within the socio-economic system or field, will be in equation form, with parameters given by the canonical analysis. The importance of these equations and empirical parameters cannot be overstated. They will provide mathematical and empirical basis for testing out the future and relative effect of socio-economic development and population policies upon the demographic change. This will give a very useful analytical and theoretical tool for population/ demographic research.

3

Analytical Models

"Make your nerves strong. What we want is muscles of iron and nerves of steel" (Swami Vivekananda, 1895, Complete Work, Centenary Volume III, 1963, p. 224).

"Fill the brain, therefore, with high thoughts, highest ideals, place them day and night before you, and out of that will come great work" (Swami Vivekananda, 1893, Complete Work, Volume II, 1963, p. 86).

Total Analytical Package

The following three steps comprise the total procedure for testing the theory (Mukherji, 1975, pp. 1-278; 1999a, pp. 1-81; 1983b, pp.1-65):

- First, three separate factor analyses are to be performed on the three data matrices: demographic behaviour (D), geo-socio-economic systems (S), and population policy (P) matrices. The principal components solution of the matrix, in each case, would systematically explore many relationships between multitudes of variables within the matrix, and would disentangle the common underlying components, or factors, describing the bases of the corresponding space. As such, matrices F_d, F_s and F_p are generated which describe "demographic behaviour types", "geo-social components", and "policy considerations", respectively. Factor analysis also generates corresponding three factor score matrices (X_d, X_s and X_p) – factor scores for each regional units or states – which become inputs in a subsequent analysis.

- Second, the geo-social Factor Score Matrix, X_s (of dimensions $n \times q$), and Population Policy Factor Score Matrix, X_p (of dimensions $n \times r$), are combined to form a New Predictor Matrix (X_s + X_p) of dimensions $n \times (q+r)$.
- Third, in the final step, a canonical analysis of these matrixes is performed, i.e., Demographic Factor Score Matrix, X_d, and the New Predictor Matrix (X_s + X_p). Thus, canonical analysis performs the tests of interdependencies between geo-socio-economic systems-cum-population policies and the resulting demographic behaviour.

It enables one to answer two interrelated basic research questions (Mukherji, 1981b, pp. 1-55; 1982, pp. 1-127):

(a) What is the overall general statistical relationship between the geo-socio-economic-cum-population policy matrix of a state (or a region) and its corresponding demographic behaviour?

(b) Given this overall relationship, what are the underlying causal relationships between a specific combination of geo-socio-economic system-cum-population policies, in the one hand, and fertility and mortality behaviour, on the other?

In short, the canonical analysis facilitates a least square fit between the two sets and uncovers causal policy-demographic linkages in the context of the geo-social-economic systems of the society (Mukherji, 1981a, pp. 1-56). First answer is given by the *trace correlation* (showing general statistical overlap, or mapping, between two matrices), and the second set of answers is given by a *series of canonical correlations* (showing the maximal correlations between matched pairs of variate from both dependent and independent matrices). The canonical model is a much higher form of the regression model, for here, instead of one dependent variable, an entire dependent matrix may be utilized, and instead of one, a whole series of canonical linkage equations can be generated (Hotelling, 1936, pp. 321-77).

Further details about the Demographic Field Theory are given in Mukherji (1977, 1979, 1981; and 1983b, pp. 1-141) and about its early proposal form, in Rummel and Mukherji (1981, pp. 1-81). Technical details about components analysis are available in Harman (1967, pp. 11-67; Rummel, 1970, pp. 51-112) and about canonical analysis in

Hotelling (1936, pp. 321-77) and in Cooley and Lohnes (1962, pp. 35-45). Further details about field theories and canonical models are given in Mukherji (1982, pp. 1-278), and about the results of the Demographic Field Theory in Mukherji (1983, pp. 1-141), Mukherji (1989, pp. 273-325) and Mukherji (1992, pp. 1-90).

Canonical Model: Final Model Linking Demographic Behaviour, Socio-Economic System, and Population Policies

Developed by Hotelling (1936, pp. 321-77), canonical analysis basically elicits maximum correlation between linear functions of two sets of variables, describing the same subject(s). Originally, he used it to connect behaviour and attributes of only *two* sets of subjects, not three. In 1974-75, the present author employed it to measure causal relationships between three (or more) data matrices of behaviour and attributes, describing, for example, migration behaviour of the individuals and their socio-economic attributes, plus place utility differences between their places of origin and destinations (as in *Mobility Field Theory*, Mukherji, 1975, pp. 1-363; 1985c, pp. 45-52; 1986a, pp. 1-20; 1986b, pp. 169-186). In 1977, I have also utilized to assess causal links between demographic behaviour of states and the combination of socio-economic characteristics of the states-cum-population policies adopted in those states (as in *Demographic Field Theory*, Mukherji, 1983, pp. 1-141).

Detailed analytic technique of canonical model and its utility, elegance, effectiveness, high statistical power, and interpretation of ensuing results are very much elaborated in successive studies made during 1970-92 by the present author (see Mukherji, 1971, 1972b, 1974, 1975, 1977b, 1979a, 1979b, 1980, 1981a, 1981b, 1982a, 1982b, 1983b, 1985c, 1986a, 1986b, 1990, 1992). Further application of Demographic Field Theory at Indian and global level were continuously made during 1995-2005 (Mukherji, 1992, 1993, 1995a, 1997a, 1997b, 1997c, 1997d, 1998a, 2001b, 2001c, 2005c). In such studies, I have successfully utilized canonical models by considering *three* data matrices simultaneously: that is, by taking one as the dependent matrix, and the combination of the other two matrices as the independent matrix. A very brief description of the canonical model and the way it is applied to the present research design is now in order.

Factor analysis is a very well-known technique, and so not elaborated here.

Canonical Analysis

Given the two sets of data on demographic behaviour of the states and socio-economic structure-cum-population policies in those states, canonical analysis may yield answers to two related basic research questions:

1. What is the overall general relationship between the demographic behaviour of the states on the one hand and socio-economic structure of those states and patterns of policies efforts therein, on the other.
2. Given that overall general relationship, what are the underlying causal relationships between specific combinations of demographic behaviour variables of those states on the one hand, and socio-economic structure-cum-population policy variables of those states, on the other.

What canonical analysis does is to delineate independent patterns in two sets of data in such a way as to ascertain maximum interrelationships between the new sets of patterns or dimensions. Just as factor analysis separates out distinct clusters of variables that vary together over a set of observations, canonical analysis uncovers clusters of patterns in two sets of observations, or matrices, by maximizing the correlation between linear combinations of variables (for details, see Mukherji, 1975, 1979a, 1979c, 1980, 1982a, 1983b). Such combinations of factors or patterns delineated in each set are independent of other patterns in the same matrix, but each is maximally correlated with a specific patterns found in the other matrix (Mukherji, 1985c, 1992) [Figures 7(a) and 7(b)].

Simultaneously, each pattern in the original matrix is independent of all, but one pattern in the second matrix. In short, each linear combination of variables becomes independent of the previously-derived linear combinations, just as factors are independent of each other in factor analysis.

The nature of canonical correlation analysis can be best explained through the algebraic model of a set of simultaneous equations (Philips, 1972, pp. 12-20):

Figure 7(a)

Steps in Canonical Analysis

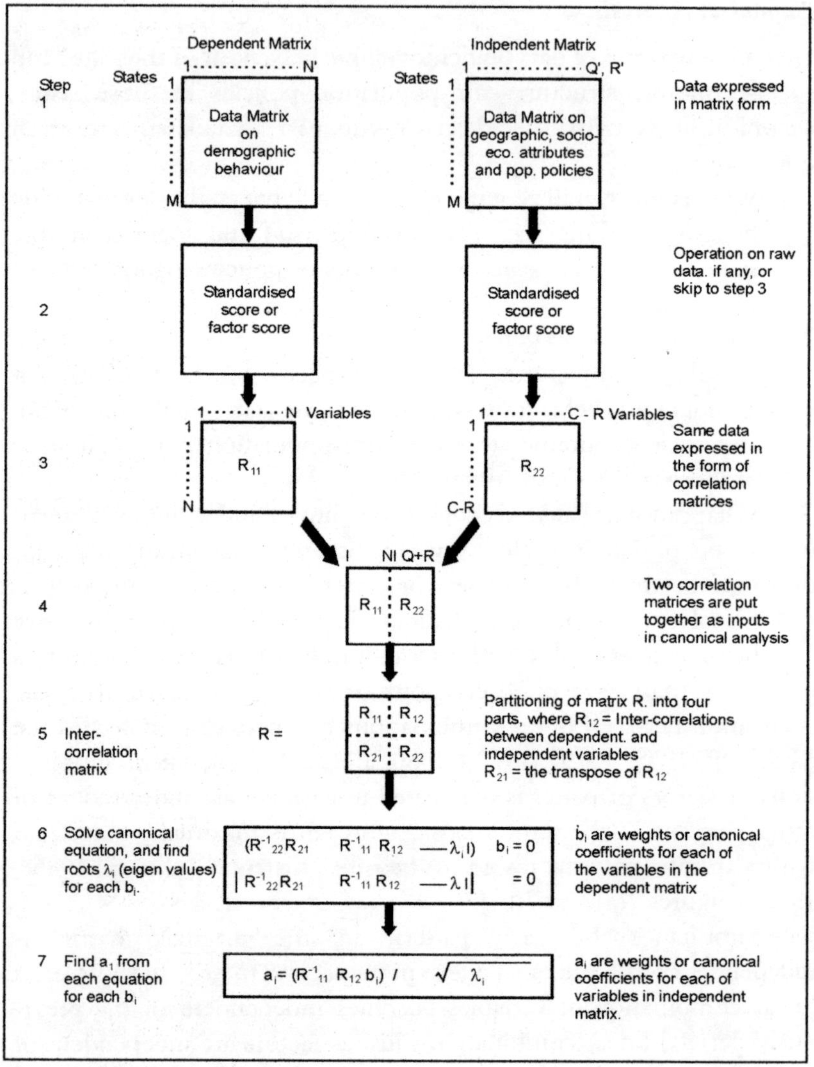

(Continued)

Figure 7 (b)
Steps in Canonical Analysis (concluded)

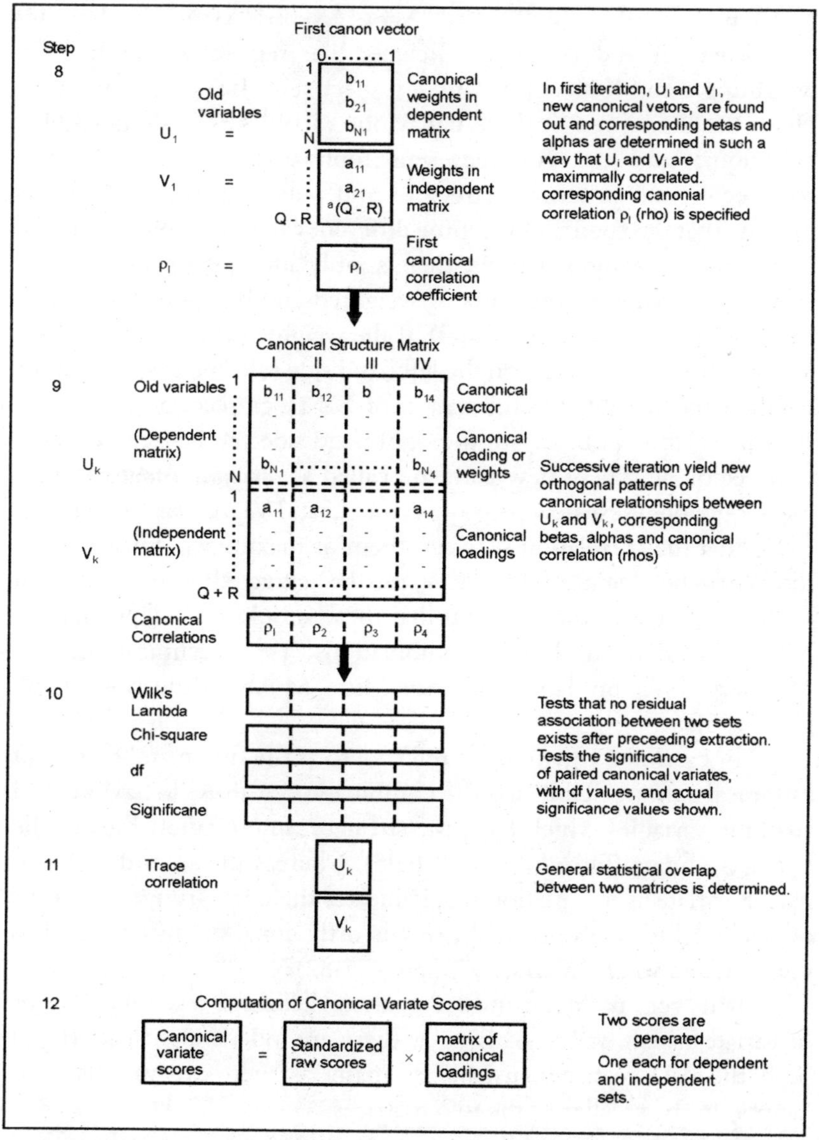

$$U_1=\beta_1Y_1+\beta_2Y_2+\beta_3Y_3=\alpha_1X_1+\alpha_2X_2+\alpha_3X_3+\alpha_4X_4=V_1 \ldots. \quad (1)$$
$$U_2=\beta_1{}^*Y_1+\beta_2{}^*Y_2+\beta_3{}^*Y_3=\alpha_1{}^*X_1+\alpha_2{}^*X_2+\alpha_3{}^*X_3+\alpha_4{}^*X_4=V_2 \ldots. \quad (2)$$
$$U_3=\beta_1{}^{**}Y_1+\beta_2{}^{**}Y_2+\beta_3{}^{**}Y_3=\alpha_1{}^{**}X_1+\alpha_2{}^{**}X_2+\alpha_3{}^{**}X_3+\alpha_4{}^{**}X_4=V_3 \ldots. \quad (3)$$

Where ß and α are coefficients like regression coefficients, weighting Y and X sets of variables, respectively, in two data matrices, Here, the Y's represent three behaviour variables (i.e., demographic behaviour) and the X's represent four attribute variables (i.e., socio-economic structure of regions and policy variables). Asterisks indicate that the coefficient assume different values in three equations. Canonical correlation analysis, then, simply attempts to *maximize* the correlations between the pairs of weighted combinations of X's and Y's. Within each equation (1 to 3), if the weighted combination of Y's (demographic behaviour) on the left hand side is termed as new vector U, then the weighted combination of X's (socio-economic system-cum-population policies) on the right hand side can be termed as the new vector, V. These new pairs are called as *canonical variate*. Within each equation, these new pairs of vectors U and V, are matched in such a way that the correlation between them, is maximized. Successively, three matched pairs of U and V can be extracted as in regression analysis, subject to the criterion that these should be independent of previously derived linear combinations (see technical details, Mukherji, 1975, pp. 1-363) (also see Mitra, Mukherji and Bose, 1980, pp. 45-75).

For example, equation (1) referred to as the first matched pair of canonical variate, delineated the combination of those behaviour and attribute variables which have the strongest interrelationships in the two sets of data (linked as a first field), whereas the second matched pair of variate as in equation (2) delineates the next strongest patterns of relationships (second field), that is orthogonal or uncorrelated to the first; and so on (Wood, 1973, pp. 477-82).

By its very nature, canonical analysis delineates a set of solutions or variate which will be as large as there are independent patterns in both the data matrices, usually as many as there are variables (or factors) in the smaller of the two matrices.

Thus, the main difference between regression analysis and canonical analysis is that in the latter both multiple dependent variables and multiple predictor variables are involved. In regression, a multiple coefficient of correlation (R) measures the strength of the relationship between one dependent and a number of independent variables. But, by comparison, in canonical analysis, a series of canonical correlations (rho's) specify the degree of interdependencies or causal interrelationships between different matched pairs of dependent and independent sets of variables, and, instead of one, a set of canonical correlations are derived (Cooley and Lohnes, 1962, pp. 45-65). Thus, in short, successive iterations linearly recombines both sets of variables (or factors) in order to uncover newer combinations, which maximizes the remaining variable. Such iteration continues until all the patterns are discovered and the matrix with the least number of variables has been exhausted (Mukherji, 1980, pp. 254-284).

Application of Canonical Model

In the present case, canonical analysis will be performed on two data matrices: behaviour (D) and attribute (A). The first matrix is of n x m dimensions (n = number of major states, 25; m = number of demographic variables). The second matrix A is of n x (S + P) dimensions (n = number of states, 25, S = number of variables related to socio-economic structure of states, and P = number of variables related to population policies/programmes). Here, matrix A is the combination of two predictor matrices – S (socio-economic matrix) and P (policy matrix).

In canonical analysis, these two (actually three) matrices are put together, considering behaviour matrix (D) as the dependent set and the predictor or attribute matrix (A) as the independent set [see Figures 7a-7b)].

Each vector of D provides a measure of an independent kind of demographic behaviour of countries, and each vector of A provides the samc for socio-cconomic structure of regions (states) and for the policy patterns. Through computer technique, canonical analysis of these two matrices transforms the vectors from D and A to an independent, uncorrelated pair of vectors, U and V, in both the matrices, without changing them. Unlike factor analysis, which maximizes the variance explained by individual factors, the canonical analysis maximizes the correlations between certain vectors of the D and A sets, while reducing other correlations to near zero. These correlations are called 'canonical correlations' between each matched pair of variate, U and V (Mukherji, 1975, pp. 65-91). These are not ordinary correlations, rather very high powered *canonical correlation coefficients*, something like regression weights (but between linear combinations of variables in two matrices, not between individual variables).

Corresponding to these correlations, R_c, are vectors of canonical coefficients b_k and a_k (*canonical loadings*, like factor loadings) that indicate which original sets of variables from D and A are maximally inter-correlated or involved in the new canonical vectors, U_k and V_k; and to what extent they determine variate scores of u_k and v_k. The new canonical vectors consist of standardized (of zero mean and unit variance) canonical variate (like factor scores) (For further technical details, see Cooley and Lohnes, 1962, pp. 45-65; Mukherji, 1979a, pp. 1-81; Mukherji, 1983b, pp. 1-145; and Schwind, 1975, pp. 1-18).

Geometrically, the canonical analysis measures the extent to which individuals (persons, cities, or nations) occupy the same relative locations in the D-dimensional demographic behaviour space as they do in (S + P) dimensional economic structure-cum-policy space. Thus, the overall correspondence between the two matrix bases is tested.

Canonical analysis provides a number of statistics for assessment of the statistical significance of the interrelationships. First is called the *trace correlation*, which indicates overall general goodness of fit between the two sets of input variables or two matrices, or, in other words, it measures the amount of variance in the one set being explained by the variance in the other set. The higher the value of trace correlation, the greater the statistical overlap between the two spaces, between behaviour and attribute sets. Usually, the trace correlation squared multiplied by 100 indicates the total amount of variance in the dependent set, which is being explained by the independent set. However, since the size of the overall trace correlation depends upon the total data sets, its magnitude can be pulled down or reduced by the presence of less significant variables, as close to the end of the analysis successive iterative cycles may keep producing less and less meaningful results and thus account for lesser amount of variance explained. Trace correlation also tests the degree of isomorphism or one-to-one relationship between the two matrices.

Generally, thus, it is more meaningful to observe the second set of statistic, that is, the successive sets of *canonical correlations* (R_c or rho), which measure the degree of interdependencies or associations between each matched pair of variate. Here, too, the square of canonical correlation times 100 indicates the amount of variance explained in the variate of the dependent set by the variate in the independent set.

The third feature of canonical analysis is the *chi-square statistic*, which indicates the statistical significance of these canonical correlations between each matched pair of variate or linear combinations of input variables (or factors).

The fourth feature is the *canonical coefficients* (similar to factor loadings), which relate each input variable to a canonical variate. Examinations of such coefficients permit precise interpretation of a canonical variate in terms of those input variables which constitute that specific variate and indicate high loadings.

The fifth statistic is *canonical variate scores*. These are standardized scores of zero mean and unit variance, and are obtained by the sum of the weights (canonical loadings) times the data products for each observations for all input variables in a specified matrix (behaviour or attribute). This gives one score each for two variate, behaviour and attributes. Plotting of these scores may reveal the geometrical mapping of relative location of each individual (cities or persons or the like) on the canonical space, defined by the given set of variate. The residuals thus obtained from plotting may be measures of unknown factors, not accounted for or not considered in the data set.

Thus, in short, this mathematical tool is a very powerful technique of assessing causal inter-connections between the economic structure of regions-cum-population policies on the one hand, and different patterns of demographic behaviour of people in those regions, on the other. The model is a general one, and can be equally applied to the study of fertility (see Mukherji, *Demographic Field Theory*, 1983b, pp. 1-141); or for migration-circulation (see Mukherji, *Mobility Field Theory*, 1975, pp. 1-362), or any other demographic research (as in Mukherji, *Spatial Field Theory*, 1993, pp. 245-75).

States Studied

Twenty-five states for which more or less complete NFHS data were available are studied. The list of states is given in Table 1. All major Indian states are considered, including Union Territory of Delhi (its urban territory). So, the findings have almost all-India coverage. Data refer to 1992-93 time-points. Total 30 relevant variables were first studied: 7 demographic, 9 socio-economic and 14 population policy variables. After initial screening, based upon strength of correlations and commonality, finally, only 21 variables are selected for analysis (4 demographic, 5 socio-economic and 12 policy variables) (Table 1). These three sets became three data matrices, and analyses were done at the matrix level.

Variables Selected for State-Level Analysis

After preliminary scanning, out of initial 30+ variables, only 21 variables are found relevant and comparable for analytic design, which are considered at the state-level analysis. Many are also not quantifiable, and could not be utilized. Finally, the following 21 variables are considered:

(a) *Four demographic variables* (like infant mortality rate (IMR), under-five child mortality rate (CMR), total fertility rate (TFR), and crude birth rate (CBR)).

(b) *Five socio-economic variables* (include female illiteracy, proportion of girls age 6-14 attending school, and other relevant aspects, like per cent of households having piped/pumped water facility, per cent of households without toilet, and proportion of women married at age below 18). Data on absence of toilet facility in the households or lack of piped/pumped water are important proxy indicators of poverty situation of the state, or the individuals. These proxy indicators are specially important, as most unfortunately, NFHS survey had not collected any income poverty data, nor economic data, nor measured the poverty condition of the respondents. This has been a great lacuna of such NFHS surveys.

    Therefore, data on female illiteracy are considered in this study as the most important surrogate or proxy indicator of the widespread poverty condition of the individual respondents and of the state.

(c) *Twelve population policy variables* were selected for which comparable data were available. These include:

1. per cent of women using contraceptives (of currently married women age 13-49),
2. proportion sterilized (male or female),
3. unmet need in family planning (per cent of currently married women who not using family planning, though do not want any more child or want to wait 2 years before the next child),
4. per cent of women who got ante-natal care (for births during last 4 years),
5. per cent of women who got tetanus toxoid (for births during last 4 years),
6. per cent of child delivery in Primary Health Centres (PHCs) (for births during last 4 years),
7. proportion of women who were assisted by health professionals (like allopathic doctors, or nurse/midwife),
8. per cent of children whom oral rehydration solution given (who had diarrhoea during past 2 weeks previous to survey),
9. proportion of children fully immunized (age 12-23 months; who got BCG, measles, and 3 doses of DPT and polio vaccines),
10. proportion of infants exclusively breastfed (age 0-3 months),
11. breastfed and mushy food also given (to infants of age 6-9 months), and
12. per cent of underweight babies (underweight is assessed by weight-for-age; undernourished babies are those having more than 2 standard deviation below the median for international reference population set by world health organization).

Out of initial 30 variables, finally, only 21 variables are found to be most relevant and considered (e.g., 4 demographic, 5 socio-economic and 12 policy variables). These are listed in Table 1 (p. 77).

Variables Selected for Individual Respondent Level Analysis in Each State

However, for individual level analysis done for all major states, the following sets of variables are considered:

Demographic Set

1. AVGCHILD (average number of children born to respective mother during her reproductive span)
2. CEB (total number of children ever born to each and respective individual mother)
3. BIRTHINT (birth interval in months between mother's age of effective marriage and her first child birth)
4. IMR (number of infant deaths occurred to her own children during one year period preceding survey)
5. CMR (number of under-five child mortality to her own children during one year period before survey)

Socio-Economic Set

1. Residenc (urban or rural residence of the women respondents)
2. Landown (whether or not she/family owns land)
3. Husoccup (husband's occupation, if he is a farmer or else)
4. Religion (religion of the women respondents, if Hindu, or other religion)
5. Illiterc (female illiteracy: is she illiterate or literate)
6. Puccahou (does she have *pucca* (brick), or kutchcha (mud/thatch-walled), or semi-*pucca* house)

Population Policy Set

1. Numfpusd (number of family planning methods used by the women respondent)
2. Femsterl (female sterilization done or not)
3. Numanc (number of ante-natal care visit made by PHC staff)
4. Numimmz (number of immunization doses given to children)
5. Brestfed (if children are breastfed)

Methodology

(a) Separate factor analyses are performed on Demographic Behaviour Matrix, Socio-economic Matrix, and Population Policy Matrix. These unraveled the main basis dimensions of the structures of those three sub-systems (i.e., demographic sub-systems, socio-economic sub-systems and population sub-systems) of the *demographic field*, and also specified relative position of each states with reference to the basis dimensions of each matrix structure (with the help of factor scores on each factor, separately for each of 3 matrices). These factor scores became inputs in further analysis (i.e., canonical model).

(b) Canonical analyses are performed between Demographic Behaviour Matrix (as dependent set) and the combination of Socio-Economic-cum-Population Policy Matrix (as predictor set). This step causally linked them, and showed interdependencies and isomorphism between demographic behaviour and socio-economic-policy factors, i.e. produced various fields that are causally linked, excluding others which did not belong to that field.

Ten Separate Models of Canonical Analysis

In this study, quantitative multivariate analyses are performed at three levels:

(a) All-India level analysis, using states as units of observation.
(b) State-level analysis, by using individual respondent level data as units of observation.
(c) State-level analysis, linking poverty index of the individual respondents and their demographic indices, and heath indicators. Besides, two high powered computer models are employed.
(a) *Factor analysis*, for identifying the main basis dimensions of massive data, and
(b) *Canonical analysis*, for finally linking the cause and effect variables within the demographic system, linking three matrices (demographic, socio-economic, and population policy matrices).

So, a total of more than 36 canonical tests are performed, and more than 40 factor analyses are also performed, by using both state-level data for all-India level analysis as well as using individual respondent level data for performing at each of 25 major Indian states. However, results of only major states are presented, due to lack of space.

Besides, numerous canonical analyses are also performed, each time linking poverty index and demographic behaviour of individual respondents (in all major states) and their policy considerations. These constitute one major contribution of this book. Although, analyses are performed for all 25 states, findings of only major states are presented, due to shortage of space. Thus, total 61 canonical analyses are performed.

In this study, thus, the following eight models of canonical analysis are performed, depending upon different set of data utilized in respective case. These are:

1. **Canonical Model I**, using all-India (total series), state level data (without first factor analysis).
2. **Canonical Model II,** using state-level rural data (without first factor analysis).
3. **Canonical Model III**, using state-level urban data (without first factor analysis).
4. **Canonical Model IV**, first doing the following separate factor analyses with three data matrices of total series data, and using their outputs in final canonical model IV, e.g.:
   (a) Factor analysis of demographic matrix of states (total series data)
   (b) Factor analysis of socio-economic matrix of states (total series data).
   (c) Factor analysis of population policy matrix of states (total series data).
   (d) Factor scores from above three factor analyses of D, S, and P matrices of states (total series data).
   (e) Then, using factor scores of three factor analyses as inputs for canonical model IV (Total series data).
5. **Canonical Model V**, similarly, first doing the following separate factor analyses with three data matrices of rural and urban data series taken simultaneously, and using their outputs in final canonical model V, e.g.:
   (a) Factor analysis of demographic matrix of states (rural and urban data series taken together).
   (b) Factor analysis of socio-economic matrix, Indian states (R-U series taken together).
   (c) Factor analysis of population policy matrix, Indian states (R-U series taken together)

(d) Factor scores from three separate factor analyses, states, rural-urban data taken together, as inputs for canonical analysis.
(e) Then, using factor scores of the above three factor analyses as inputs for canonical analysis model V (rural and urban series together).

6. **Canonical Model VI,** similarly, first doing the following separate factor analyses with three data matrices of rural data series only, and using their outputs in final canonical model VI, e.g.:
   (a) Factor analysis of demographic matrix of states (rural data only).
   (b) Factor analysis of socio-economic matrix of states (rural data only).
   (c) Factor analysis of population policy matrix of states (rural data only).
   (d) Factor scores on various dimensions of the three matrices (rural data only).
   (e) Then, factor scores of three factor analyses are used as inputs for canonical model VI (rural data only).
7. **Canonical Model VII,** similarly, first doing the following separate factor analyses with three data matrices of urban data series only, and using their outputs in final canonical model VII, e.g.:
   (a) Factor structure of demographic matrix of Indian states (urban data only).
   (b) Factor structure of socio-economic matrix of Indian states (urban data only).
   (c) Factor structure of population policy matrix of Indian states (urban data only).
   (d) Factor scores from three separate factor analyses of state level data (urban parts only).
   (e) Similarly, factor score of three matrices used as inputs for final canonical model VII (urban parts only).
8. **Canonical Model VIII,** described below.
9. **Canonical Model IX:** Measuring Poverty Index and linking it with fertility and mortality behaviour (using individual level data).

10. **Canonical Model X:** Canonical analysis of 1998-99 data set performed.

State-Level Analysis, Taking Individuals as Units

Canonical Model VIII: 21 separate canonical analyses are performed for each major Indian state by using Individual level data of women respondents' demographic, socio-economic and policy data matrices (sometimes such data matrices exceeds 5,000 or more cases for a large state)(Chapter VII).

Canonical Model IX: Finally, Poverty Index is measured for each female respondents, and such scores are canonically linked with fertility and mortality rates, and using individual level data. Performed for all major states (Chapter VIII).

Factor Analytic Models

Besides, the following two kinds of factor analyses are also performed which have revealed remarkable results:

1. **Factor Model I**: Done at all-India level, using state level data series of all major variables of demographic matrix, socio-economic matrix and population matrix of states, considered all variables and matrices simultaneously (rural and urban series taken together). Factor scores are also generated on all those dimensions which showed crucial interrelationships between demographic, socio-economic, and population policy variables. Findings offered very crucial interrelationships and results. Relative position of each state and their rural-urban parts are graphically shown in Figure 19. The dimensions are clusters of interrelated variables and they together depict the main structure of the demographic system across all states.
2. **Factor Model II**: 21 separate factor analyses are also performed on 21 major states of India, by using individual respondent level micro data on the three matrices (demographic, socio-economic, and policy). These 21 factor outputs also unraveled crucial inter-relationships between those three sub-systems of demographic fields for each state separately. However, these factor outputs are

not presented due to shortage of space, and also because they form intermediate steps for final canonical models (presented).

Elegance and Utility of Canonical Analysis in Demographic and Geographic Research

Canonical model yields a series of canonical interrelationships, every time linking a particular set of socio-economic-cum-policy variables with a particular set of demographic behaviour variables, maximally correlating only those factors or variables which belonged to that particular demographic field, while reducing other to near zero value which did not belong to that field, or system. In this way, through successive iterations, every time a very specific and independent causal relation between demographic behaviour and socio-economic-cum-policy variables has emerged, orthogonal and independent of previously derived canonical linkages in the earlier iterations. And, instead of one single solution (as in regression model), a series of solutions has emerged in the canonical model, each time independent and orthogonal of previous linkages. Therefore, successive canonical correlations provided many measures of interdependence between them (Mukherji, 1979c, pp. 234-249).

Furthermore, trace correlation also provided a measure of interdependence and isomorphism between the entire demographic behaviour matrix and the entire socio-economic-plus-policy matrix – a general statistical overlap between the two sets, two sub-systems. Thus, the demographic field theory and canonical model can perform a higher level of analysis, which cannot be done through other multivariate models, like regression model as they can handle only one dependent variable, not a matrix of dependent variables; and can yield only one solution, not a series of independent solutions.

One Very Notable Aspect of Canonical Model and Demographic Field Theory

Thus, this is one of the most elegant and most useful ways of assessing independent contribution of family planning upon fertility decline in different states, distinct from contribution of socio-economic-cultural factors and development measures. The demographic field theory and canonical model, thus, can perform a higher level of social analysis, which usual multivariate models cannot achieve.

Conceptually linking demographic matrix with socio-economic-policy matrix, and verifying it through canonical model, provides a much higher level analysis, which cannot be done by regression or simultaneous equations. Thus, both methodologically and conceptually, the present canonical model is capable of making a new, novel, and a very useful contribution to demographic, population, geographic and policy research.

Besides, the Demographic Field Theory is a unique and a novel theory, and like a general systems theory, it can also be applied to investigate any systems, health system or demographic system, mobility system, socio-economic system, or political system, and can be performed at any level, the individuals, settlements, cities, regions, or nations!

4

Demographic, Socio-Economic and Population Policy Situation in India

"Let each one of us pray day and night for the downtrodden millions in India who are held fast by poverty, priest-craft, and tyranny – pray day and night for them" (Swami Vivekananda, 1895, Complete Work, Centenary Volume V, 1963, p. 480).

"Serve as worship of the Lord Himself in the poor, the miserable, the weak" (Swami Vivekananda, 1896, Complete Work, Centenary Volume IV, 1963, p. 246).

"No need looking behind. FORWARD! We want infinite energy, infinite zeal, infinite courage, and infinite patience, then only great things be achieved" (Swami Vivekananda, 1894, Complete Work, Centenary Volume, VI, 1963, p. 384).

Introduction

Table 1 provides detailed demographic, socio-economic, and policy data of Indian states, based on NFHS-I survey of 1992-93. Table 2 and Table 3 provide data for rural parts and urban parts, respectively. In canonical analysis (as in Table 4), the first four variables of Table 1 are treated as dependent matrix, and the next 17 variables, as comprising of independent matrix. Names of variables are given in Table 1.

Demographic situation of all major states of India (rural and urban components combined) are illustrated in Figures 8 to 10. Corresponding socio-economic situations are depicted in Figure 8. Finally, all-India health situations are shown in Figures 11 and 12. On the other hand, the demographic and socio-economic conditions in rural India are illustrated in Figures 13 to 15, while the corresponding situations in urban India are presented through Figures 16 to 18. Most such maps are self-explanatory, and not elaborated much.

All-India Situation

All-India picture is depicted in Table 1 and several maps (Figures 8 to 12).

Female Illiteracy or Poverty in India

Figure 8 presents female illiteracy or poverty situation in India during 1992-93 (Table 1). Almost entire northern India, from Rajasthan to Andhra Pradesh, had very high female illiteracy (60% to 80%) among adult eligible women (age 15-49). Rajasthan ranked first (75%), followed by Bihar (71%), Uttar Pradesh (69%), Madhya Pradesh (66%) and Andhra Pradesh (62%). This has been the heartland of abject poverty and very high female illiteracy zone of India (Mukherji, 1996b, pp. 1-15). Surrounding this, came the second belt of high female illiteracy (40% to 60%), which included Orissa (59%), Assam (49%), West Bengal (45%), Arunachal Pradesh (58%), Maharashtra (45%), Karnataka (54%), Tamil Nadu (44%), Gujarat (49%), Punjab (48%), Haryana (54%), Himachal Pradesh (43%) and Jammu & Kashmir (48%). That comprised almost 90 per cent of India, which suffered from acute female illiteracy of over 40 per cent, or similar degree of abject poverty. This has been the basic socio-economic context in which the *demographic field* of India is imbedded, and unless this 'field', or socio-economic context, is tremendously improved, nothing can be hoped for! Neither for India's demography, nor its society, nor economy!

Total Fertility Rates in India

Figure 9 illustrates fertility situation over Indian states (1992-93). Total fertility rates ranged between 4 to 5 children per mother over

Figure 8

India (All-India), Female Illiteracy (Females age 15-49), 1992-93

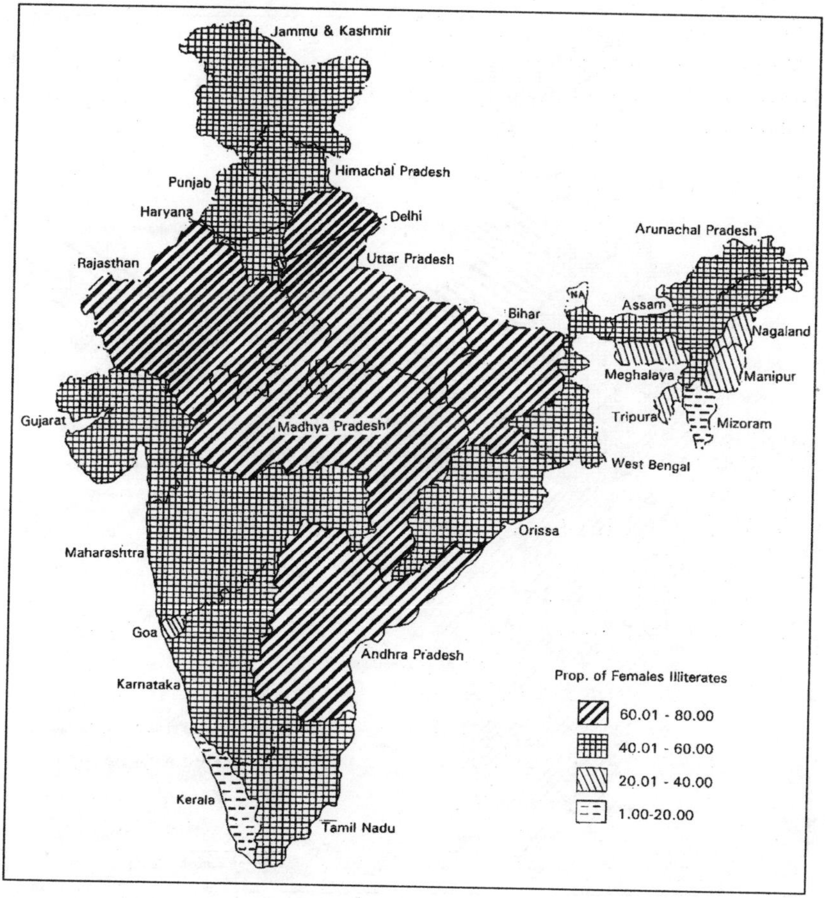

Figure 9

India (All-India), Total Fertility Rate, 1992-93

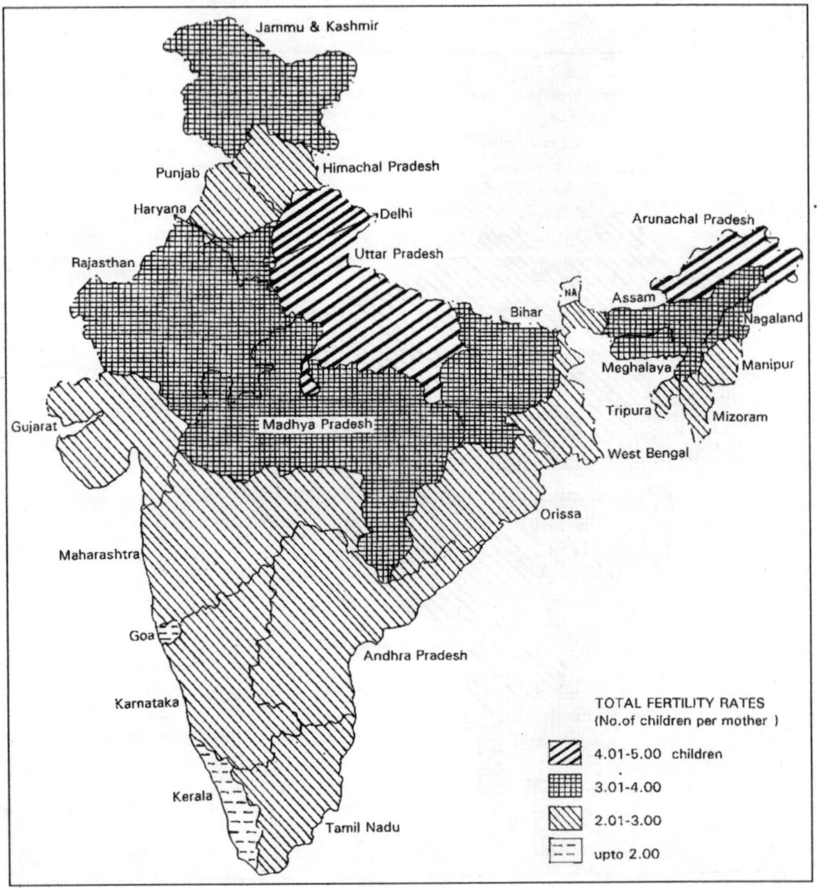

Figure 10

India (All-India), Infant Mortality Rate, 1992-93

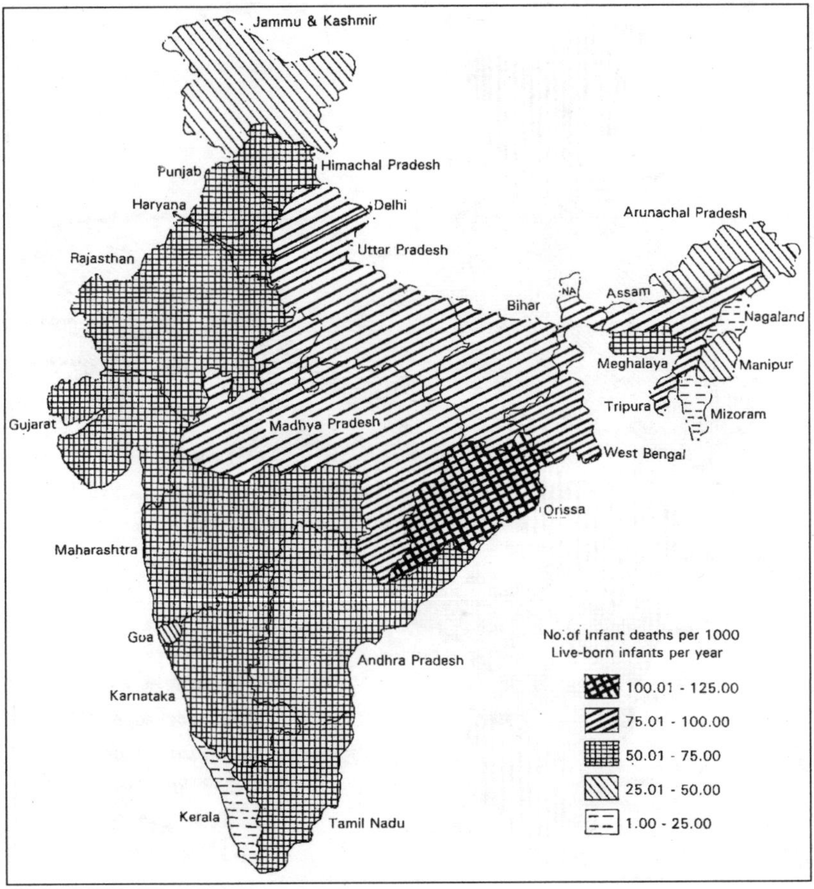

Figure 11

India (All-India), Proportion of Children Fully Immunized (children age 12-23 months), 1992-93

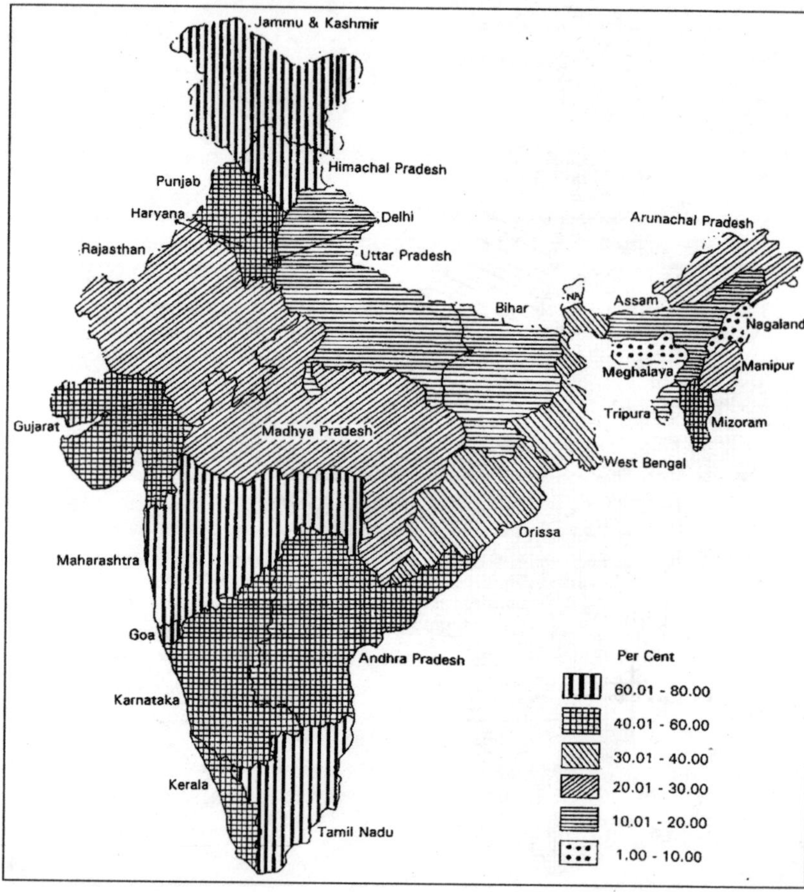

Figure 12

India (All-India), Per cent Sterilized (Male or Female), 1992-93

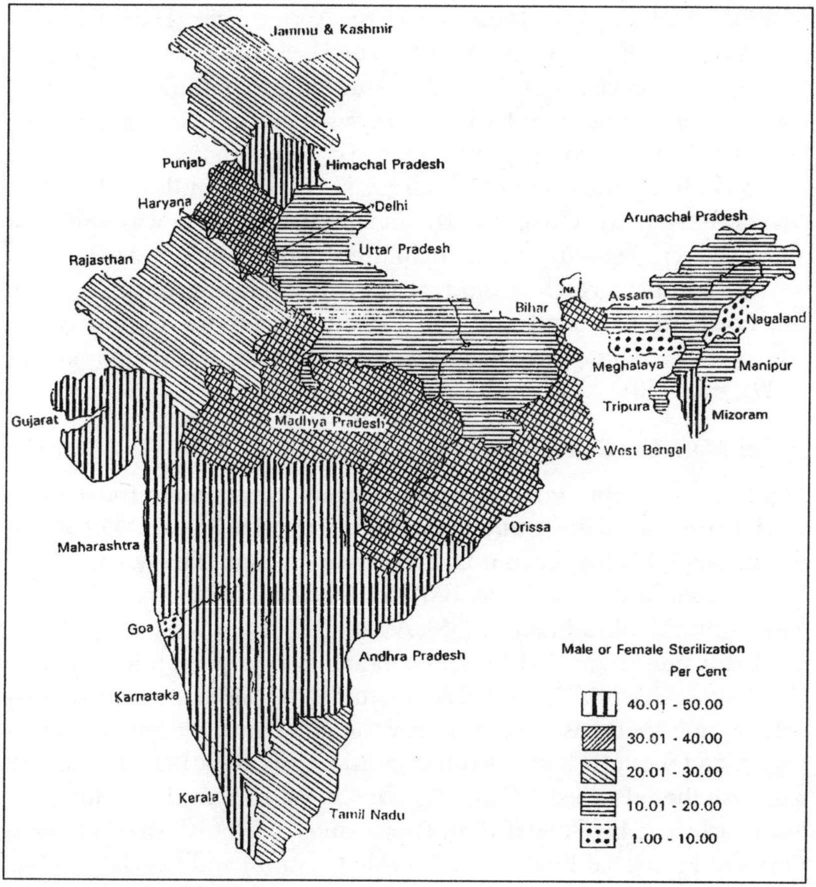

most of northern India (Table 1). Uttar Pradesh had the highest fertility (4.8 children). Rest of the heartland also had high fertility, varying between 3 to 4 children; for instance, Bihar (4.0 children), Madhya Pradesh (3.9), Rajasthan (3.6), Assam (3.5), Haryana (4.0), and Jammu & Kashmir (3.1). This entire heartland needs revamping of poverty alleviation and family planning programmes. However, southern and eastern India had comparatively less fertility, ranging between 2 to 3 children per mother, e.g., West Bengal (2.9), Orissa (2.9), Andhra Pradesh (2.6), Karnataka (2.9), Tamil Nadu (2.5), Maharashtra (2.9), Gujarat (3.0), and Punjab (2.9). It was still high above the replacement level (2.1 children). Fortunately, Goa (1.9) and Kerala (2.0) have reached the replacement level of fertility. So, both the northern heartland and the Deccan region need tremendous efforts for demographic development and fertility decline (Mukherji, 1999a, pp. 1-20).

Infant Mortality Rates in India

Figure 10 and Table 1 depict infant mortality condition in India. First, Orissa had the highest infant mortality rate (IMR), i.e., 112 infant deaths per 1,000 live-born infants per year. Second, this was followed by northern heartland (80 to 100), for instance, Uttar Pradesh (100), Bihar (89), Madhya Pradesh (85), Assam (89), even West Bengal (75). Unfortunately, high IMR is very conducive to raise high fertility also (Chandrasekhar, 1972, pp. 1-25). So, this is the domain where the war against high IMR has to be seriously fought. Third, the entire Deccan region and western India also had considerably high IMR (50 to 75), e.g., Andhra Pradesh (70), Karnataka (65), Tamil Nadu (68), Maharashtra (51), Gujarat (69), Rajasthan (73), Punjab (54), Haryana (73) and Himachal Pradesh (56). Only Goa (32) and Kerala (24) had low IMR, and consequently, low TFR. Reduction of IMR, thus, is a moral and medical responsibility of health administration and entire nation. Any effort in this crucial domain will pay high demographic dividends in the form of reduced IMR, as well as reduced fertility.

Child Immunization Situation

Map 11 and Table 1 show very wide spatial variations in child immunization in India. On the one hand, while we notice substantial immunization in Maharashtra (64% of children of age 12-23 months

Table 1

Demographic, Socio-Economic, and Population Policy Variables of Indian States, All-India (Total Series of Data), NFHS-I, 1992-93

Variables	*1*	*2*	*3*	*4*	*5*	*6*	*7*	*8*	*9*	*10*	*11*	*12*	*13*	*14*	*15*	*16*	*17*	*18*	*19*	*20*	*21*
Andhra Pradesh	70.4	91.2	24.2	2.59	61.5	54.8	68.6	63.4	75.6	47.0	44.8	10.4	86.3	74.8	32.8	49.3	32.5	45.0	70.5	47.8	49.1
Arunachal Pradesh	40.0	72.0	34.6	4.25	57.9	65.3	43.9	75.8	26.4	23.6	10.7	20.4	48.9	31.9	19.9	21.3	33.3	22.5	73.9	35.8	39.7
Assam	88.7	142.2	30.4	3.53	49.3	66.0	44.4	43.2	50.4	42.8	14.4	21.7	49.3	34.9	11.1	17.9	35.2	19.4	65.0	39.2	50.4
Bihar	89.2	127.5	32.1	4.00	71.4	38.3	69.1	63.6	83.5	23.1	18.6	25.1	36.8	30.7	12.1	9.0	23.0	10.7	51.6	18.1	62.6
Delhi	65.4	109.3	26.6	3.02	29.2	86.3	28.7	99.5	15.9	60.3	23.3	15.4	82.4	72.5	44.3	53.0	39.4	57.8	20.0	25.1	41.6
Goa	31.9	38.9	17.2	1.90	26.9	92.5	7.2	92.5	56.5	47.8	30.5	15.7	95.4	83.4	86.8	88.4	41.4	74.9	10.8	33.9	35.0
Gujarat	68.7	104.0	27.2	2.99	48.7	68.4	33.4	75.1	64.2	49.3	41.0	13.1	75.7	62.7	35.6	42.5	20.7	49.8	36.3	22.9	50.1
Haryana	73.3	98.7	32.9	3.99	54.1	74.7	57.3	73.0	73.1	49.7	34.8	16.4	72.7	63.3	16.7	30.3	19.5	53.5	37.5	38.5	37.9
Himachal Pradesh	55.8	69.1	28.2	2.97	42.6	87.6	24.2	57.6	87.4	58.4	45.8	14.9	76.0	47.4	16.0	25.6	44.9	62.9	36.4	39.9	47.0
Jammu of J.K.	45.4	59.1	27.9	3.13	48.2	79.6	20.5	57.3	80.9	49.4	29.7	17.5	79.5	68.9	21.9	31.2	44.4	65.7	16.9	44.8	44.5
Karnataka	65.4	87.3	25.9	2.85	53.5	64.4	51.2	75.6	68.8	49.1	42.5	18.2	83.5	69.8	37.5	50.9	34.0	52.2	65.6	38.2	54.3
Kerala	23.8	32.0	19.6	2.00	17.6	94.8	19.3	21.0	29.1	63.3	48.3	11.7	97.3	89.8	87.8	89.7	37.8	54.4	59.2	69.3	28.5
Madhya Pradesh	85.2	130.3	31.6	3.90	65.7	54.8	73.3	55.8	78.7	36.5	31.5	20.5	52.1	42.8	15.9	30.0	33.0	29.2	31.4	27.7	57.4
Maharashtra	50.5	70.3	26.3	2.86	44.1	76.6	53.9	78.5	59.2	53.7	46.1	14.1	82.7	71.0	43.9	53.2	41.7	64.1	37.1	25.0	54.2
Manipur	42.4	61.7	24.4	2.76	37.0	86.8	14.3	47.0	16.9	34.9	13.8	21.7	63.4	48.0	23.0	40.4	63.1	29.1	70.4	50.0	30.1
Meghalaya	64.2	86.9	31.9	3.73	39.8	75.7	28.1	47.6	45.7	20.7	10.0	25.1	51.8	30.0	29.6	36.9	40.7	9.7	18.0	56.3	45.5

Contd...

Contd...

Mizoram	14.6	59.3	20.8	2.30	11.1	88.5	13.3	40.1	17.0	53.8	44.6	11.9	88.9	42.5	48.9	61.5	24.5	56.4	45.5	64.3	28.1
Nagaland	17.2	20.7	31.3	3.26	28.2	89.0	16.4	72.1	20.7	13.0	6.4	26.7	39.3	33.0	6.0	22.2	24.6	3.8	61.1	43.5	28.7
Orissa	112.1	131.0	26.5	2.92	58.6	62.0	45.5	50.9	87.8	36.3	31.6	22.4	61.6	53.8	14.1	20.5	41.1	36.1	45.7	30.2	53.3
Punjab	53.7	68.0	25.0	2.92	48.0	77.8	14.9	98.6	63.3	58.7	34.0	13.0	87.9	82.7	24.8	48.3	32.7	61.9	3.3	37.3	45.9
Rajasthan	72.6	102.6	27.0	3.63	74.6	40.6	69.5	57.3	80.2	31.8	27.7	19.8	31.2	28.3	11.6	21.8	22.7	21.1	65.9	9.4	41.6
Tamil Nadu	67.7	86.5	23.5	2.48	43.9	78.7	36.1	74.6	70.6	49.8	39.5	14.6	94.2	90.1	63.4	71.2	27.1	64.9	55.8	56.5	48.2
Tripura	75.8	104.6	23.1	2.67	35.6	76.7	41.1	44.1	20.6	56.1	19.1	13.5	64.9	58.7	30.7	33.5	00.0	19.0	47.9	65.0	48.8
Uttar Pradesh	99.9	141.3	35.9	4.82	68.5	48.2	63.9	74.3	77.1	19.8	13.1	30.1	44.7	37.4	11.2	17.2	22.7	19.8	60.3	19.4	59.0
West Bengal	75.3	99.3	25.5	2.92	44.8	62.9	56.4	84.9	59.6	57.4	30.6	17.4	75.3	70.4	31.5	33.0	74.7	34.2	40.0	53.6	56.8

List of Variables

1. IMR (Infant Mortality Rate) (per 1000 live-born infants during 5 years previous to survey)
2. CMR (Child Mortality Rate) (per 1,000 live births during 5 years previous to survey)
3 CBR (Crude Birth Rate) (based on births to women age 15-49 during 3 years previous to survey)
4 TFR (Total Fertility Rate) (based on births to women age 15-49 during 3 years previous to survey)
5. Proportion of female illiterates (age 15-49)
6. Girls age 6-14 going to school
7. Proportion women married at age <18
8. Proportion households with water facility
9. Proportion households without toilet (sanitary)
10. Proportion of women using contraceptives (per cent of currently married women age 13-49)
11. Proportion sterilized (male or female)
12. Unmet need in FP (per cent of currently married women who not using family planning, though do not want more child or to wait 2 years before next child.
13. Proportion got ante-natal care (for births during last 4 years)

Contd...

Contd...

14. Proportion got Tetanus Toxoid (for births during last 4 years)
15. Proportion of delivery in PHC (for births during last 4 years)
16. Proportion assisted by health professionals (allopathic doctors, or nurse/midwife)
17. Per cent Oral Re-hydration Solution given (of children who had diarrhoea during past 2 weeks)
18. Proportion children fully Immunized (age 12-23 months; who got BCG, measles, and 3 doses of DPT and polio vaccines)
19. Proportion children exclusively breastfed (age 0-3 months)
20. Breastfed + mushy food given (age 6-9 months)
21. Per cent underweight babies (underweight assessed by weight-for-age; undernourished are those more than 2 standard) deviations apart from the measure, set by World Health Organization (WHO).

Note: No Survey done in Kashmir part of Jammu-Kashmir.

covered), Tamil Nadu (65%), Jammu & Kashmir (65%), Gujarat (50%), Karnataka (52%) and Andhra Pradesh (45%), on the other hand, also exist states of very low immunization like Uttar Pradesh (20%), Bihar (19%), Madhya Pradesh (29%), Orissa (36%), West Bengal (34%) and Rajasthan (21%). Owing to such low child immunization rates, IMR and under-five child mortality rate (CMR) were so high in Orissa (112 and 131, respectively), Madhya Pradesh (85, 130), Rajasthan (73, 102), Uttar Pradesh (100, 141), Gujarat (69, 104) and Bihar (89, 103), Hence, child mortality situation is terrible in India. It has not improved adequately, as to be examined later. Even recently, UNICEF (2005) lamented that India ranks a dismal 131 out of 193 countries in the under-five child mortality ranking (U5MR), a critical indicator of the well-being of the children, and needs drastic steps for such sad human condition.

Female Sterilization Situation

Female sterilization is quite high in some states (Figure 12, Table 1), like Himachal Pradesh (46%), Gujarat (41%), Karnataka (48%), Tamil Nadu (40%) and Kerala (43%) (Table 1). It is only at moderate level in West Bengal (31%), Orissa (32%), Madhya Pradesh (32%), Punjab (34%), Haryana (35%) and Andhra Pradesh (45%). On the other hand, it is very low in Uttar Pradesh (13%) and Bihar (14%). Consequently, fertility level is also very high there, compounded with massive poverty and female illiteracy. Besides, massive female illiteracy also fails to motivate them to seek female sterilization and the small family norm. Hence, positive strategies are required both for alleviating poverty/illiteracy, as well as for family planning methods.

Rural India's Picture

Rural India's situation is shown in Table 2, and illustrated in Figures 13 to 15. Maps are not discussed in details, since these are self-explanatory.

Female Illiteracy or Poverty in Rural India

Highest female illiteracy was found in Rajasthan (82%) (Figure 13, Table 2), followed by a very vast belt of high female illiteracy (60% to 80%) that spanned from Haryana in the west to Bihar in the east, and

Figure 13

India (Rural), Female Illiteracy (age 15-49), 1992-93

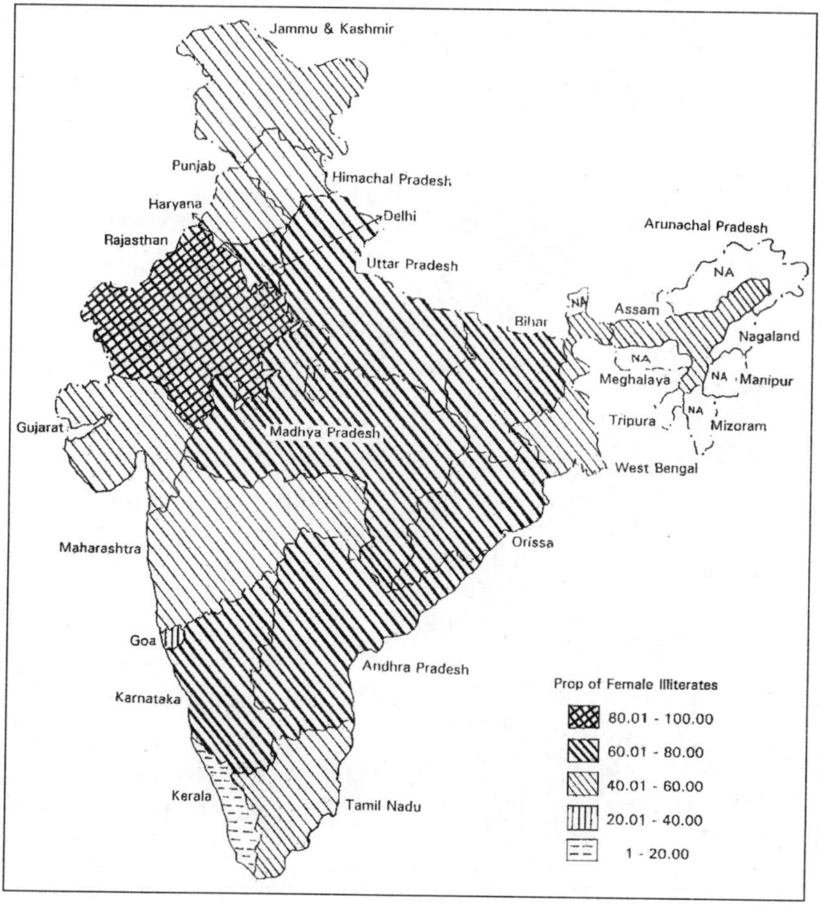

Figure 14
India (Rural), Total Fertility Rate, 1992-93

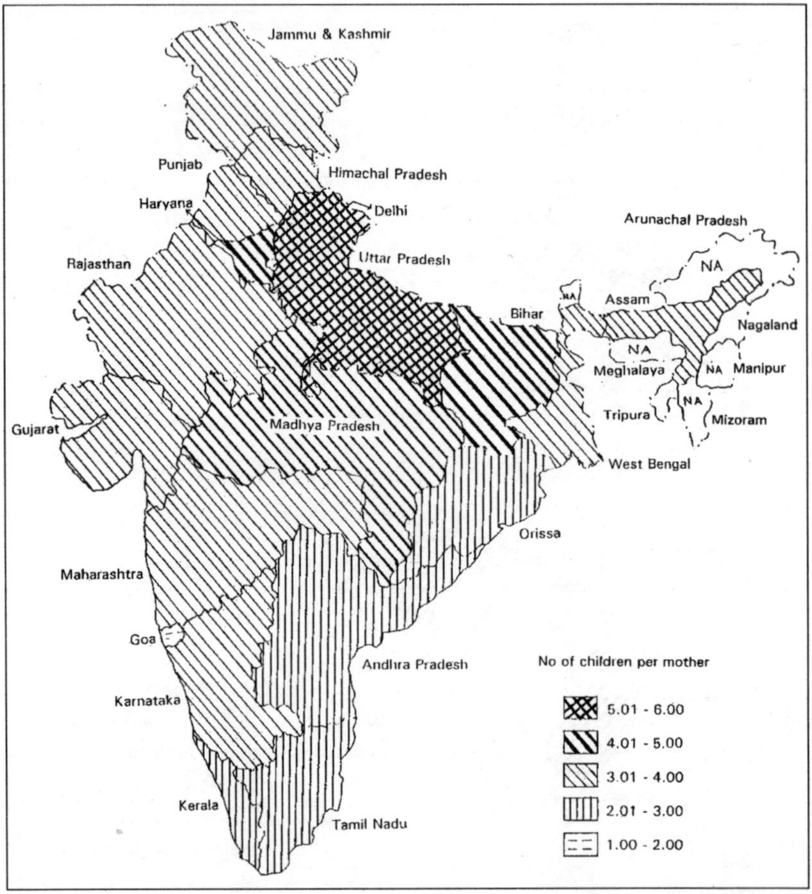

Table 2

Demographic and Socio-economic Data of Indian States, Rural Parts, NFHS Data (1992-93)

States	*IMR*	*CMR*	*CBR*	*TFR*	*Female illiteracy*	*Female going school*	*HH no toilet*	*No use of contrace-ptives*	*Steriliza-tion*	*No ANC care*	*TT given*	*Health profe-ssional assisted*	*Immuniza-tion*	*Pucca houses*
Andhra Pradesh	72.3	97.1	24.7	2.67	72.4	42.5	91.8	43.6	42.4	14.1	71.4	39.7	39.7	19.4
Assam	90.8	146.1	31.4	3.68	52.5	52.5	56.6	40.1	13.3	53.7	31.8	14.1	17.4	0.8
Bihar	93.8	132.7	32.9	4.15	77.3	33.2	92.7	19.8	16.6	66.8	26.4	15.0	9.1	7.6
Goa	29.1	38.0	17.8	1.99	32.7	88.2	68.9	44.4	33.6	3.3	81.0	86.8	75.2	35.0
Gujarat	70.2	108.2	28.4	3.17	57.0	51.4	83.3	47.5	42.6	27.4	56.4	32.0	46.2	19.5
Haryana	79.6	107.0	35.1	4.32	62.6	53.7	90.8	46.7	37.0	27.3	59.4	24.1	52.1	24.4
Himachal Pradesh	56.4	71.0	29.0	3.07	45.1	86.5	95.6	57.1	46.6	25.5	46.2	22.2	61.3	17.4
Jammu (of J&K.)	46.5	61.2	29.3	3.36	53.5	59.8	93.7	46.2	30.1	23.2	66.3	25.4	62.8	22.2
Karnataka	67.7	94.4	27.5	3.09	63.4	57.6	90.8	47.7	43.5	17.3	66.4	40.3	49.9	5.4
Kerala	28.7	38.5	20.3	2.09	18.7	88.7	34.3	61.4	47.5	2.4	88.9	87.6	54.0	15.8
Madhya Pradesh	92.9	145.2	33.3	4.11	74.9	39.5	95.2	33.4	30.7	52.0	36.7	22.1	25.6	3.1
Maharashtra	60.8	81.1	28.4	3.12	56.5	67.7	90.2	54.3	50.8	21.8	65.4	37.6	65.6	7.3
Orissa	116.9	135.1	27.0	3.00	62.7	58.0	95.0	34.2	30.5	39.7	50.7	15.6	34.7	5.3
Punjab	57.2	71.8	26.5	3.09	53.9	52.8	78.8	57.2	35.4	13.6	81.0	44.7	57.7	39.6
Rajasthan	73.4	107.5	28.1	3.87	81.8	29.5	93.2	28.2	25.1	70.6	23.8	17.4	16.1	25.1
Tamil Nadu	71.4	98.0	23.6	2.54	52.9	79.6	91.3	49.2	42.2	6.9	87.4	59.7	60.3	13.6
Uttar Pradesh	108.2	152.2	38.0	5.19	75.9	32.4	93.4	16.7	12.4	59.6	32.4	11.6	17.4	6.9
West Bengal	77.4	104.0	28.4	3.25	52.3	58.4	80.1	55.7	32.6	26.7	68.1	23.1	31.3	9.4

Source: National Family and Health Survey, All-India Report, International Institute of Populations Sciences, Mumbai, 1995

Note: Description of variables are same as given below Table 1.

from Uttar Pradesh in the north down to Karnataka in the south (excluding Maharashtra). The next belt of illiteracy (40% to 60%) covered Gujarat, Maharashtra, Tamil Nadu, West Bengal, Assam, Punjab, Himachal Pradesh and Jammu. Goa had lower illiteracy (20% to 40%), and Kerala enjoyed the lowest female illiteracy (less than 20%).

Indeed, all-India female illiteracy map (Figure 8) is a replica of rural female illiteracy map (Figure 13), as India truly lives in the villages. Hence, this widespread rural female illiteracy (i.e., massive poverty), which posits as the main stumbling block to demographic transition in India, and exactly here lies the key to the solution to this war on rural female illiteracy and rural poverty.

Total Fertility Rates in Rural India

Likewise, Figure 9 is an epitome of Figure 14, that is, all-India fertility map is almost a mirror image of rural fertility map, albeit in modified form (Table 2). In both, Uttar Pradesh has the highest fertility (above 4 children), followed by other states of northern heartland (except Rajasthan). In both the maps, the Deccan region and the eastern region have less fertility. Again, in both, Kerala and Goa have the lowest fertility. The essential corollary is that, we need to attack rural fertility levels first, before all-India fertility would come down. The crux of the matter lies in rural India. Thus, rural poverty alleviation is a must, before rural fertility will decline, and all-India fertility transition would also set in!

However, this is easier said than done. In India, the people and the academia seem to have limited understanding of these. Plans are almost always made against the poor. In India, there is no such thing as "Plan for the Poor"! It appears that always a pro-urban development bias in planning is advocated, and instead of "Garibi Hatao" (poverty alleviation) programme, we have actually succeeded in "Garib Hatao" (banishing the poor from villages, towns, slums of India, and from prosperity). Otherwise, precious sixty years after independence would not have been wasted. And, long ago, poverty, illiteracy, high fertility, high infant mortality, misery, agony, humiliation, severe exploitation and extreme corruption in public life would have been wiped out from

Figure 15
India (Rural), Infant Mortality Rate, 1992-93

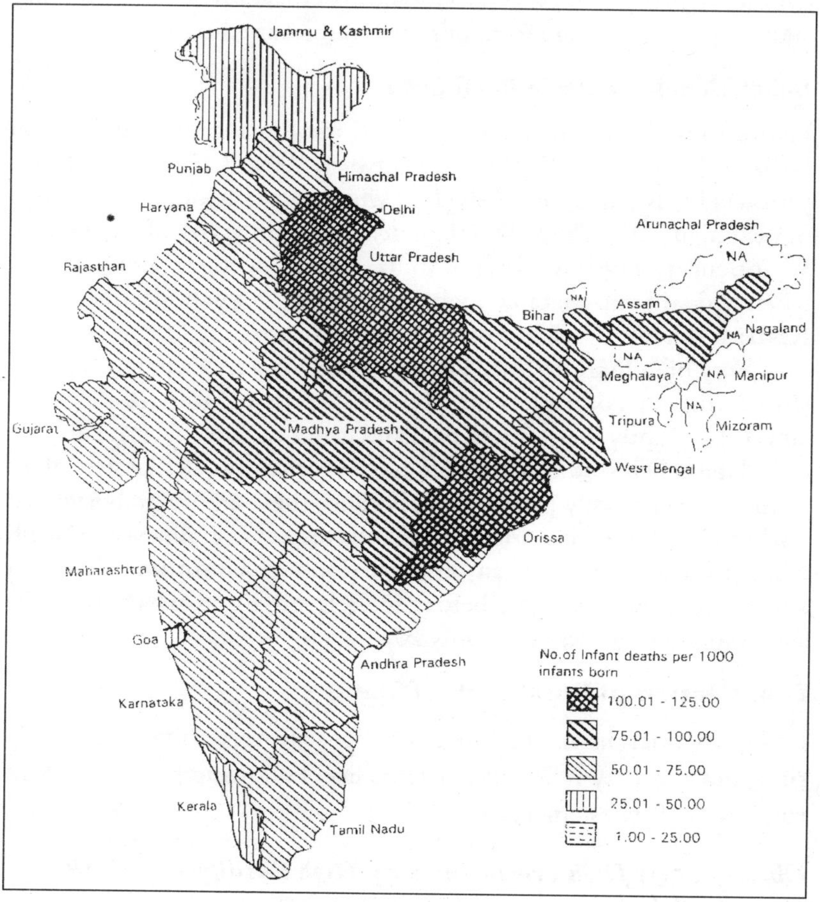

surface of India. Such very basic and crucial reality of the country would have been very easily understood and acted upon by all concerned people long before. The series of maps on poverty, illiteracy and inequality just stare us in our face, and testify the truth.

Infant Mortality Rates in Rural India

Figure 15 illustrates the pathetic condition of infant mortality rates in India (Table 2). Rural IMR ranged between 100 to 125 infant deaths in Orissa (117) and Uttar Pradesh (108) which were surrounded by a zone of next high IMR (75 to 100 infant deaths) in Bihar, Madhya Pradesh, West Bengal and Assam. Rest of India, both its northern and southern parts, had still considerably high IMR (50 to 75 infant deaths). Only Kerala and Jammu had less than 25 infant deaths.

Very high IMR in Uttar Pradesh and Orissa tells a poignantly sad story of millions of hapless new-born babies dying in India each year, and consequently their untold pain and miseries. No cold statistics can ever depict such sordid state of affairs. Majority of such massive infant deaths are very easily preventable, because these are water-borne and air-borne diseases like diarrhoea and respiratory illnesses. Death control must be undertaken on a war footing. Unfortunately, India still has a long way to go, before IMR level falls at what Sri Lanka achieved long ago (less than only 20).

Four Clusters of Rural Parts of States

Only very brief discussions are made, specially regarding situations in rural India as they reflect the true reality. Following four clusters of rural parts of states emerge:

Cluster 1: Very High Female Illiteracy-High Fertility-High IMR States (with little access to health services)

Typically, this is represented by highly populous and high growth states of Bihar, Uttar Pradesh, Rajasthan, and Madhya Pradesh, where very high female illiteracy or poverty (74% to 82%) causes very high fertility (4 or more children/mother), and high IMR (90 infants or more dying per 1,000 born per year). Because of very high female illiteracy, use of contraceptives is less than 20 per cent, and so also female sterilization and over 66 per cent of eligible mothers do not get AN care. These states need very urgent attention. They are the most problematic states for ensuring demographic transition.

Cluster 2: Considerably High Female Illiteracy-Moderate Fertility States (slightly more health services)

Characterized by quite high female illiteracy or poverty (57% to 63%) causing moderately high fertility (3 to 4.32 children/mother), and quite high IMR (67 to 79 infants dying per 1,000 born). Owing to quite high female illiteracy, use of contraceptives is still low (34% to 47%); likewise, also female sterilization (25% to 43%). One-third of eligible mothers do not have access to ANC (17% to 39%). Child immunization also needs serious attention. This cluster is represented by rural parts of Karnataka, Orissa, Haryana and Gujarat, and they need sustained efforts.

Cluster 3: Moderate Illiteracy-Moderate Fertility (moderately high use of health services)

Represented by Maharashtra, Punjab, Jammu, Assam, West Bengal and Andhra Pradesh. These are in transitory stage, characterized by moderately high female illiteracy or moderate poverty (52% to 72%), moderate fertility (2.7 to 3.7 children/mother), moderate IMR (46 to 90 infant deaths), moderate utilization of health services (child immunization, 17% to 65%) or female sterilization (13% to 55%). It is primarily due to moderately high level of female illiteracy, that health utilization rates are also moderate, and consequently, fertility and infant mortality are also moderate, not vice versa. Evidently, given more female education, female employment and better health services, these states will also achieve fertility decline. Policy prescriptions must be made accordingly.

Cluster 4: Low Illiteracy-Low Fertility States (quite high use of health services)

Fourth cluster has already experienced demographic transition, and is characterized by quite low female illiteracy (19% to 52%) and which has substantially dampened fertility (1.99 to 3.07 children/mother), and IMR is also quite low (28 to 71 infants dying per 1,000 infants). Due to relatively low female illiteracy (or less poverty), the use of contraceptives is quite high (44% to 61%). Similarly, female sterilization is higher (33% to 48%). Owing to high female literacy, very high proportion of mothers do get ANC. Likewise, access to child immunization is quite high (54% to 75%). This cluster is represented by rural Kerala, Goa, Tamil Nadu and Himachal Pradesh. These progressive states may serve as models of demographic decline for India.

Urban India Scenario

Urban India's situation is presented in Table 3, and illustrated in Figures 16 to 18.

Female Illiteracy or Poverty in Urban India

Obviously, female illiteracy in urban parts of the states is considerably less (Figure 16). Still some states have quite high female illiteracy, e.g., Uttar Pradesh (42%), followed by Bihar (38%), Madhya Pradesh (37%) and Orissa (36%). Even relatively developed states like Punjab and Gujarat have more than one-third women illiterate. Andhra Pradesh, Haryana and Rajasthan also have over 30 per cent women illiterate. Adverse effects of such a large burden of female illiteracy is reflected, in turn, on very low ANC rates; for instance, no ANC care is given to 29 per cent of eligible women in Uttar Pradesh, 34 per cent in Bihar and 23 per cent in Madhya Pradesh. Likewise, performance rates are also very much depressed regarding female sterilization, CPR rates and child immunization in such states. Evidently, causal linkages between female illiteracy and low utilization rates of various health services popped out very distinctly.

Total Fertility Rates in Urban India

Consequent to moderately high female illiteracy in urban components of states, total fertility rates are also moderately high (Figure 17). An almost 'one-to-one correspondence' between two features is manifest. For example, Uttar Pradesh has 42 per cent female illiteracy and 3.58 children per mother, followed by Bihar (with corresponding figures of 38 and 3.25). This in turn are followed by Madhya Pradesh (37 and 3.3.), Haryana (31 and 3.1), Rajasthan (32 and 2.8), Gujarat (33 and 2.7), Orissa (36 and 2.5), down to Tamil Nadu (28 and 2.36), Goa

Table 3

Demographic and Socio-economic Data of Indian States, Urban Parts, NFHS Data (1992-93)

States	IMR	CMR	CBR	TFR	Female illiteracy	Female going school	HH no toilet	No use of contrace-ptives	Sterili-zation	No ANC care	TT given	Health profess-ional assisted	ORS given	Immu-nization	% breast fed
Andhra Pradesh	64.6	73.7	22.3	2.35	32.7	76.2	29.6	56.6	51.3	6.6	84.9	78.3	50.0	58.3	18.0
Assam	66.8	101.0	23.2	2.53	25.9	75.7	7.6	62.3	22.7	19.4	66.2	56.8	58.1	40.0	29.1
Bihar	59.3	92.9	27.5	3.25	38.4	69.7	32.2	42.5	30.7	34.3	58.7	52.0	21.4	21.5	25.7
Delhi	65.4	83.1	26.7	3.02	29.2	79.1	15.9	60.3	23.2	17.6	72.5	53.0	39.4	57.8	21.5
Goa	34.9	39.8	16.4	1.80	20.4	92.0	34.5	51.7	27.4	5.1	86.1	90.1	23.8	74.6	19.7
Gujarat	65.4	94.2	24.7	2.65	33.2	74.5	29.0	52.7	38.1	15.9	76.7	65.7	25.0	57.0	17.7
Haryana	51.6	70.7	26.7	3.14	31.1	71.4	29.3	58.0	28.5	31.2	76.8	52.5	21.7	58.0	21.9
Himachal Pradesh	48.8	48.8	20.2	2.03	17.2	95.6	21.6	70.4	38.7	5.1	62.6	67.4	65.5	81.5	16.2
Jammu (of J & K)	39.2	46.5	21.2	2.13	22.8	82.0	23.1	64.4	27.5	3.9	84.8	67.2	57.1	84.8	18.0
Karnataka	60.0	70.6	22.7	2.39	25.4	80.1	26.1	52.0	40.4	12.1	78.2	77.2	34.0	57.6	21.3
Kerala	9.5	13.1	18.0	1.78	14.6	91.9	15.7	68.2	50.4	0.5	92.3	95.7	43.3	55.7	23.7
Madhya Pradesh	54.7	72.6	27.2	3.27	37.1	68.4	26.7	47.7	34.6	24.4	66.9	61.1	45.6	43.0	21.2
Maharashtra	33.3	52.4	24.4	2.54	27.2	84.3	18.4	52.9	39.5	9.8	79.8	77.8	43.5	61.6	22.7
Orissa	84.5	107.2	23.9	2.53	36.1	77.8	32.5	47.4	37.2	22.4	71.6	48.7	50.0	43.8	24.7
Punjab	42.3	55.5	21.0	2.48	33.7	62.3	12.5	62.7	30.3	7.2	88.6	60.1	33.3	75.6	18.4
Rajasthan	68.6	77.7	22.3	2.77	32.5	69.1	42.4	47.1	38.1	48.8	52.7	45.2	14.2	45.9	21.7
Tamil Nadu	61.2	64.7	23.4	2.36	27.7	87.3	26.2	50.9	34.7	3.0	94.9	92.8	24.3	73.3	14.1
Uttar Pradesh	59.1	88.8	28.6	3.58	41.8	60.5	30.5	32.0	15.8	29.3	62.1	44.2	21.4	32.9	24.3
West Bengal	68.2	83.3	18.5	2.14	27.0	80.9	34.6	61.8	25.4	17.7	78.1	66.5	47.9	44.1	27.3

Source: National Family and Health Survey (NFHS),All-India Report, International Institute of Population Sciences, Mumbai, 1995.

Note: Description of variables are same as given below Table 1.

Figure 16

India (Urban), Female Illiteracy (age 15-49), 1992-93

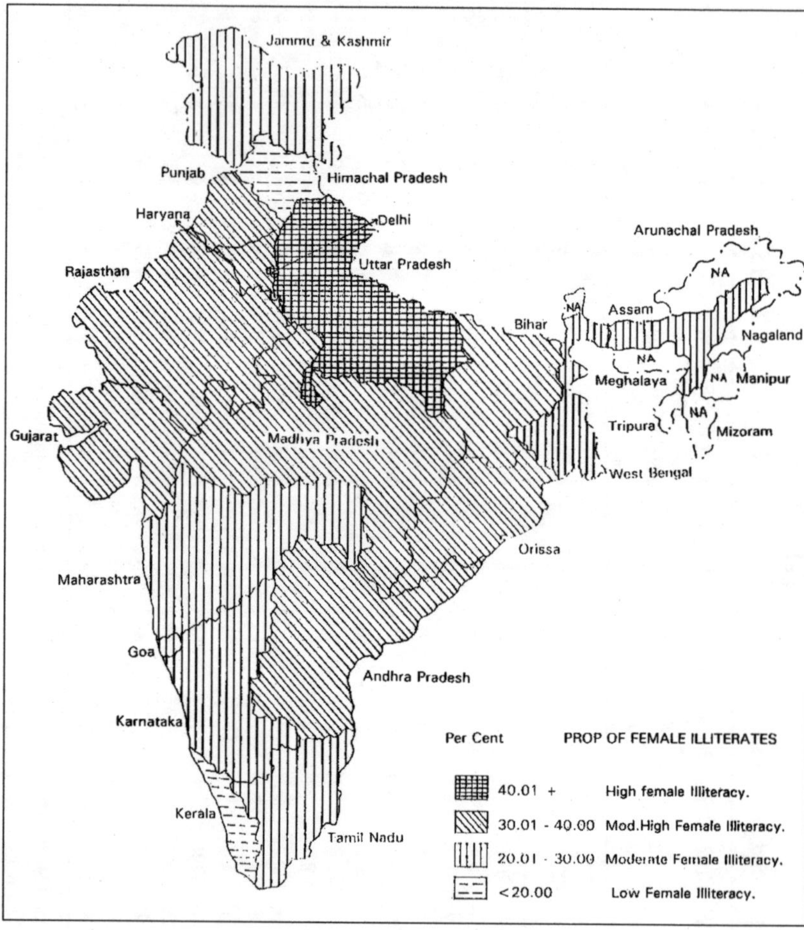

Figure 17
India (Urban), Total Fertility Rate, 1992-93

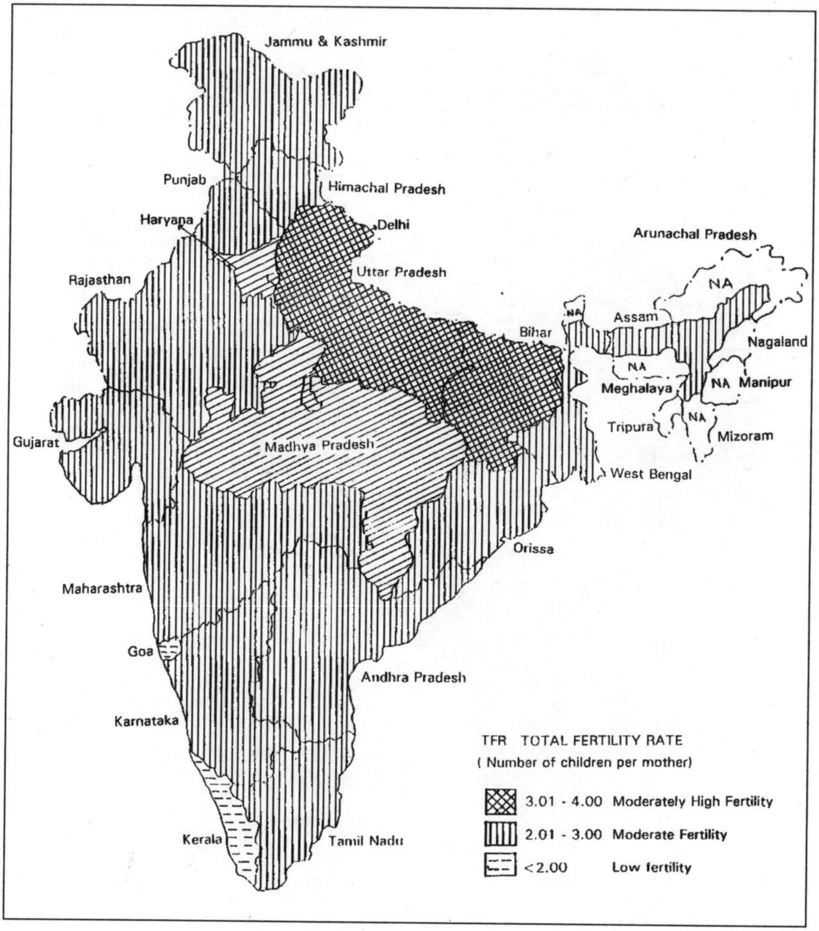

Figure 18
India (Urban), Infant Mortality Rate, 1992-93

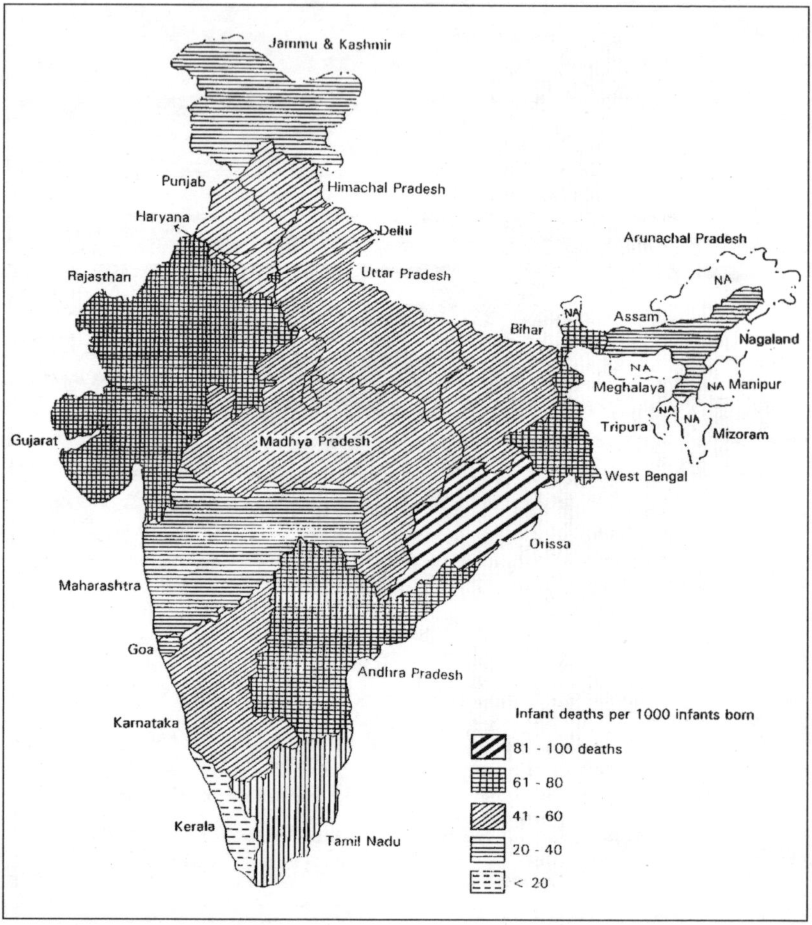

(20.4 and 1.8) and Kerala (14.6 and 1.78). Such a unique step-like pattern has emerged, of course, with some knick-points. The fact that such a wonderful 'one-to-one relationship' or 'isomorphism' has occurred, is itself very remarkable. In social sciences, even in physical sciences, such a strong and clear isomorphism is very rarely achieved!

Infant Mortality Rates in Urban India

The poignantly sad story of high infant mortality levels, even in urban India, is very depressing (Figures 18). IMR is highest even in urban Orissa (84 infant deaths). It lies between 61 to 80 infant deaths in urban parts of West Bengal, Andhra Pradesh, Gujarat and Rajasthan. IMR is also very high (between 41 and 60 infant deaths) in entire Hindi heartland (urban components of Uttar Pradesh, Bihar, Madhya Pradesh, Punjab, Haryana, and Himachal Pradesh) – where female illiteracy is very widespread, and consequently, child immunization, ANC care, and institutional child delivery are all very dismal. The causal bonding between very high female illiteracy and very high infant mortality is rampant everywhere! Because the mothers are poor and illiterate, they do not have easy and effective access to health care services, and as a resultant of the two, IMR is also very high. Causal relations here must be understood and appreciated in this crucial direction not vice versa.

5

Findings of Direct Canonical Analysis of Demographic, Socio-Economic and Population Policies of India: Models I, II, and III

"Say, the ignorant Indian, the poor and destitute Indian, the Brahmin Indian, the Pariah Indian is my brother" (Swami Vivekananda, 1896, Complete Work, Centenary Volume IV, 1963, p. 480).

"Tell the truth boldly, whether it hurts or not" (Swami Vivekananda, 1893, Complete Work, Centenary Volume VII, 1963, p. 79).

"Stand as a rock; you are indestructible" (Swami Vivekananda, 1894, Complete Work, Centenary Volume II, 1963, p. 236).

Introduction

Recapitulation of Demographic Field Theory

The Demographic Field Theory does not visualize demographic phenomena in isolation, rather views them as a *gestalt*, in a holistic approach, in a system way, within a field theoretic schema, all varied elements seen in their causal relations, and as an organized and structured whole (Mukherji, 1989b, pp. 343-373). Briefly speaking, it verbally states and also mathematically verifies that:

(a) demographic behaviour sub-system (i.e., fertility and mortality behaviour of states/regions, or the individuals);
(b) their respective socio-economic-cultural-political sub-system; and
(c) their population policies or programmes sub-system, consciously or unconsciously followed (like family planning, or ante-natal care, child immunization, etc.).

All are causally related; all these three sub-systems are interdependent parts of the larger *demographic system,* or the *demographic field*, within which any change in one part would generate corresponding changes in other. It also states that demographic behaviour of any region (country, or society, or any individual) is a linear function of its respective socio-economic-cultural-political attributes-cum-population policies or programmes that are followed/ adopted.

The Theory states and also proves that these three sub-systems, i.e., demographic matrix (D), socio-economic matrix (S), and population policy matrix (P), are interdependent and isomorphic, and changes in one sub-system will bring corresponding changes in other. The theory and its notion of causal relations and interdependence of matrices and their elements can be tested with canonical model. In this study, the theory is verified by performing canonical correlation tests upon three data matrices, narrated above, by using NFHS data (see Mukherji, 1989). Canonically, the Demographic Field Theory can be shown as, D = (S + P).

Further verifications of the Demographic Field Theory and findings were also presented elsewhere (Mukherji, 1992, pp. 1-91; 2005a, pp. 1-75; 2005b, pp. 1-38; and 2005c, pp. 38-75).

Demographic and Socio-Economic Maps of India

In the last chapter, we have seen that Figures 8 to 12 present maps of demographic, socio-economic and population programme situations of India or all major states (rural and urban parts combined). Conversely, Figures 13 to 15 provide the same for rural parts of all major states, and Figures 16 to 18 present the picture of urban India. Most such figures are self-explanatory, and not elaborated further (see also Tables 1 to 3, Chapter 4).

Findings of All-India (Total) State-Level Canonical Analysis (Model I)

Final canonical linkages are generated between demographic, socio-economic and population policy matrices. Table 4 presents all findings of canonical analysis. Here, data of 25 states are analyzed (taking total series, i.e., rural-urban series combined). As a result, four canonical linkages are generated, every time causally linking only those variables from the dependent and the independent set that are causally linked – which belong to that particular *demographic field* or *demographic system*, while reducing others to near zero, which do not belong to that specific field. Important canonical loadings or weights are shown in bold letters in all tables. In Table 1, following four canonical linkage pairs, or causal links, have emerged in Table 4, and all of them are statistically very highly significant (Mukherji, 2000d, pp. 1-145).

Canonical analysis usually yields a set of solutions as large as there are patterns in D (demographic) and S+ P (socio-economic plus policy) matrices, whichever has the smaller number of dimensions. Since there were only four variables in D matrix, then, only four pairs of canonical vectors or canonical variates are extracted successively from D and S + P, with decreasing order of predictability in the same manner as in principal components analysis. As can be seen from each such canonical interrelationships, a specific type of socio-economic-cum-policy variables are causally linked, and in each case the canonical correlations between the pair of vectors maximized.

With reference to Canonical Structure Matrix (Table 4), the following points are noteworthy:

1. *Canonical variates* are separate patterns of relationships between input factors (or variables).
2. *Canonical loadings* are degree and direction of relationship of specific variables with canonical variate pattern.
3. *Canonical correlation* is statistical dependence between each matched pair of variates.
4. *Trace Correlation* is general statistical overlap between two sets, dependent and independent.

Very Highly Statistically Significant and Meaningful Findings

The overall statistical overlap or *trace correlation* is also very high, i.e., 0.90; the independent set has thus explained 81 per cent of total variance in the dependent set. Besides, successively four very highly significant relations have also emerged, with canonical values as high as 0.99, 0.96, 0.86, or 0.78. These are not only very highly statistically powerful results, but also very meaningful findings, having great policy implications.

Table 4

Canonical Structure Matrix – All-India (Total Series Data), State Level, NFHS Data, 1992-93

	Canonical Variate			
	1	*2*	*3*	*4*
A. *Demographic Matrix (Dependent Set)*		*Canonical Weights*		
1. IMR (Infant Mortality Rate)	**.73**	-.38	-.33	.38
2. CMR (Child Mortality Rate)	**-.61**	**.46**	-.27	**-.44**
3. CBR (Crude Birth Rate)	.14	**-.55**	-.35	**-.57**
4. TFR (Total Fertility Rate)	.25	**.56**	**.82**	**.56**
B. *Socio-economic-cum-Policy Matrix (Independent Set)*		*Canonical Weights*		
5. Femilliteracy (prop. female illiterates)	**.52**	.06	**.43**	.33
6. Femtoschool (girls age 6-14 going school)	.37	**-.53**	.11	-.29
7. Married<18 (prop. women married at age <18)	.09	.04	-.04	-.24
8. Hhwithwater (prop. HH with water facility)	.05	-.05	.16	.09
9. Hhnotoilet (prop. HH without toilet)	.01	-.21	-.32	.10
10. Secontracept (prop. using contraceptives)	.07	**.42**	-.09	.27
11. Sterilization (prop. sterilized)	.14	**-.25**	**.34**	.11
12. Unmetneedfp (unmet need in FP)	.28	.22	.17	.23
13. ANC Care (prop. got ante-natal care)	**.33**	.02	**-.48**	**-.53**
14. GOT TT (Prop. got tetanus toxoid)	-.01	**-.35**	-.01	.25
15. Deliveryinphc (prop. of delivery in PHC)	.24	-.04	.23	.23
16. Assistedbyhp (prop. assisted by health prof.)	**-.37**	.32	-.18	.13
17. Orsgiven (per cent oral rehydr. solution given)	-.05	-.07	-.01	.00
18. Child immunized (prop. children immunized)	**-.35**	.33	.27	.00
19. Breastfed (prop. children breastfed)	-.09	-.06	-.10	-.09
20. Breastfed+ Food (breastfed + mushy food)	.00	.01	.27	.22
21. Underweight (per cent underweight babies)	-.09	-.07	-.15	**-.29**

Contd...

Contd...

C. *Canonical Correlation*			**.99** **.97**	**.86** **.79**
D. *Meaning of Canonical Linkage Pair*	High IMR due to high female illiteracy, and also due to less child immunization and less assisted by health professional	High TFR due to less females going to school, & also less sterilization, and less TT for mothers.	High TFR due to female illiteracy, little ANC care, and inspite of some sterilization.	Less CMR due to fewer underweight babies who are breastfed and got solid, mushy food. TFR also moderately high due to less ANC care.

E.	*Trace Correlation*	= **.904** (that is, general statistical overlap between dependent and independent sets is about 82% (trace correlation (.90) squared times 100)
	Wilks Lambda	= .000175
	Chi Square	= 121.098
	Significance	= *0.0001*

The interdependence of the demographic behaviour and social policy matrices is tested by such a significant value of 'trace correlation'. Given that most multivariate tests in social science research have correlations ranging only around 0.4 or 0.5, this value of trace correlation must be considered very high.

Interpretation of Canonical Variates

Corresponding canonical loadings describing the correlations of the variables are also given for behaviour (i.e., demographic) and attribute (socio-economic-cum-policies) sets. These canonical loadings or coefficients indicate the degree of correlations of variables (or factors) with canonical variates.

Comparison of the loadings for all variables (or factors) with the pair of variates permits the identification of these socio-economic-cum-policy variables (or factors) that are most highly related to a particular demographic behaviour(s) (Important loadings are shown with bold face in Table 4 and all other tables in Chapters 5 to 8 and 10) (read each column from up-downwards).

For instance, in the first column, the above-mentioned causal factor from socio-economic matrix, defined as high female illiteracy, with canonical loading of 0.52, is intimately linked with one variable of demographic matrix, i.e., 'high IMR' with canonical loading of (0.73), while other variables reduced to near zero. In short, these two variables are found to be 'canonically matched', or highly causally linked. Amidst multitudes of data, observations and relationships, this particular relationship is of greatest importance. Corresponding canonical correlation is remarkably high, i.e., 0.986, which indisputably testifies that in the present-day India, to wage war against high female illiteracy will be the most required socio-economic developmental effort needed to dampen high IMR. These two variables, together, have emerged as a 'demographic field'; a specific socio-demographic linkage equation; a system, *a gestalt*.

For those unfamiliar with canonical interpretations, following elaboration of this pair of variates may be helpful. When factor analysis is done before canonical analysis, and since each behaviour (dependent set) and attribute (independent set) variate are linear combinations of the vectors of earlier behaviour and attribute (socio-economic-cum-policy) matrices, then, interpretations of relationships between two canonical vectors become all the more complicated. Because a few original variables have formed a 'factor', then a few factors from both the sets have formed canonical pair, or 'a field'. Many such smaller fields together make the total demographic field, or the system. To illustrate these points, the following kinds of relationships can be shown for new canonically-transformed scores (u and v), written with respect to first pair of behaviour (demographic) and attribute (socio-economic-plus-policies) variates (see Table 4):

u_1 = **0.73** (IMR) - **0.61**(CMR) + 0.14(CBR) + 0.25 (TFR)

v_1 = **0.52** (female illiteracy) + 0.37 (girls age 6-14 going to school) + 0.09 (women married at age < 18) + 0.05 (households with water) + 0.005 (households without toilet) +0.07(use contraceptives) + 0.14 (sterilized) + 0.28 (unmet need in FP) **+ 0.35** (ANC care given) - 0.003 (got TT) + 0.24 (delivery in PHC) **- 0.37** (assisted by health professionals) - 0.05 (ORS given) **- 0.35** (child immunized) - 0.09 (breastfed) + 0.00 (breastfed plus mushy food given) - 0.09 (underweight babies).

Noteworthy feature is that while a few specific factors (with higher loadings, usually greater than 0.30) are picked-off from both attribute (predictor) and behaviour (dependent) sets to show their maximal relationships, the relations with other variables are reduced close to zero. That is, *a particular demographic field is identified*, amidst masses of data and relationships – which we cannot easily intuit or cognize. Thus, a system, a field, an organic whole, a gestalt, a causal relation, or a socio-economic-demographic cause-and-effect linkage equation is generated by such analysis – specifically linking only those factors which belong to that particular field, excluding others which do not belong to that particular demographic field.

In this sense, only canonical analysis can permit generating and identifying such causal relations, which cannot be found through ordinary regression analysis, or factor analysis. Here lies profound utility and elegance of field theory-cum-canonical model.

The above complicated canonical linkage equation now can be rewritten as follows, based on *only high loadings:*

0.73 (IMR) = **0.52** (female Illiteracy) + **0.33** (ANC care given) - **0.35** (assisted by health professional) - **0.35** (child immunized)

This can easily and meaningfully be interpreted that, for the first largest set of canonical variates, the attribute, 'female illiteracy' increases 'high IMR', specially when health assistance and child immunization are lacking (and even when some ANC care given). Canonical correlation between this matched pair of canonical variates is **0.99**, indicating that 97 per cent (correlation squared times 100) of variance in this set of variate pair has been explained by such specific attribute-bahaviour indicators. That is, one single factor, widespread and universal female literacy will be greatly conducive to reduce infant mortality in underdeveloped and neglected states of India.

This single factor has emerged as the strongest determinant of demographic behaviour, amidst a total 21 variables, including masses of data, entities and interrelationships. Conspicuous absence of many other important variables (specially female sterilization or CPR of family planning) in the first fundamental canonical linkage is also very noteworthy. That is, compared to female illiteracy factor in determining fertility rate, other factors turned out to be near zero (Mukherji, 2000e, pp. 10-15).

Some salient points regarding interpretations require mention. First, mostly, interpretations of canonical linkages are easy and straight-forward, which can be obtained by just identifying and causally linking the more highly loaded canonical weights (usually above 0.40), with each specific variable(s) (shown with bold face in Table 4 and all Tables in Chapter 5 to 8 and 10). Second, however, sometimes, interpretations become very complex, particularly when third or fourth pair of canonical variates indicate 'bi-polar' or 'complex' relations. In such cases, only the most clearer picture among the two poles that emerges, is to be considered (sometimes ignoring another bi-polarity). Third, the importance is primarily given to the 'positive' canonical weights, ignoring the 'negative' weights, whenever these do not make sense and blur the picture. Fourth, whenever one variable/factor indicates high canonical weights on two (or more) canonical variate pairs, then, only that specific canonical variate pair is considered with which that particular variable is loaded relatively highest, ignoring the lower weights. Regarding such canonical interpretations, more details are given in Pyle (1974, pp. 21-141) and Wood (1973, pp. 477-82).

In like manner, successive canonical correlations, loadings, and corresponding patterns of causal relationships between demographic behaviour set and socio-economic attribute-cum-policy set can be easily interpreted (Table 4). The three remaining canonical relationships are briefly stated below.

All these canonical linkage equations are not only statistically highly significant, but also practically very meaningful (Mukherji, 2000b, pp. 1-35). Each of them has emerged as a separate demographic field, orthogonal and independent of the previous one. Their interpretations and policy implications are very apparent. All the four canonical linkages mainly emphasize upon the need for enhancing developmental components (like universal female literacy programmes), side by side with great need for improvement of health services, nutrition development, and women's employment and development as useful policy instruments, apart from continuation of current family welfare programmes and spread of contraception.

These are interpreted as follows:

1. High IMR occurs in India due to high female illiteracy, and also due to less immunization and less assisted in child delivery by health professionals (canonical correlation: 0.987).

2. High total fertility rate and high level of child mortality occur, because of less girls are attending schools, and also less sterilization and less tetanus toxoid are given to the mothers (canonical correlation: 0.965).
3. Very high level of total fertility rate occurs, due to high female illiteracy, and also due to little ante-natal care given, in spite of some sterilization (canonical correlation: 0.867).
4. Less child mortality occurs due to less proportion of underweight babies, who were breastfed and also got solid/mushy food. Besides, TFR is also moderately high due to less ante-natal care given (canonical correlation: 0.787).

Significance of All-India (Total Series) Findings of Model I

The implications of these very crucial findings are very clear. Here, in this study, illiteracy is considered as the surrogate or proxy indicator of widespread poverty in India. The findings thus show that it is the widespread poverty that is most responsible for high levels of fertility and high levels of infant mortality in India, specially in the backward and neglected states of UP, MP, Bihar, Rajasthan, and others. The evil and unjust syndrome between poverty and high fertility must be delinked very urgently in India, if we are indeed soulfully concerned about fertility decline in this country (Mukherji, 1998a, pp. 250-270).

The findings therefore emphasize upon the great need for providing universal and general education to all the girls as well as to all the adult women in India, if we are really desirous of on-setting fertility decline in these Indian states, and also to bring down infant mortality rates. This step alone will do the miracle. Without fighting out massive illiteracy among the Indian women, specially in rural areas (of UP, MP, Bihar and Rajasthan where it exceeds 80%), nothing can be changed, no matter how much we may try to motivate the women and men to adopt the small family norm (Mukherji, 2000h, p. 4). This is the greatest requirement.

Secondly, there is also the great need to enhance the family planning programmes, as well as ANC care, child immunization, MCH care, and all other aspects of the reproductive health. There is a great need to activate all these crucial aspects of primary health services, specially in rural, backward, and hitherto neglected and inaccessible regions. Thus, socio-economic development efforts and programmes for providing safe motherhood and child survival programmes and catering reproductive health should go simultaneously.

Thirdly, the crucial relationship between illiterate mothers and very high level of infant deaths has emerged time and again; so also the causal relations between high TFR and widespread female illiteracy. These evil syndromes between fertility, infant mortality and female illiteracy (which is indeed an index of abject poverty) must be delinked, before demographic decline will set in all parts of India, firmly and securely. Without such essential changes, very little can be achieved. These findings are confirmed by mathematically very high-powered canonical findings, as detailed in the table.

Female Illiteracy Emerged as the Most Important Cause of Fertility and Infant Mortality

In this section, the Demographic Field Theory is applied by performing canonical analysis upon the three data matrices (D, S, and P), mentioned above. Recent NFHS data of 25 major states are used, taking rural and urban components separately. Two separate canonical analyses are thus made, separately for rural and urban parts of India. The variables taken are shown in Tables 2 and 3. The canonical findings are shown in Table 5 and 6. Very many notable results are generated. These findings emphatically indicate that female illiteracy has emerged as the most important cause of fertility and infant mortality in India. These results are not only statistically very highly significant, but they are also very meaningful findings having great policy import.

In this context, we may also examine the findings of some other studies. For instance, Parasuraman, Roy et al. (1999, p. 135) found that "the educated women initiate use of contraception early in their reproductive life. Compared to illiterates, educated women desire to have less number of children and they implement this desire more efficiently". Here, the lacuna of the study is that the researchers did not probe into the actual socio-economic 'processes' and 'forces' behind such 'desire' for less children among the educated women vis-à-vis the illiterate and poor women. The underlying causes must be found, and which are explained in the present study.

Table 5

Canonical Structure Matrix for Rural India, Using All-India NFHS Data, 1992-93

Variables	*Canonical Variate Pair*			
	I	*II*	*III*	*IV*
A. *Demographic Matrix (Dependent set)*	*Canonical Loadings*			
1. Infant Mortality Rate (IMR)	.11	.31	**-.64**	.12
2. Child Mortality Rate (CMR)	.17	-.25	**.65**	**-.78**
3. Crude Birth Rate (CBR)	**-.65**	**.68**	.29	.17
4. Total Fertility Rate (TFR)	**.72**	**-.61**	-.28	**.58**
B. *Socio-economic-cum-Policy Matrix (Independent Set)*	*Canonical Loadings*			
1. Female illiteracy rate	**.55**	-.01	-.06	**-.57**
2. Prop. females attending school	.34	.17	-.36	**-.54**
3. Prop. no toilet in houses	-.26	-.16	.12	.19
4. Prop. using contraceptives	-.32	**-.33**	.42	.02
5. Prop. used sterilization	-.03	.23	-.24	.01
6. No ante-natal care given	**.39**	-.31	-.28	.40
7. Tetanus toxoid given to women	**.44**	.20	**-.56**	.02
8. Assisted during child delivery	-.18	**-.79**	**.38**	-.01
9. Prop. children immunized	-.10	.01	.12	**.41**
10. Prop. *pucca* houses	.05	-.06	-.18	.02
C. *Canonical Correlation*	**0.96**	**0.94**	**0.83**	**0.69**
D. *Meaning of Canonical Linkage Pair*	Because of high female illiteracy, high fertility occurs (TFR), also as not much ANC care given, though TT given.	Less contraceptives, so high CBR, specially when not helped by health professionals.	IMR is low because female illiteracy is low, not because contraceptive use is less and assistance from health professional during delivery also available.	CMR is low, as immunization is much. High TFR, also as less females are attending school.

E. *Trace Correlation*	**0.861** (indicates 0.86 squared times hundred = 74% of total variance in dependent set is explained by independent set)
Wilks Lambda	0.001
Chi Square	67.59
Significance	*0.0001*

That study further argued that "illiterate women desire to have more children, and though they too implement their desire by using contraceptives, they lack the necessary will or are not properly equipped to implement it at an appropriate junction. Therefore, with education, demand for children reduces and also the capacity to implement the desire also improves" (Parasuraman, Roy, et al., 1999, pp. 135-36). However, the study did not delve into the real 'causal reasons' behind the illiterate women's so-called 'lack of will' or 'not properly equipped' implementation of contraceptives; nor untangled the 'cause and effect relationship' between poverty and high fertility. As if, such incapacities are the actual causes, they themselves are not the very consequences of widespread and abject poverty among illiterate women!

Findings of Rural India, State-Level Analysis (Model II)

Table 5 presents the findings of canonical analysis with reference to rural components of the states. Here data of rural parts of 24 major Indian states are considered (Delhi obviously had no rural part and so excluded). Consequently, four canonical linkages are generated, every time causally linking only those variables from the dependent and the independent sets that are causally related. That is, only those variables are picked-up in each iteration which belong to that specific *demographic system* or *demographic field*, while reducing other variables to near zero which do not belong to that particular system or field. Noteworthy canonical loadings or weights are shown in bold face in Table 5. The technical details of canonical model is available in Cooley and Lohnes (1962, pp. 45-65); and the way it is integrally used in Demographic Field Theory is given in earlier studies (Mukherji, 1983b, pp. 1-65; 1989b, pp. 342-73).

The following four canonical linkage pairs, or causal links, have emerged, and all of them are found to be statistically of very high value. The general statistical overlap or mapping or *Trace correlation* is also found to be remarkably high, i.e., 0.8614; thus, 81 per cent of total variance in the dependent matrix has been explained by the independent matrix. Moreover, successively, there also emerged four very highly significant canonical linkages, with canonical values as high as 0.96, 0.94, or, 0.83, or 0.69. It is exceptionally rare to find either in physical or social sciences successively such high values of canonical correlations, specially in a single test. The canonical linkage pairs are not only statistically very powerful findings, but are also practically very meaningful interrelations. These crucial canonical linkages have great policy implications.

These are as follows:

1. Because of high female illiteracy, high total fertility occurs; this is also because ante-natal care is not given, though sometimes tetanus toxoid is given to mothers (canonical correlation is 0.9557).
2. Because less contraceptives are used, high level of Crude Birth Rate occurs, specially when help of health professionals is not available for child deliveries (canonical correlation is 0.9414).
3. Infant mortality is found to be low because female illiteracy is low in certain states; also because contraceptive use is moderately high and assistance from health professionals during child delivery is also available (canonical correlation is 0.8250).
4. Child mortality rate is low because child immunization is considerably high. Also Total Fertility Rate is high owing to the fact that less proportion of females are attending schools (proportion of girls attending school education appears to have an indirect, but definite, dampening effect upon the fertility levels in the households/states) (canonical correlation is 0.6983).

Findings of Urban India, State-Level Analysis (Model III)

Table 6 presents the findings of urban components of 25 major states of India (including urban Delhi). The variables remained almost the same in both the sets, except only two variables in the independent set (like oral rehydration solution (ORS) given to the children, and proportion of children breastfed were found to be more relevant in the urban data and included).

Here also, the following four pairs of canonical linkages, or causal relations, are generated by canonical analysis, and all of them are statistically of very high value. The overall statistical mapping or *trace correlation* is also exceptionally high, i.e., 0.8274; 69 per cent of total variance in the demographic set is thus being explained by the

Table 6

Canonical Structure Matrix for Urban India, Using All-India NFHS Data, 1992-93

Variables	*Canonical Variate Pair*			
	I	*II*	*III*	*IV*
A. *Demographic Matrix (Dependent Set)*		*Canonical Loadings*		
1. Infant Mortality Rate (IMR)	-.19	**.44**	-.55	.21
2. Child Mortality Rate (CMR)	**.40**	-.48	**.58**	**.63**
3. Crude Birth Rate (CBR)	-.52	**.65**	.37	.04
4. Total Fertility Rate (TFR)	**.72**	-.38	-.45	**-.73**
B. *Socio-economic-cum-policy Matrix (Independent Set)*		*Canonical Loadings*		
1. Female illiteracy rate	**.67**	-.06	**.35**	**.61**
2. Prop. females attending school	-.18	.28	**.45**	**.46**
3. Prop. no toilet in houses	.02	-.21	**-.46**	.29
4. Prop. using contraceptives	.33	-.25	-.15	**.34**
5. Prop. used sterilization	-.29	.00	.16	.01
6. No ante-natal care given	-.02	**.46**	-.39	-.32
7. Tetanus toxoid given to women	**-.40**	.38	.00	-.04
8. Assisted during child delivery	.23	-.24	-.28	-.19
9. Oral rehydration Solution given	-.21	.24	-.22	.02
10. Prop. children immunized	-.12	**-.30**	-.04	.00
11. Prop. children breastfed	.18	**-.48**	.32	.23
C. *Canonical Correlation*	**0.99**	**0.91**	**0.75**	**0.60**
D. *Meaning of Canonical Linkage Pair*	Because of high female illiteracy, so high fertility (TFR), inspite of contraceptive use. And mod. high CMR, as TT not given.	High IMR, as little immunization, no ANC care, and no breastfeeding done. CBR is also quite high.	CMR is high as only mod. ANC given, little breast-feeding, female illiteracy quite high inspite of some females attend school.	When females attend school, TFR is low; and though female illiteracy high. Contraceptive use also contribute much. CMR is high.

E. *Trace Correlation*	**0.827** (indicates 0.83 squared times hundred = 69% of total variance in dependent set is explained by independent set)
Wilks Lambda	.0006
Chi Square	80.05
Significance	**0.0001**

combined set of socio-economic-cum-policy variables. Besides, in successive iterations, four very highly significant canonical linkages are also generated, having canonical values as high as 0.99, 0.91, 0.75, or 0.60. It is simply very remarkable to obtain successively such a series of high values of canonical correlations in social sciences. It is also heartening to note that these canonical linkages are not only statistically of high values, but they also have very pragmatic meaning. They also appeal to the common sense. Evidently, such canonical findings have great policy import. These results include:

1. High total fertility rate (TFR) occurs because of high female illiteracy. This occurs in spite of some contraceptive use among the females. Moderately high child mortality also occurs, because often Tetanus Toxoid is not given to mothers (i.e., child often surviving in the first year, but remains weak, and dies later, thus increasing child mortality) (canonical correlation is 0.9928).
2. High infant mortality occurs because little immunization is provided to children, no ante-natal care, nor breast-feeding is given. Crude birth rate is also high (canonical correlation is 0.9083).
3. Child mortality rate is high as only to some extent ante-natal care is given, little breast-feeding is practised, and female illiteracy is quite high, although some females attend school (canonical correlation is 0.7508).
4. Total fertility rate (TFR) is low, because females attend school (and this have a negative effect upon fertility), although female illiteracy is quite high in some states. Contraceptive use also contributes in dampening the fertility. However, due to high level of female illiteracy, child mortality is also high (canonical correlation is 0.6032).

Significance of Findings of Rural and Urban India Level Analysis

One of the most fundamental findings that clearly emerges, for both rural and urban India, is that it is primarily the widespread female illiteracy that has caused very high fertility in various states of India. Canonical linkage shows almost a one-to-one relationship between the two. It clearly emphasizes that in India it is the widespread female illiteracy, which is the '*cause*' and fertility is the '*effect*'; not vice versa. As Tables 1 and 2 demonstrate, compared with female illiteracy factor, other variables contribute much less in determining the fertility, often insignificant.

Most frequently, very many conventional thinkers argue that the relationship between female illiteracy and fertility is already known, or the relationship is bi-polar, or that we do not yet know which one is the cause and which is the effect variable; or some may also say – what is new about it? So on and so forth. They argue in these ways (over millennium!), and thereby try to de-emphasize the great importance and policy and social significance of such a crucial causal relationship, so that we will never need to take a very serious and soulful concern of this oppressive phenomena! Nor ever need to take actions to relieve such pitiable situation! Some development economists and population specialists still argue lately in the opposite direction that high contraceptive use, more family planning and sterilization is the best way of poverty reduction (Gillespie, 2004, pp. 34-38), without ever resolving the eternal egg-and-chicken questions: What is the basic 'cause' and what is the ultimate 'effect?' Why excess number of children are born ONLY among the poor, and never among the rich and affluent? What is the fundamental root cause? Are deprivation and abject poverty not compelling them to give births to excessive number of children??? Such very crucial issues must be resolved soon. But my life-long all efforts were in vain. And, river Ganga quietly flows on… and on... over time… and space…

And, in the meantime, sixty years (1947-2006) of precious Indian demographic time and economic history have elapsed without changing the lot of the downtrodden and their fertility/mortality levels. Evidently, such conventional and pseudo-scientific thinking will not perform the serious task of the time!

In this study, at least, very high powered canonical linkages have repeatedly demonstrated and confirmed the truth, that is, widespread female illiteracy is the primary cause of high fertility and high infant mortality in India, and that crucial battle against this evil syndrome must be fought out (Mukherji, 2000c, pp. 1-5).

Policy import of these very fundamental causal relations are crystal clear. It highlights the most urgent need for providing universal and massive (functional) education to all the girls and to all the adult women of India, if we are truly serious about on-setting fertility decline in the hitherto neglected and lagging Indian states, and for reducing infant mortality rates. Such a massive education programme alone will perform the miracle (Mukherji, ibid., pp. 4-5). It will definitely and substantially bring down the levels of fertility and infant and child mortality, as various canonical linkages have clearly demonstrated. Without waging a war against the widespread illiteracy among the Indian women, especially in rural areas (particularly in Bihar, MP, UP, Rajasthan, where it exceeds even 85%), no dent upon the demographic scenario of India can be made, no matter how much we may vainly try to motivate the pauperized and illiterate women (and men) to adopt the family planning and the contraceptives. This is the greatest need of the hour. Sooner we soulfully understand and act upon this finding, the better for us and for the country (Mukherji, 2005c, pp. 38-75).

In a recent study, the notable demographer Srinivasan (2006, pp. 23-32) has also concluded that "in retrospect it is found that programmes that combine social and economic benefits with family planning services for poor women encouraging them to have fewer children and enhance their prospects of achieving a different, less dependent kind of life are likely to be more acceptable, effective and less controversial".

Secondly, as many canonical linkages have testified, both in rural and urban India, there is an urgent need to revamp the family planning programmes, as well as augment the ANC care, child immunization programmes, MCH care, and all other aspects of the reproductive health. There is also great and immediate requirement to activate all these crucial aspects of primary health services, specially in rural, backward, and hitherto neglected, and remote and inaccessible tracts. This is equally true for urban India, as now urban poverty has swelled in many mega cities and large urban centres of India. Therefore, both the programmes for socio-economic upliftment of the poor and the illiterates and the programmes for providing safe motherhood, child survival, and reproductive health should go simultaneously.

Thirdly, the crucial relationship between illiterate mothers and very high level of infant deaths has emerged time and again; so also the causal relations between high TFR and widespread female illiteracy. These evil syndromes between fertility, infant mortality, and female illiteracy – which is indeed an index of abject poverty – must be broken, before demographic decline will occur in all parts of India, conclusively and permanently. Without such fundamental essential changes in the Indian society and economy, very little can be achieved. We need to act now. Without any further dilly dallying. Without any further waste of time (Mukherji, 2005a, pp. 1-95).

6

Findings of Factor-cum-Canonical Analysis of Three Systems: Models IV to VII

"Love the poor, the miserable, the downtrodden, and the Lord will bless you" (Swami Vivekananda, 1893, Complete Work, Centenary Volume V, 1963, p. 23).

"Be good and have mercy on those who suffer" (Swami Vivekananda, 1893, Complete Work, Centenary Volume II, 1963, p. 181).

"Work on: be lions; and the Lord will bless you. I shall work incessantly until I die, and even after death I shall work for the good of the world" (Swami Vivekananda, 1894, Complete Work, Centenary Volume V, 1963, p. 64)

In this chapter, all the analyses are performed in two parts: first, by performing three separate factor analyses on three matrices (demographic, socio-economic, and policy), and secondly, by performing canonical analysis on the factor scores generated from the previous step. Therefore, these are called factor-cum-canonical analyses. All analyses are performed at *state level*. Moreover, the entire analysis is performed on four data series, as follows. In successive four major sections, the findings of these four canonical models (IV to VII) are very briefly presented:

1. For all-India (total series data): *Canonical Model IV*
2. For rural and urban series taken together: *Canonical Model V*
3. For rural data only: *Canonical Model VI*
4. For urban data only: *Canonical Model VII*

Findings of Three Separate Factor Analyses, Using Total Series Data: Inputs for Model IV

The data is presented in Table 1, in the beginning of Chapter 4. First four variables and variables V21 are treated as comprising of demographic matrix (D); the variables V5 to V9 and variable V20 are considered as comprising of the socio-economic matrix (S), and the remaining variables, V10 to V19, are treated as consisting of population policy matrix (P). These three separate data matrices were indeed joined together to present as the total data set, given in Table 1. The same set is now split into three separate data matrices for three separate factor analyses (of D, S, and P matrices). The list of variables is also given in Tables 7 to 9. Each factor analysis has uncovered the latent roots of the data structure and has yielded the main basis dimensions of the factor structure. These analyses have yielded very meaningful basic dimensions of each respective data matrix. Throughout discussions, the terms '*factors*' or '*dimensions*' are used interchangeably (meaning the same).

As usual, identification and naming of factors is largely done by examining the variables most closely associated with a factor and the concept expressed by that cluster of interrelated variables. This is also supplemented by meticulously examining the factor scores on respective factor, especially when interpreting a more complex dimension.

Demographic Matrix

Factor analysis is performed on the demographic data matrix of all the states of India, and it has generated two main factors, denoted as follows, with eigen-values greater than 1, and explaining about 92.8 per cent of total variance in the data sets (Table 7). The factors are identified as:

1. High IMR, high CMR, and many underweight babies (explains 69.9% of variance).
2. High TFR, high CBR (explains another 22.9%).

Table 7

Rotated Factor Structure of Demographic Matrix of Indian States, (Total Series Data), 1992-93

Variables	*Factor 1*	*Factor 2*
	High IMR, high CMR, many underweight babies	*High TFR, high CBR*
V1 IMR (Infant Mortality Rate)	**.94**	.23
V2 CMR (Child Mortality Rate)	**.89**	.31
V3 CBR (Crude Birth Rate)	.21	**.96**
V4 TFR (Total Fertility Rate)	.28	**.94**
V21 Prop. of underweight babies	**.89**	.17
Eigen-value	3.49	1.14
Per cent variance explained (Pct Var)	69.90	22.90
Cumulative per cent variance (Cum Pct Var)	69.90	92.80

The first factor has identified the mortality segment of the demographic picture, while the second factor has captured high fertility condition in the country, still prevailing in many Indian states. Together, they have captured the most profound characteristics of demographic scenario of India, that have been happening even in the 1990s.

The noteworthy point is that in the first factor, which, as a rule, describes the first principal axis of the entire demographic system of India, both the mortality indices appear to have very intimately linked and clustered, emerging into one single basic dimension.

Socio-Economic Matrix

Factor analysis of socio-economic matrix has yielded two main basis dimensions, with eigen-values greater than unity, and explains about 82.6 per cent of total variance (Table 8). These factors are:

1. Female illiteracy, girls (age 6 to 14) not attending school, households without toilet, and infant children are neither breastfed, nor given any mushy food, and women married at young age (explains 62.9% of variance).

2. Water facility is available in households, but very young children are not breastfed, nor given any mushy food (explains another 19.7%).

Is it not very sad and very unfortunate that these two dimensions have emerged as the basic fundamental structure of socio-economic condition in India, even in the decade of 1990s, after so much tall claims of India's economic development after 60 years of planned development? The data and the findings of factor analysis unravel the hollowness of such claims. Indeed, this is the true picture of India. Plagued by widespread illiteracy, abject poverty, and very dismal socio-economic situation (here, the variable, proportion of children breastfed plus given mushy food is taken as an indirect indicator of socio-economic condition).

Table 8

Rotated Factor Structure of Socio-Economic Matrix of Indian States, (Total Series Data), 1992-93

Variables	*Factor 1*	*Factor 2*
	Female illiteracy, girls (age 6-14) not attending school, households without toilet, children not breastfed, nor given mushy food, women married at young age	*Water facility available in HH, but children not breastfed, nor given mushy food*
V5 FEMILLITERACY (prop. female illiterates)	**.94**	.19
V6 FEMINSCHOOL (girls age 6-14 going to school)	**-.95**	-.04
V7 MARRIED <18 (prop. females married age <18)	**.91**	-.02
V8 HHWITHWATER (households with water facility)	-.02	**.95**
V9 NOTOILET (households without sanitary toilets)	**.73**	.24
V20 BREASTFEDFOOD (breastfed + mushy food)	**-60**	**-.64**
Eigen-value	3.77	1.18
Pct Var	62.90	19.70
Cum Pct Var	62.90	82.60

As a result of factor analysis of the socio-economic matrix (of six variables by 25 states), two independent orthogonally rotated principal components with eigen-values greater than 1, were successively extracted and identified, with decreasing order of predictability, explaining about 82.6 per cent of the total variance. These two dimensions define the underlying and unknown complex web of socio-economic forces in the social field of entire India and describe the bases of the socio-economic structure of these states (Table 8).

These two socio-economic dimensions are identified as stated above. Most such dimensions speak for themselves. The first principal axis forms a tremendously compact cluster of majority of the variables, indicating an underdeveloped situation, and in relation to which individual states show maximum variations. The poor states like Uttar Pradesh or Bihar show large positive factor scores with reference to this axis, while more developed states like Kerala or Gujarat show large negative factor scores.

Population Policy Matrix

Factor analysis of the population policy matrix, on the other hand, generated two new factors, with eigen-values greater than 1 and explaining about 74 per cent of total variance (Table 9). These factors are:

1. Contraceptives used, sterilization done, children are immunized, ante-natal care given, Tetanus Toxoid given, and health services provided (explains about 64.10 of variance).
2. Oral rehydration solution is given, but young infants are not breastfed, nor mushy food given to infant children (explains about 11.10% of variance).

These factors may appear to be good enough, and may also portray the main features of the population policies and programmes of India. However, negative factor scores on these two dimensions, actually may reveal that these factors are conspicuous by their absence, rather than their presence, in most states. So, the health facilities are indeed just not available in the majority of the states.

These factors can be termed as 'major policy components' or considerations that are found to be relevant in policy-demographic mix of India. These dimensions are identified as above.

Table 9

Rotated Factor Structure of Population Policy Matrix of Indian States, (Total Series Data), 1992-93

Variables	*Factor 1*	*Factor 2*
	Contraceptives used, sterilization done, child immunized, ANC care given, TT given, and health services provided	*ORS given, not breastfed, nor mushy food given to children*
V10 Usecontracept (prop. using contraceptives)	**.85**	.18
V11 Sterilization (prop. sterilized)	**.83**	-.02
V12 Unmetneedin FP (unmet need in FP)	**-.90**	.05
V13 Anccare (prop. got ante-natal care)	**.93**	.27
V14 Got TT (prop. got Tetanus Toxoid)	**.86**	. 26
V15 Deliveryin PHC (prop. delivery in PHC)	**.79**	.13
V16 Assistedbyhp (prop. assisted by health professional)	**.84**	. 15
V17 Orsgiven (prop.oral rehydration solution given)	-.02	**.83**
V18 Childimmunized (prop. children immunized)	**.85**	.32
V19 Breastfed (prop. children breastfed)	-.25	**-.61**
Eigen-value	6.30	1.11
Pct Variance	63.10	11.10
Cum Pct Variance	63.10	74.20

Taken all these factors together, the most pitiable and sad picture of India's demographic, socio-economic and population policy systems becomes very clear. Not much to be described. Table 10 provides the factor scores of all these six factors, generated from three separate factor analyses.

Table 10

Factor Scores from Three Factor Analyses of D, S, and P Matrices of Indian States, (Total Series Data), Inputs for Canonical Analysis

States	*Demographic Matrix*		*Socio-economic Matrix*		*Population Policy Matrix*	
	FS_1	FS_2	FS_3	FS_4	FS_5	FS_6
Andhra Pradesh	.50	-.88	1.09	-.59	.95	-1.04
Arunachal Pradesh	-1.24	1.98	.07	.36	-1.03	-.67
Assam	1.05	.42	.37	-.94	-.96	-.34
Bihar	1.24	.85	1.78	.07	-1.35	-.66
Delhi	.17	-.15	-1.23	1.85	.51	1.03
Goa	-.87	-1.82	-1.37	1.68	1.19	1.38
Gujarat	.50	-.22	.07	.89	.69	-.70
Haryana	-.35	1.40	.38	.27	.31	-.53
Himachal Pradesh	-.25	.03	-.28	.04	. 26	.56
Jammu of J&K	-.65	.21	-.16	-.14	.07	1.41
Karnataka	. 50	-.51	.42	.34	.64	-.50
Kerala	-1.45	-1.31	-1.17	-2.2	1.86	-.42
Madhya Pradesh	1.03	.79	1.42	-.40	-.58	.16
Maharashtra	. 04	-.36	.05	.85	.85	.42
Manipur	-1.06	-.29	-.98	-.75	-.85	1.03
Meghalaya	-.25	1.03	-.36	-1.01	-1.3	1.12
Mizoram	-1.41	-.93	-1.59	-1.41	1.03	-.84
Nagaland	-2.32	1.14	-1.30	.42	-1.61	-.63
Orissa	1.68	-.65	.87	-.34	-.60	.42
Punjab	-.22	-.37	-.66	1.66	.73	.97
Rajasthan	.09	.34	1.87	.06	-.82	-1.32
Tamil Nadu	.43	-1.02	-.29	.06	1.36	-.55
Tripura	.77	-.99	-.47	-1.55	.33	-1.92
Uttar Pradesh	1.14	1.93	1.33	.56	-1.42	-.51
West Bengal	. 90	-.60	.15	.23	-.20	2.12

Note: Negative score on a particular factor for a state means that that particular facility/characteristic is *not* available to that state. For example, -1.42 factor score for UP on FS 5 means that "contraceptives used, child immunized, and health services available" (which depicts that particular factor or dimension, F_5) is *not at all available* in UP.

Canonical Model IV: All-India Analysis Using State-Level Data (Total Series)

Canonical analysis is performed on six factor scores of those three matrices, which have generated the following two very crucial canonical interrelationships, with very high statistical power and meaningfulness. These are identified as (Mukherji, 1997d, pp. 1-35; 2005c, p. 38-75):

1. High fertility rate occurs, because of high female illiteracy and also due to very little contraceptives used, and high IMR exists due to little or no immunization (canonical correlation is 0.879).
2. Less female illiteracy, so less infant mortality rate occurs, and high total fertility rate occurs due to less contraceptives used (canonical correlation is 0.665).

Trace correlation is very high 0.78, explaining about 63 per cent the total variance in the dependent set. Not only this is remarkably very high, but also yields two very meaningful canonical linkages, with great policy import.

Second one is a bipolar canonical variate. We can emphasize only upon the clearer negative polarity of this linkage equation, i.e., focusing only upon negative signs. It means that IMR is less, because less female illiteracy prevails in certain states. Besides, we can also interpret that TFR is also high in some states, in spite of some contraceptives are used, and slight ANC care also available.

These findings are new, novel, meaningful, and show causal relations in precise mathematical forms, which are very rarely done in the majority of population or demographic studies. Most such studies are descriptive and vague; neither analytic nor synthetic. Most such studies deal with decimal demography, explaining demographic patterns in terms of very minute differences in decimal and insignificant differences in percentages. Contrarily, the present set of canonical analyses ascertain the cause-and-effect relations between poverty (or illiteracy) and fertility in precise mathematical terms. Nothing is left to vague imagination or slipshod thinking. This is the great elegance of canonical models presented, and of the Demographic Field Theory, evolved and discussed.

Table 11

Canonical Structure Matrix, All-India (Total Series Data), 1992-93

	Variables/Factors	*Canonical Variate*	
		1	*2*
A.	*Demographic Variables (Factors) (Dependent Set)*	*Canonical Weights*	
1.	High IMR, high CMR, much underweight babies	**.60**	**-.79**
2.	High TFR, and high CBR	**.79**	**.60**
B.	*Socio-Economic-cum-Policy Variables (Factors) (Independent Set)*		
1.	High female illiteracy, girls not attending school, women married young, houses without toilet, and breast-feeding not done	**.54**	**-.68**
2.	Breast-feeding and mushy food not given, though water facility available	.21	.14
3.	Contraceptives used, sterilization done, ANC care given, children immunized	**-.63**	**-.65**
4.	ORS given, some immunization, breast-feeding not done	-.05	-.29
C.	*Canonical Correlation*	**.88**	**.67**
D.	*Meaning of Canonical Linkage Pair*	High fertility, because high female illiteracy, high IMR, and no immunization and very little contraceptives used.	Less female illiteracy, so less IMR, and less contraceptives, and high TFR.
E.	*Trace Correlation*	**0.779** (i.e., independent set explains about 64% of variance in dependent set)	
	Wilks Lambda	.1261	
	Chi Square	44.502	
	Significance	0.0001	

Interrelationships between Demographic, Socio-Economic and Population Policy Variables (All-India and States)

For such delineation, a factor analysis is performed on all the main and common variables of rural and urban parts of all states of India (data as in Table 12), which has generated two main factors or dimensions of the entire data structure of these matrices, with eigen-values greater than 1 and explaining about 81.6 per cent of the total variance (Tables 12, 13, and 14; and Figure 19). The factor structure of these results is

Table 12

Rural and Urban Data Series Taken Together for Demographic, Socio-Economic and Policy Matrices, 1992-93, Indian States, for Three Separate Factor Analyses

States	IMR	CMR	CBR	TFR	Fem illiteracy	Fem in school	HH no toilet	Use contra	Steri-lized	No ANC care	TT given	Health prof. assisted	Immuni-zed
1. Andhra Pradesh (R)	72.3	97.1	24.7	2.67	72.4	42.5	91.8	43.6	42.4	14.1	71.4	39.7	39.7
2. Andhra Pradesh (U)	64.6	73.7	22.3	2.35	32.7	76.2	29.6	56.6	51.3	6.6	84.9	78.3	58.3
3. Assam (R)	90.8	146.1	31.4	3.68	52.5	52.5	56.6	40.1	13.3	53.7	31.8	14.1	17.4
4. Assam (U)	66.8	101.0	23.2	2.53	25.9	75.7	7.6	62.3	22.7	19.4	66.2	56.8	40.0
5. Bihar (R)	93.8	132.7	32.9	4.15	77.3	33.2	92.7	19.8	16.6	66.8	26.4	15.0	9.1
6. Bihar (U)	59.3	92.9	27.5	3.25	38.4	69.7	32.2	42.5	30.7	34.3	58.7	52.0	21.5
7. Delhi (U)	65.4	83.1	26.7	3.02	29.2	79.1	15.9	60.3	23.2	17.6	72.5	53.0	57.8
8. Goa (R)	29.1	38.0	17.8	1.99	32.7	88.2	68.9	44.4	33.6	3.3	81.0	86.8	75.2
9. Goa (U)	34.9	39.8	16.4	1.80	20.4	92.0	34.5	51.7	27.4	5.1	86.1	90.1	74.6
10. Gujarat (R)	70.2	108.2	28.4	3.17	57.0	51.4	83.3	47.5	42.6	27.4	56.4	32.0	46.2
11. Gujarat (U)	65.4	94.2	24.7	2.65	33.2	74.5	29.0	52.7	38.1	15.9	76.7	65.7	57.0
12. Haryana (R)	79.6	107.0	35.1	4.32	62.6	53.7	90.8	46.7	37.0	27.3	59.4	24.1	52.1
13. Haryana (U)	51.6	70.7	26.7	3.14	31.1	71.4	29.3	58.0	28.5	31.2	76.8	52.5	58.0
14. Himachal Pradesh (R)	56.4	71.0	29.0	3.07	45.1	86.5	95.6	57.1	46.6	25.5	46.2	22.2	61.3
15. Himachal Pradesh (U)	48.8	48.8	20.2	2.03	17.2	95.6	21.6	70.4	38.7	5.1	62.6	67.4	81.5
16. Jammu (R)	46.5	61.2	29.3	3.36	53.5	59.8	93.7	46.2	30.1	23.2	66.3	25.4	62.8
17. Jammu (U)	39.2	46.5	21.2	2.13	22.8	82.0	23.1	64.4	27.5	3.9	84.8	67.2	84.8

Contd...

Contd...

18. Karnataka (R)	67.7	94.4	27.5	3.09	63.4	57.6	90.8	47.7	43.5	17.3	66.4	40.3	49.9
19. Karnataka (U)	60.0	70.6	22.7	2.39	25.4	80.1	26.1	52.0	40.4	12.1	78.2	77.2	57.6
20. Kerala(R)	28.7	38.5	20.3	2.09	18.7	88.7	34.3	61.4	47.5	2.4	88.9	87.6	54.0
21. Kerala (U)	9.5	13.1	18.0	1.78	14.6	91.9	15.7	68.2	50.4	0.5	92.3	95.7	55.7
22. Madhya Pradesh (R)	92.9	145.2	33.3	4.11	74.9	39.5	95.2	33.4	30.7	52.0	36.7	22.1	25.6
23. Madhya Pradesh (U)	54.7	72.6	27.2	3.27	37.1	68.4	26.7	47.7	34.6	24.4	66.9	61.1	43.0
24. Maharashtra (R)	60.8	81.1	28.4	3.12	56.5	67.7	90.2	54.3	50.8	21.8	65.4	37.6	65.6
25. Maharashtra (U)	33.3	52.4	24.4	2.54	27.2	84.3	18.4	52.9	39.5	9.8	79.8	77.8	61.6
26. Orissa (R)	116.9	135.1	27.0	3.00	62.7	58.0	95.0	34.2	30.5	39.7	50.7	15.6	34.7
27. Orissa (U)	84.5	107.2	23.9	2.53	36.1	77.8	32.5	47.4	37.2	22.4	71.6	48.7	43.8
28. Punjab (R)	57.2	71.8	26.5	3.09	53.9	52.8	78.8	57.2	35.4	13.6	81.0	44.7	57.7
29. Punjab (U)	42.3	55.5	21.0	2.48	33.7	62.3	12.5	62.7	30.3	7.2	88.6	60.1	75.6
30. Rajasthan (R)	73.4	107.5	28.1	3.87	81.8	29.5	93.2	28.2	25.1	70.6	23.8	17.4	16.1
31. Rajasthan (U)	68.6	77.7	22.3	2.77	32.5	69.1	42.4	47.1	38.1	48.8	52.7	45.2	45.9
32. Tamil Nadu (R)	71.4	98.0	23.6	2.54	52.9	79.6	91.3	49.2	42.2	6.9	87.4	59.7	60.3
33. Tamil Nadu (U)	61.2	64.7	23.4	2.36	27.7	87.3	26.2	50.9	34.7	3.0	94.9	92.8	73.3
34. Uttar Pradesh (R)	108.2	152.2	38.0	5.19	75.9	32.4	93.4	16.7	12.4	59.6	32.4	11.6	17.4
35. Uttar Pradesh (U)	59.1	88.8	28.6	3.58	41.8	60.5	30.5	32.0	15.8	29.3	62.1	44.2	32.9
36. West Bengal (R)	77.4	104.0	28.4	3.25	52.3	58.4	80.1	55.7	32.6	26.7	68.1	23.1	31.3
37. West Bengal (U)	68.2	83.3	18.5	2.14	27.0	80.9	34.6	61.8	25.4	17.7	78.1	66.5	44.1

presented in Table 13. These two dimensions are identified as follows (details in Mukherji, 1998a, p. 250-270):

1. "High female illiteracy, poverty, high TFR, high IMR, and little availability of health services" dimension (explaining 71.8% of variance).
2. "Prosperity, low TFR, Low IMR, more health services and more contraceptive use" dimension (explains another 9.8%).

It is indeed extremely remarkable that these two factors have been very successful to capture the essence of the socio-economic-demographic-cum-policy structure of the present-day India: that is, depicting that about 72 per cent of Indians suffer, both socially and spatially, from acute illiteracy, poverty, high TFR, and IMR, and a complete lack of health services, on the one hand, and about 10 per cent of people and regions somewhat enjoy the privileges of prosperity, good health services, contraceptives, sterilization, ANC care, child immunization and so forth, and consequently, manifest a low TFR and low IMR, on the other. Indeed, this picture correctly manifests India at present.

On the one hand, while results of this factor analysis are remarkably successful and profoundly useful to unravel the underlying socio-economic-political nexus in India, prevailing even in 1992-93, on the other hand, this portrays a very dismal and sordid socio-economic situation, which urgently calls for vast systems transformation and for the promotion of much more egalitarian and much less poverty-stricken society. These factors should act as profound eye-openers to the conventional social scientists and population specialists, and to the complacent policy makers and bureaucrats. Indeed, we very urgently need to do a great deal of action-oriented social work and economic regeneration for uplifting the masses of the poor, the illiterate, the humiliated, and the downtrodden.

The factor scores generated on these two dimensions are shown in Table 14, and is illustrated in Figure 19. This illustration is a unique and most useful diagram, which depicts the relative position of various states, specially their rural and urban parts on this two-dimensional socio-economic-cum-demographic-cum-population policy space. Each state is shown by a vector (with specific length and a specific direction with the X-axis), according to its score on each of the two

Table 13

Rotated Factor Matrix of All Variables of Demographic Matrix, Socio-economic Matrix and Population Matrix of Indian States (Rural and Urban Data Series Together)

Variables	*Factor 1*	*Factor 2*
	High female illiteracy, girls not going school, no toilets in houses, poverty, and so high TFR, high IMR, high CMR, no TT and ANC, no health assistance, no immunization, no use of contraceptives	*Low female illiteracy, girl attending school, fewer house without toilet, so less household poverty, also contraceptives used, child immunized, ANC care and TT given, also health prof assistance given*
IMR (Infant Mortality Rate)	**.61**	**-.56**
CMR (Child Mortality Rate)	**.64**	**-.64**
CBR (Crude Birth Rate)	**.74**	**-.47**
TFR (Total Fertility Rate)	**.70**	**-.58**
FEM-ILLT (female illiteracy)	**.92**	-.28
Girl-School(girls age 6-14 not in school)	**-.75**	**.50**
No toilet (Prop. houses without toilet)	**.93**	.05
Use-Cont (Prop. use contraceptives)	**-.59**	**.61**
Steriliz (Prop. sterilized)	.07	**.88**
Noanccar (Prop. no ANC care given)	**.55**	**-.75**
Tt-Given (Prop. tetanus toxoid given)	**-.61**	**.65**
Heal-Prof (health professionals assisted)	**-.80**	**.46**
Immunized (Prop. children immunized)	**-.46**	**.73**
Eigen-value	9.33	1.28
Pct Variance	71.80	9.80
Cum. Variance	71.80	81.60

Table 14

Factor Scores on Dimensions showing Crucial Interrelationships between Demographic, Socio-Economic, and Policy Variables, All Variables, Indian States (R-U Data Series Taken Together)

States	FS_1	FS_2
	High female illiteracy, girls not going school, no toilets in houses, poverty, and so high TFR, high IMR, high CMR, no TT and no ANC, no health assistance, immunization, no use of contraceptives	*Low female illiteracy, girl also attending school, fewer houses without toilet, so less household poverty, also contraceptives used, child immunized, ANC care and TT given, also health prof assistance given*
1. Andhra Pradesh (R)	1.31	.95
2. Andhra Pradesh (U)	-. 21	.98
3. Assam (R)	.05	-2.19
4. Assam (U)	-1.34	-1.14
5. Bihar (R)	1.10	-1.92
6. Bihar (U)	-.45	-1.01
7. Delhi (U)	-1.00	-.72
8. Goa (R)	-.62	.93
9. Goa (U)	-1.49	.23
10. Gujarat (R)	1.15	.55
11. Gujarat (U)	-.43	.07
12. Haryana (R)	1.49	.39
13. Haryana (U)	-.65	-.37
14. Himachal Pradesh (R)	1.07	1.19
15. Himachal Pradesh (U)	-1.04	.62
16. Jammu (R)	.82	.58
17. Jammu (U)	-1.19	.34
18. Karnataka (R)	1.23	1.00
19. Karnataka (U)	-.71	.24
20. Kerala (R)	-.82	1.07
21. Kerala (U)	-1.23	1.27
22. Madhya Pradesh (R)	1.52	-.75
23. Madhya Pradesh (U)	-.42	-.36
24. Maharashtra (R)	1.35	1.54

Contd...

Contd...

25. Maharashtra (U)	-.84	.38
26. Orissa (R)	1.08	-.49
27. Orissa (U)	-.32	-.29
28. Punjab (R)	.65	.84
29. Punjab (U)	-.89	.26
30. Rajasthan (R)	1.23	-1.20
31. Rajasthan (U)	-.26	-.41
32. Tamil Nadu (R)	.68	1.24
33. Tamil Nadu (U)	-.93	.38
34. Uttar Pradesh (R)	1.31	-2.14
35. Uttar Pradesh (U)	-.67	-1.59
36. West Bengal (R)	.68	.01
37. West Bengal (U)	-1.18	-.51

dimensions. The relative position of each state (their rural-urban parts) can be easily understood, relative to the two main factors and dimensions. Distances between a pair of states can also be found out. Their nearness or distances enable them to cluster, according to their essential characteristics. Accordingly, the following four main clusters are found out.

Out of 37 regions of India, thus studied, only 12 are much developed on all the three dimensions (D, S, P), demographically, socio-economically, and health-wise (Cluster 1). These regions/states are: Kerala (Urban), Kerala (Rural), Goa (Urban), Goa (Rural), Maharashtra (Urban), Gujarat (Urban), Punjab (Urban), Andhra Pradesh (Urban), Himachal Pradesh (Urban), Delhi (Urban), Jammu (Urban) and Rajasthan (Urban).

Another nine are on the incipient demographic transition, and may show some substantial improvement in the next 5 to 10 years (Cluster 2). They include: Haryana (Urban), West Bengal (Urban), Tamil Nadu (Urban), Madhya Pradesh (Urban), Assam (Urban), Uttar Pradesh (Urban), Bihar (Urban), Rajasthan (Urban) and Orissa (Urban). They are just on the threshold of development.

But, on the other hand, there still exist about eight regions, viz., Tamil Nadu (Rural), Gujarat (Rural), Haryana (Rural), Maharashtra (Rural), Himachal Pradesh (Rural), Andhra Pradesh (Rural), Jammu & Kashmir (Rural), and Punjab (Rural) – which show much female

Figure 19

Clusters of States and State Vectors on Two-dimensional Space, showing Inter-relationships between Demographic, Socio-Economic, and Policy Variables (1992-93)

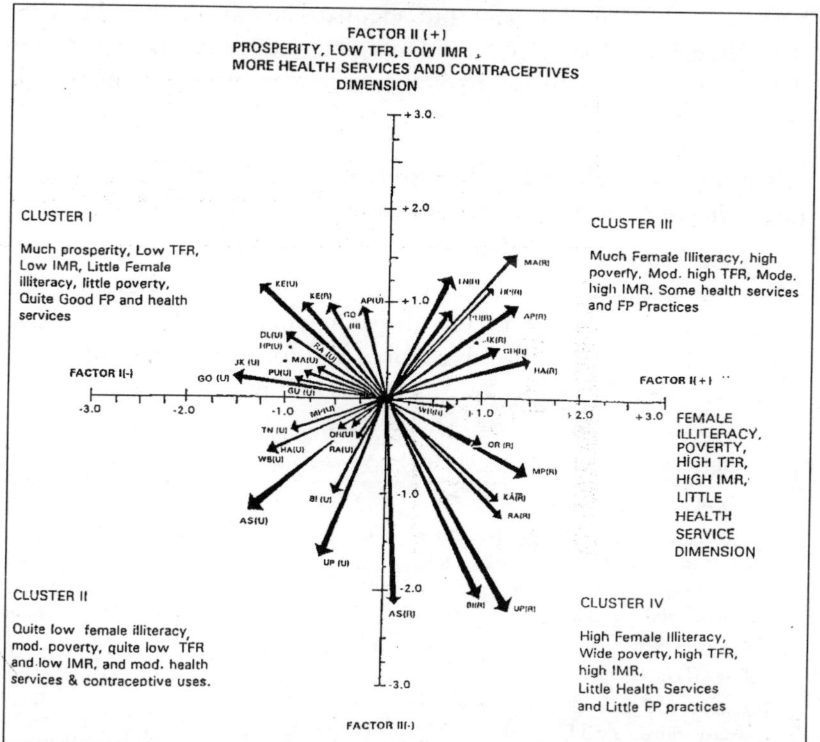

illiteracy, widespread poverty, moderately high TFR, moderately high IMR, and only slight health services and family planning practices. These states and regions need considerable revamping of their health services as well as sincere and sustained efforts for poverty alleviation (Cluster 3).

Finally, the hardcore areas of severe underdevelopment lie in such states as Uttar Pradesh (Rural), Bihar (Rural), Madhya Pradesh (Rural), Rajasthan (Rural), West Bengal (Rural), Orissa (Rural), Karnataka (Rural) and Assam (Rural). These regions suffer from very high female illiteracy, widespread poverty, high TFR, high IMR, little health services, and little family planning practices. These are very large and highly populous states, and these needs very urgent action-oriented programmes for demographic transition and employment generation. Verily, these are the most crucial regions which need urgent poverty alleviation programmes and all concerted efforts for both economic development and adequate health services. Priority-wise, these hitherto neglected and marginalized regions must be given the top-most attention for economic regeneration and demographic decline (Cluster 4).

Clusters of Developed and Underdeveloped States *(according to Demographic, Socio-Economic and Health Situations)*

Based on the above interrelationships between the three matrices, the following four clusters of states can be delineated. These clusters indicate the states and their sub-parts which need more urgent attention for providing health services and for fertility and mortality reduction (total 37 regions considered, as in Table 12):

	Cluster Characteristics	*States/Rural-Urban Parts in the Cluster*
1.	*Cluster I (Most Developed)*	*12*
	Depicting much prosperity, low TFR, low IMR, little female illiteracy, little poverty, quite good family planning services and health services. Need persisted efforts.	Kerala (U), Goa (U), Goa (R), Kerala (R), Maharashtra (U), Delhi (U), Andhra Pradesh (U), Gujarat (U), Himachal Pradesh (U), Punjab (U), Jammu (U), Rajasthan (U)
2.	*Cluster II (In Transition)*	*9*
	Quite low female illiteracy, moderate poverty, quite low TFR, and low IMR, and moderate health services and contraceptive use. Need further action.	Tamil Nadu (U), Haryana (U), West Bengal (U), Orissa (U), Assam (U), Uttar Pradesh (U), Bihar (U), Rajasthan (U), Madhya Pradesh (U)
3.	*Cluster III (Underdeveloped)*	*8*
	Much female illiteracy, widespread poverty, moderately high TFR, moderately high IMR, some health services and family planning practices. Need urgent attention.	Tamil Nadu (R), Gujarat (R), Haryana(R), Maharashtra (R), Himachal Pradesh (R), Andhra Pradesh (R), Jammu (R), Punjab (R)
4.	*Cluster IV (Most Underdeveloped)*	*8*
	High female illiteracy, widespread poverty, high TFR, high IMR, little health services, and little family planning practices. Need greatest attention and urgent action.	Uttar Pradesh (R), Bihar (R), Madhya Pradesh (R), Rajasthan (R), West Bengal (R), Orissa (R), Karnataka (R), Assam (R)

Inputs for Canonical Model V: Demographic and Socio-Economic-cum-Policy Factors

First, the selected variables are separately factor analyzed (see Table 15 (A), 15 (B), 15 (C)); then the factor scores for the states are used as inputs in the final linking canonical model (shown in Table 16).

Demographic Matrix (4 important variables)

Table 15 (A) portrays the findings of this factor analysis. All seven demographic variables are clustered into one single, very tightly-organized dimension, titled as 'high fertility, high mortality, high maternal mortality and less urbanization' dimension. Very high factor loadings are noteworthy. Eigen-value is 4.95, and this single factor alone explains 70.7 per cent of total variance of demographic system of India. This is simply remarkable. It fundamentally emphasizes that fertility, infant mortality, child mortality, maternal mortality in rural-traditional-less urbanized context, in fact, just operates as a single whole, as a single system, as a gestalt; no matter what the population scientists and demographers conventionally tend to treat them as separate variables. They are very intimately linked, and must be seen that way. It also means that for onsetting fertility decline, infant mortality and child mortality control is a mandatory step.

Table 15 (A)

Factor Structure of Demographic Matrix of Indian States (R-U Series Together)
(Separate Factor Analysis, before Canonical Analysis)

Variables	*Factor 1* *High IMR, high CMR, and high TFR Dimension*
IMR (Infant Mortality Rate)	**.89**
CMR (Child Mortality Rate)	**.94**
CBR (Crude Birth Rate)	**.92**
TFR (Total Fertility Rate)	**.92**
Eigen-value	3.41
Pct Var	85.2
Cum Pct	85.2

That is, the connections between infant mortality rate and total fertility rate appear as one single organized whole; as a system; not isolated. This indicates that for onsetting fertility decline in India, we must first ensure decline in infant mortality and child mortality, before we can expect dampening fertility. The finding emerging from this study thus calls forth that much greater attention should be given to this factual relationship between fertility and mortality than casually and academically attended so for.

Socio-Economic Matrix (3 important variables)

Table 15 (B) provides the findings of factor analysis of socio-economic matrix. Ten variables collapsed into only one basic dimension, explaining together 72.6 per cent of variance. This principal axis is:

Table 15 (B)

Factor Structure of Socio-Economic Matrix, Indian States (R-U Series Together) (Separate Factor Analysis, before Canonical Analysis)

Variables	*Factor 1*
	Very high female illiteracy, girls (age 6-14) are also not attending school, houses are without any sanitary toilet facility
FEM-ILLT (female illiteracy)	**.99**
GIRL-SCHOOL (girls age 6-14 going school)	**-.91**
NOTOILET (households without sanitary toilet)	**.89**
Eigen-value	2.63
Pct Var	87.70
Cum Var	87.70

This factor, or principal axis, emerged as the most important characteristics of the socio-economic nexus of Indian society, with reference to which different states are relatively positioned on the advantageous-disadvantageous scale. UP or Bihar has positive factor score on this dimension, while Kerala or Tamil Nadu has highly negative factor score, with Maharashtra or Karnataka lying in between.

Population Policy Matrix (6 important variables)

Table 15 (C) presents the findings of the factor structure of policy matrix. Eight policies have collapsed into three main policy dimensions, explaining 61.3 per cent of total variance.

Table 15 (C)

Factor Structure of Population Policy Matrix, Indian States (R-U Series Together) (Separate Factor Analysis, before Canonical Analysis)

Variables	*Factor 1*
USE-CONT (prop. use contraceptives)	**.85**
STERILIZ (prop. sterilized)	**.62**
NOANCCAR (prop. no. ANC care given)	**-.96**
TT-GIVEN (Tetanus Toxoid given)	**.93**
HEA-PROF (health prof. assisted)	**.85**
IMMUNIZE (prop. children immunized)	**.87**
Eigen-value	4.43
Pct of Var	73.80
Cum Pct	73.80

Factor Scores as Inputs

Factor scores from three factor analytic Tables 15(A), (B) and (C) are extracted and shown in Table 16. These are utilised as inputs for final linking canonical model (shown in Table 17).

Table 16

Factor Scores from Separate Factor Analyses, Indian States, Rural-Urban Data Series Taken Together, 1992-93, as Inputs for Canonical Analysis (Model V)

States	*Demographic Matrix (high IMR, TFR and CMR dimension)*	*Socio-Economic Matrix (poor female illiterates, without basic household facility)*	*Policy Matrix (health and FP services given, like sterilization,. contraceptives., immunization, etc.)*
	FS_1	FS_2	FS_3
1. Andhra Pradesh (R)	. 07	1.46	.01
2. Andhra Pradesh (U)	-.46	-.63	1.05
3. Assam (R)	1.43	. 50	-1.78

Contd...

Contd...

4. Assam (U)	-.09	-.98	.03
5. Bihar (R)	1.61	1.75	-2.34
6. Bihar (U)	.24	-.36	-.64
7. Delhi (U)	.10	-.90	.25
8. Goa (R)	-1.56	-.44	.85
9. Goa (U)	-1.62	-1.12	.93
10. Gujarat (R)	.52	.90	-.24
11. Gujarat (U)	-.04	-.59	.50
12. Haryana (R)	1.40	1.04	-.30
13. Haryana (U)	-.11	-.57	.18
14. Himachal Pradesh (R)	.04	.11	-.05
15. Himachal Pradesh (U)	-1.09	-1.39	1.01
16. Jammu (R)	-.03	.77	-.16
17. Jammu (U)	-1.13	-1.01	1.06
18. Karnataka (R)	.29	.98	.09
19. Karnataka (U)	-.50	-.88	.67
20. Kerala (R)	-1.39	-1.10	1.19
21. Kerala (U)	-2.07	-1.44	1.48
22. Madhya Pradesh (R)	1.71	1.61	-1.42
23. Madhya Pradesh (U)	.01	-.42	-.01
24. Maharashtra (R)	.16	.64	.38
25. Maharashtra (U)	-.83	-1.01	.76
26. Orissa (R)	1.17	1.01	-1.07
27. Orissa (U)	.21	-.56	.01
28. Punjab (R)	-.07	.76	.45
29. Punjab (U)	-.91	-.52	.92
30. Rajasthan (R)	.79	1.92	-2.07
31. Rajasthan (U)	-.23	-.36	-.50
32. Tamil Nadu (R)	-.03	.35	.71
33. Tamil Nadu (U)	-.51	-.98	1.15
34. Uttar Pradesh (R)	2.60	1.75	-2.24
35. Uttar Pradesh (U)	.38	-.13	-.86
36. West Bengal (R)	.60	.63	-.34
37. West Bengal (U)	-.62	-.78	.33

Note: (Table 16): Negative score on a particular factor for a state (either rural or urban part) means that that particular facility/characteristic is *not* available to that part of the state. For example, -2.24 factor score for UP (Rural) on FS_3 means that "Health and FP Services" (which depicts that particular factor or dimension) F_3 is *not at all available* in rural parts of UP.

Results of Canonical Model V, Using Rural and Urban Series of States Together

Table 17 presents the findings of this final canonical structure matrix. Findings of this table may be considered as one of the pinnacle of entire study, as it forms the apex of entire screening process, and final linkage formulation (details in Mukherji, 2000d, pp. 1-145).

Table 17

Canonical Structure Matrix of Indian States, Rural and Urban Data Series Together, 1992-93

Factors/Variables		*Canonical Variate Pair*
		1
A. *Demographic Factors(Dependent Set)*		*Canonical Weight*
1. Very high IMR, high CMR, and very high TFR dimension		**.99**
B. *Socio-Economic-cum-Policy Factors (Independent Set)*		
2. Poor, female illiterates, girls not attending school, and houses without sanitary toilet facilities		**.44**
3 Health services given, like immunization, sterilization, contraceptives, etc		**-.89**
C. *Canonical Correlation*		**.90**
D. *Meaning of Canonical Linkage Pair*	Very high TFR and very high IMR occur in the states, because they are poor illiterate females, without minimum sanitary facilities, and without any kind of health and FP services given to them.	
E. *Trace Correlation*	**.903** (i.e., this explains 0.90 squared, times 100 = 81% of variance in dependent set is explained by independent set).	
Wilks Lambda	.1835	
Chi Square	59.33	
Significance	.0001	

The testing and application of the Demographic Field Theory started initially with 30 variables. After successive screening and testing, 13 variables with higher canonical loadings were found to be more relevant and significant. Thus, three separate factors analyses of these three matrices were done which generated a set of only three factors: one demographic factor, one socio-economic factor, and one policy factors. These three factors are independent among themselves as well as across three matrices, as each matrix was separately analyzed. These are unbiasedly treated.

When these independent factors, taken from three separate analyses, are put together in the final integrative canonical model, and are found to have very high powered interrelationships, then, that must be considered as manifesting the true reality.

Table 17 presents such hard facts and true reality. All three factors have collapsed into only one single canonical variate, one canonical vector, one profound canonical linkage equation. This final linkage can be expressed as:

0.999 (high fertility, high IMR, and high child mortality dimension)

=**0.448** (high female illiteracy, poverty, and girls not attending school)

- 0.894 (contraceptives used, immunization given, ante-natal care given, sterilization services and health assistance for delivery available)

The meaning of this final canonical interrelationship is crystal clear: very high total fertility and very high level of infant mortality as well as child mortality rate occur in Indian states primarily because of very high female illiteracy, both among the adult women and among young girls, and very widespread poverty among them, as well as due to utter lack of health services and family planning services, specially contraceptives, child immunization and ante-natal care for the mothers. It poignantly tells a story of complete chaos and utter neglect of the poor and downtrodden, specially in pauperized villages and urban slums.

Corresponding canonical correlation is wonderfully high, i.e., **0.903**. Trace correlation is also equally high, 0.903. Evidently, because here trace correlation and canonical correlation remain the same.

In short, the above-mentioned canonical variate pair, as well as the trace correlation between the two data sets, have explained 81 per cent of the total variance (0.903 squared times 100) in the original variables of demographic matrix. Such a high powered explanation is simply unbelievable, both in physical and social sciences. It is unthinkable specially in social sciences.

This finding should be considered as the great eye-opener for all concerned: academicians, policy makers, administrators, and everybody else. We have wasted most valuable sixty years after India's independence in utter complacency and total neglect of the need of the poor people who are reeling under abject poverty, inequity, and unjust exploitation. The above crucial findings are reiterating the same hard reality time *and again* (Mukherji, 2000d, ibid.).

It is well to remember that we started with 13 variables, and all those informations are contained in those three factors, as well as in the final canonical results. Thus, in reality, 81 per cent of the original matrix of 13 main variables are explained.

These results are not only statistically very highly significant, but are also practically very meaningful. The above result reiterates upon the tremendous importance of combating widespread female illiteracy, raising the levels of living of the poor people, freeing them from the clutches of bondage and humiliation, and tremendously improving health services for family planning, child and maternal health, if we are really desirous of achieving quick and effective decline in the present-day high fertility and high infant mortality in the Indian states.

In this relationships, very high TFR, IMR and CMR occur, because they are poor, illiterate females, without minimum sanitary facilities, and without any health and FP services (Table 17).

Results of Rural India State-Level Factor and Canonical Analysis

Table 18 provides the raw data for factor analysis of rural India. Table 19 (a), (b), and (c) provides separate results of three factor analysis. The factor scores from these three factor analyses become inputs for Canonical Model VI (rural India only) (not shown). Table 20 finally presents the canonical results for Canonical Model VI (rural India). These tables are self-explanatory, hence not elaborated (details in Mukherji, 1998a, pp. 250-270; 2000d, pp. 65-85).

Table 18

Data of Seventeen Demographic, Socio-Economic, and Policy Variables of Indian States (Rural Data Only)

States	*1*	*2*	*3*	*4*	*5*	*6*	*7*	*8*	*9*	*10*	*11*	*12*	*13*	*14*	*15*	*16*	*17*
Andhra Pradesh	72.3	97.1	24.7	2.67	72.4	42.5	91.8	43.6	42.4	10.3	14.1	71.4	39.7	39.7	30.3	52.1	19.4
Assam	90.8	146.1	31.4	3.68	52.5	52.5	56.6	40.1	13.3	22.6	53.7	31.8	14.1	17.4	31.0	51.8	0.8
Bihar	93.8	132.7	32.9	4.15	77.3	33.2	92.7	19.8	16.6	25.9	66.8	26.4	15.0	9.1	29.0	64.1	7.6
Goa	29.1	38.0	17.8	1.99	32.7	88.2	68.9	44.4	33.6	16.7	3.3	81.0	86.8	75.2	15.7	36.2	35.0
Gujarat	70.2	108.2	28.4	3.17	57.0	51.4	83.3	47.5	42.6	13.2	27.4	56.4	32.0	46.2	21.6	45.8	19.5
Haryana	79.6	107.0	35.1	4.32	62.6	53.7	90.8	46.7	37.0	16.8	27.3	59.4	24.1	52.1	24.9	39.4	24.4
Himachal	56.4	71.0	29.0	3.07	45.1	86.5	95.6	57.1	46.6	15.3	25.5	46.2	22.2	61.3	22.7	48.3	17.4
Jammu	46.5	61.2	29.3	3.36	53.5	59.8	93.7	46.2	30.1	18.6	23.2	66.3	25.4	62.8	23.5	46.8	22.2
Karnataka	67.7	94.4	27.5	3.09	63.4	57.6	90.8	47.7	43.5	19.3	17.3	66.4	40.3	49.9	26.0	57.3	5.4
Kerala	28.7	38.5	20.3	2.09	18.7	88.7	34.3	61.4	47.5	11.9	2.4	88.9	87.6	54.0	26.1	30.6	15.8
Madhya Pradesh	92.9	145.2	33.3	4.11	74.9	39.5	95.2	33.4	30.7	20.2	52.0	36.7	22.1	25.6	26.9	59.4	3.1
Maharashtra	60.8	81.1	28.4	3.12	56.5	67.7	90.2	54.3	50.8	13.3	21.8	65.4	37.6	65.6	25.5	57.5	7.3
Orissa	116.9	135.1	27.0	3.00	62.7	58.0	95.0	34.2	30.5	22.3	39.7	50.7	15.6	34.7	29.7	34.7	5.3
Punjab	57.2	71.8	26.5	3.09	53.9	52.8	78.8	57.2	35.4	13.7	13.6	81.0	44.7	57.7	19.0	47.4	39.6
Rajasthan	73.4	107.5	28.1	3.87	81.8	29.5	93.2	28.2	25.1	20.9	70.6	23.8	17.4	16.1	28.0	41.1	25.1

Contd...

Contd...

Tamilnadu	71.4	98.0	23.6	2.54	52.9	79.6	91.3	49.2	42.2	14.0	6.9	87.4	59.7	60.3	21.2	52.1	13.6
Uttar Pradesh	108.2	152.2	38.0	5.19	75.9	32.4	93.4	16.7	12.4	31.0	59.6	32.4	11.6	17.4	28.3	50.5	6.9
West Bengal	77.4	104.0	28.4	3.25	52.3	58.4	80.1	55.7	32.6	17.7	26.7	68.1	23.1	31.3	34.6	60.4	9.4

List of Variables

1. IMR (Infant Mortality Rate)
2. CMR (Child Mortality Rate)
3 CBR (Crude Birth Rate)
4. TFR (Total Fertility Rate)
5. Prop. female illiterates
6. Girls age 6-14 going to school
7. Prop. HH without sanitary toilet
8. Prop. using contraceptives
9. Prop. sterilized
10. Unmet need in FP
11. Prop. without ante-natal care visit
12. Prop. got Tetanus Toxoid
13. Prop. assisted by health professional
14. Prop. children immunized
15. Prop. children breastfed
16. Per cent underweight babies
17. Prop. pucca houses

Table 19 (A)

Factor Structure of Demographic Matrix of Indian States (Rural Data Only)

Variables	*Factor 1*
	High IMR, high CMR, high TFR, and high underweight babies
IMR (Infant Mortality Rate)	**.89**
CMR (Child Mortality Rate)	**.93**
CBR (Crude Birth Rate)	**.92**
TFR (Total Fertility Rate)	**.90**
UNDERWT (underweight babies)	**.54**
Eigen-value	3.64
Pct Var	72.80
Cum Pct	72.80

Table 19 (B)

Factor Structure of Socio-Economic Matrix of Indian States (Rural Data Only)

Variables	*Factor 1*
	High female illiteracy, also girls not attending school, and houses are without sanitary toilet facility (indicating poverty)
FEM-ILLT (prop. female illiterates)	**.99**
GIRL-SCHOOL (girls age 6-14 in school)	**-.88**
NOTOILET (prop. houses without toilets)	**. 80**
Eigen-value	2.41
Pct Var	80.40
Cum Var	80.40

Table 19 (C)

Factor Structure of Population Policy Matrix of Indian States (Rural Data Only)

Variables	*Factor 1*	*Factor 2*
	Contraceptives used, ANC and TT given, sterilization done, prof assistance given, little unmet need in FP, etc	*Pucca houses, breastfeeding not done, some health assistance given*
USE-CONT (prop. use contraceptives)	**.91**	.13
STERILIZ (prop. sterilized)	**.90**	.11
UNMETFP (prop. unmet need in FP)	**-.87**	-.22
NOANCCAR (prop. without ANC care)	**-.88**	**-.38**
TT-GIVEN (prop. Tetanus Toxoid given)	**.83**	**.38**
HEA-PROF (prop. health professional assisted)	**.61**	**.53**
IMMUNIZE (prop. children immunized)	**.73**	**.56**
BREASFED (prop. children breastfed)	-.22	**-.89**
PUCCAHO (prop. pucca houses)	.14	**.86**
Eigen-value	6.17	1.25
Pct Var	68.60	13.90
Cum Var	68.60	82.50

Table 20

Canonical Structure Matrix using Factor Scores on Demographic Matrix, Socio-Economic Matrix, and Population Policy Matrix, of Indian States (Rural Data Only Model VI)

	Factors	*Canonical Variate*
A.	*Demographic Matrix (Dependent Set)*	*Canonical Weight*
1.	Very high IMR, high CMR, very high TFR.	**.99**
B.	*Socio-Economic-cum-Policy matrix (Independent Set)*	
2.	Female illiteracy, poverty, also girls not attending school	**.53**
3.	Contraceptives used, immunized. health facility given	**-.60**
4.	Pucca house, not breastfed, some health facility	**-.59**
C.	*Canonical Correlation*	**.91**

Contd...

Contd...

D.	*Meaning of Canonical Linkage Pair*	High female illiteracy, poverty, girls not attending school, health facilities not given, nor immunization, nor FP services; so TFR is very high, IMR is very high, also CMR very high.
E.	*Trace Correlation*	**.914**
	Wilks Lambda	.1630
	Chi Square	28.07
	Significance	.0001

Results of Urban India State-Level Factor and Canonical Analysis (Model VII)

Likewise, for urban India (Canonical Model VII), factor results are given in Table 21 (in three parts), their factor scores are taken from these three analyses (scores not shown), and final canonical results are given in Table 22 (Mukherji, 2000d, ibid.). All these tables are self-explanatory, and hence are not further elaborated.

Table 21 (A)

Factor Structure of Demographic Matrix of Indian States (Urban Data Only)

Variables	*Factor 1: High IMR, high TFR, high CMR dimension*
IMR (Infant Mortality Rate)	**.79**
CMR (Child Mortality Rate)	**.90**
CBR (Crude Birth Rate)	**.86**
TFR (Total Fertility Rate)	**.86**
Eigen-value	2.96
Pct Var	74.10
Cum Var	74.10

Table 21 (B)

Factor Structure of Socio-Economic Matrix of Indian States (Urban Data Only)

Variables	*Factor 1: Female illiterates girls, also not going to school, and no toilet facility in houses (urban poverty)*
FEM-ILLT (Prop female illiterate)	**.96**
GIRL-SCHOOL (prop. girls 6-14 in school)	**-.91**
NOTOILET (prop. houses without toilet)	**.46**
Eigen-value	1.99
Pct Var	66.50
Cum Var	66.50

Table 21 (C)

Factor Structure of Population Policy Matrix of Indian States (Urban Data Only)

Variables	*Factor 1: Sterilized, ANC and TT given, health assistance given, and immunized*	*Factor 2: ORS, Contraceptives and ANC given*
USE-CONT (contraceptives used)	.34	**.81**
STERILIZ (prop. sterilized)	**.48**	.11
NOANCCAR (no ANC care given)	**-.77**	**-.51**
TT-GIVEN (prop. Tetanus Toxoid given)	**.82**	.18
HEA-PROF (health assistance given)	**.83**	.18
ORS (oral rehydration solution given)	-.02	**.93**
IMMUNIZE (prop. children immunized)	**.79**	.30
BREASFED ((prop. children breastfed)	**-.79**	.15
Eigen-value	4.20	1.41
Pct Var	52.50	17.70
Cum Pct	52.50	70.20

Table 22

Canonical Structure Matrix using Factor Scores on Demographic Matrix, Socio-Economic Matrix, and Population Policy Matrix, of Indian States (Urban Data Only) (Model VII)

Factors		*Canonical Variate Pair*
A. *Demographic Factors (Dependent Set)*		*Canonical Loadings*
1. High IMR, High TFR, and High CMR		**.99**
B. *Socio-Economic-cum-Policy Factors (Independent Set)*		
1. Female illiterates, girls not going school, and no toilet in houses (poverty)		**.85**
2. Sterilization, ANC, TT and immunization given		**-.53**
3. ORS, contraceptives, ANC given		-.05
C. *Canonical Correlation*		**.84**
D. *Meaning of Canonical Linkage Pair*	High IMR, high CMR, high TFR occur even in urban India, because very high female illiteracy, and virtually no health services nor FP services given to females and children.	
E. *Trace Correlation*	**.845**	
Wilks Lambda	.2853	
Chi Square	20.69	
Significance	0001	

Relation between education and fertility was studied, however, in another investigation, using NFHS-I data. The authors stated: "Education brings about a substantial change in demands for child. The urge to adhere to small family norm increases considerably with education. It is significant that even marginal increase makes a sizable difference" (Parasuraman, Roy, et al., 1999, p. 135). However, the study did not explore how the denial of minimum education to the masses of poor and illiterate women is forcing them to urge for more children, as sheer hands of labour, and increasing their fertility.

7

Results of Canonical Analysis of Individual Level Data of States: Model VIII

"Bring light to the poor; and bring more light to the rich, for they require it more than the poor" (Swami Vivekananda, 1895, Complete Work, Volume III, 1963, p. 247).

"Your country requires heroes; be heroes!" (Swami Vivekananda, 1894, Complete Work, Volume V, 1963, p. 51).

"We must rouse India and the whole World" (Swami Vivekananda, 1894, Complete Work, Volume VI, 1963, pp. 61-62).

Summary Results of Analysis of Individual Level Data of Women and their Demographic Behaviour

As elaborated in Chapter 3, a series of canonical analyses were also performed for each major state, using individual level data of women respondents, and to explain their demographic behaviour as well as its relation to female illiteracy and poverty situation. Table 23 provides the summary of such findings. Tables 24 to 38 present results of each of 15 major states. These canonical linkage results yield a wealth of important findings. Most of them are explained within respective table, and hence are not further elaborated due to shortage of space (for details see, Mukherji, 2000d, pp.80-145).

Table 23

Summary Table of Canonical Findings of States, Using Individual Level Data

States	*Canonical Variate Pair* 1	2	3
1. Andhra Pradesh			
A. Meaning of Canonical Linkage Pair	More ANC, less CEB	More br.fed, less IMR	More fem. illiterates, ANC available, less Av child per rep.span
B. Trace Correlation	=	.40	
2. Assam			
A. Meaning of Canonical Linkage Pair	More br.fed, less IMR	More ANC, less CEB	Urban residents, less Av child/span
B. Trace Correlation	=	.40	
3. Bihar			
A. Meaning of Canonical Linkage Pair	More br.fed, less IMR	More fem.illiterate, more CEB, some fem. sterilizaion and less ANC	High Av No of child; in rural area, inspite of sterilization
B. Trace Correlation	=	.28	
4. Goa			
A. Meaning of Canonical Linkage Pair	More ANC, less CEB	Less br.fed, more IMR	Urban resi., less Av child per rep.span
B. Trace Correlation	=	.37	
5. Gujarat			
A. Meaning of Canonical Linkage Pair	More ANC given, less CEB	More br.fed, less IMR	More fem. sterilization, less CEB, but more Av child/span
B. Trace Correlation	=	.39	
6. Haryana			
A. Meaning of Canonical Linkage Pair	Less br.fed, higher IMR	High fem. illiterates, higher CEB, inspite of fem. sterilization	Less Av child/rep span, due to ANC given, in spite of fem. illiteracy
B. Trace Correlation	=	.37	

Contd...

Contd...

7.	Himachal Pradesh			
A.	Meaning of Canonical Linkage Pair	More ANC, less CEB	High br.fed, less IMR	High fem. illiterates, higher Av child/span
B.	Trace Correlation	=	.37	
8.	Jammu			
A.	Meaning of Canonical Linkage Pair	More ANC, less CEB	Less br.fed, more IMR	More fem. illiterates, more av child per repro. span among rural people inspite of ANC given
B	Trace Correlation	=	.36	
9.	Karnataka			
A.	Meaning of Canonical Linkage Pair	Less br.fed, more IMR	Less ANC, more CEB, inspite of sterilization	Urban resi, less Av child rep.span
B.	Trace Correlation	=	.45	
10.	Kerala			
A.	Meaning of Canonical Linkage Pair	More br. fed, less IMR	More ANC, less CEB	More fem. illiterates, more Av child
B.	Trace Correlation	=	.40	
11.	Madhya Pradesh			
A.	Meaning of Canonical Linkage Pair	More br. fed, less IMR	High CEB,due to fem. illiteracy, inspite of sterilization	Inspite of fem.sterilization, high Av child/span
B.	Trace correlation	=	.31	
12.	Maharashtra			
A.	Meaning of Canonical Linkage Pair	More br.fed, less IMR	More ANC, less CEB	Inspite of fem. sterilization, Av child/span is high
B.	Trace Correlation	=	.47	
13.	New Delhi			
A.	Meaning of Canonical Linkage Pair	ANC care given, low CEB	More br. fed, low IMR	Not significant
B.	Trace Correlation	=	.34	

Contd...

Contd...

14. Orissa			
A. Meaning of Canonical Linkage Pair	More ANC, less CEB, though little sterilization	More br.fed, less IMR. Also more ANC, less CEB.	Not Significant
B. Trace Correlation	=	.31	
15. Punjab			
A. Meaning of Canonical Linkage Pair	More ANC, less CEB, though little sterilization	More br. fed and less illiteracy, so less IMR	In urban areas, less Av. number of children
B. Trace Correlation	=	.32	
16. Rajasthan			
A. Meaning of Canonical Linkage Pair	More br. fed, less IMR	High CEB, mod. fem. illiteracy, as little ANC, in spite of sterilization	Less Av. number of child in urban areas, though high illiteracy
B. Trace Correlation	=	.35	
17. Tamil Nadu			
A. Meaning of Canonical Linkage Pair	More br. fed, less IMR	Less ANC, high CEB in spite of high fem. sterilization	Though high illiteracy and low sterilization still low Av child/span
B. Trace Correlation	=	.46	
18. Uttar Pradesh			
A. Meaning of Canonical Linkage Pair	More br. fed, less IMR	More ANC, less CEB	Rural residents, high Av child/rep.span
B. Trace Correlation	=	.34	
19. West Bengal			
A. Meaning of Canonical Linkage Pair	More br. fed, less IMR	Less ANC, more CEB inspite of mod. fem.steril	Rural resi, have Av child/rep.span.
B. Trace Correlation	=	.38	

Note: Av = Average, br.fed = Breast-fed, CEB=Children Ever Born, Rep. span = Reproductive span, Mod.=Moderate, ANC = Ante-natal Care, fem=females, Resi=Residence.

Note: Kashmir was not surveyed due to political disturbances.

Socio-Economically and Demographically Least Developed States

This group of states includes Rajasthan, Bihar, Uttar Pradesh and Madhya Pradesh. They are characterized by very high female illiteracy, very high fertility, and very little health services (Mukherji, 2000d, pp. 100-120). They also indicate some common canonical (causal) relationships, such as: (a) more breastfeeding, so less infant mortality rate; (b) high female illiteracy rates and consequently higher number of children ever born per mother, sometimes in spite of some female sterilization or ANC given; and (c) higher average number of children during reproductive span of mother(s) in rural areas, sometimes in spite of some practice of slight female sterilization or ANC utilization (for details, see Tables 24 to 27).

Table 24

Canonical Structure Matrix, Rajasthan

Variables		*Canonical Variate*		
		1	*2*	*3*
A. *Demographic Matrix (Dependent Set)*			*Canonical Weights*	
1. Avchild (average number of children/repro. span)		.06	-.07	**-.98**
2. CEB (Children Ever Born)		.10	**.98**	.18
3. IMR (Infant Mortality Rate)		**-.99**	.15	-.06
B. *Socio-Economic-cum Policy Matrix (Independent Set)*				
4. Residence (urban residence)		.05	-.01	.35
5. Femilliteracy (prop. female illiterates)		.01	**.32**	**.82**
6. Femsterilization (female sterilization)		.22	**.81**	-.43
7. Ancgiven (ante-natal care given)		.04	-.43	-.01
8. Breastfed (children breastfed)		**.97**	-.18	.04
C. *Canonical Correlation*		**.46**	**.37**	**.12**
D. *Meaning of Canonical Linkage Pair*		More breast-fed, less IMR	High CEB, mod. female illiteracy, as little ANC, in spite of sterilization.	Less av. No of children in urban areas, though high illiteracy.
E. *Trace Correlation*	**.3506**			
Wilks Lambda	.6661			
Chi Square	596.6			
Significance	.0001			

Table 25

Canonical Structure Matrix, Bihar

Variables		*Canonical Variate*	
	1	2	3
A. *Demographic Matrix (Dependent Set)*		*Canonical Weights*	
1. Avchild (No. av child/repro. span)	.06	-.25	**.99**
2. CEB (Children Ever Born)	-.11	**.95**	.09
3. IMR (Infant Mortality Rate)	**-.99**	-.13	.02
B. *Socio-Economic-Cum-Policy Matrix (Independent Set)*			
4. Residence (Urban residence)	.06	-.01	.11
5. Femilliteracy (Prop. female illiterates)	-.15	**.48**	-.57
6. Femsterilization (Female sterilization)	-.03	**.66**	**.80**
7. Ancgiven (Antenatal care given)	.12	**-.53**	-.01
8. Breastfed (Children breastfed)	**.97**	.19	-.11
C. *Canonical Correlation*	**.37**	**.31**	.08
D. *Meaning of Canonical Linkage Pair*	More breastfed, less IMR	More female illiterates, more CEB. Some fem. sterilization and less ANC	High av No of child; in rural areas, in spite of female sterilization.
E. *Trace Correlation*	= **.287**		

Table 26

Canonical Structure Matrix, Uttar Pradesh

Variables		*Canonical Variate*	
	1	2	3
A. *Demographic matrix (Dependent Set)*		Canonical Weights	
1. Av child (No. av child/repro. span)	.04	.25	**.99**
2. CEB (Children Ever Born)	-.01	**-.96**	.07
3. IMR (Infant Mortality Rate)	**-.99**	-.04	.06
B. *Socio-Economic-Cum-Policy Matrix (Independent Set)*			
4. Residence (Urban Residence)	.14	.03	**-.93**
5. Femilliteracy (Prop. female illiterates)	-.10	-.56	-.21
6. Femsterilization (Female sterilization)	-.02	-.52	.28
7. Ancgiven (Antenatal care given)	.05	**.61**	.05
8. Breastfed (Children breastfed)	**.98**	-.11	-.03
C. *Canonical Correlation*	**.52**	**.28**	.08

Contd...

Contd...

D.	*Meaning of Canonical Linkage Pair*	More Breastfed, Less IMR	More ANC, Less CEB	Rural residents, high Av child/ Rep. span
E.	*Trace Correlation*	**.3463**		
	Wilks Lambda	.6642		
	Chi Square	954.3		
	Significance	.0001		

Table 27

Canonical Structure Matrix, Madhya Pradesh

	Variables		*Canonical Variate*	
		1	*2*	*3*
A.	*Demographic Matrix (Dependent Set)*		*Canonical Weights*	
1.	Av child (No. av child/repro. span)	.13	-.15	**.99**
2.	CEB (Children Ever Born)	-.01	**.98**	-.06
3.	IMR (Infant Mortality Rate)	**-.99**	.01	.12
B.	*Socio-Economic-Cum-Policy Matrix (Independent Set)*			
4.	Residence (Urban residence)	.13	.22	-.06
5.	Femilliteracy (Prop. female illiterates)	-.07	**.38**	-.74
6.	Femsterilization (Female sterilization)	.05	**.76**	.62
7.	Ancgiven (Antenatal care given)	.01	-.45	.20
8.	Breastfed (Children breastfed)	**.98**	-.01	-.10
C.	*Canonical Correlation*	**.43**	**.32**	.06
D.	*Meaning Of Canonical Linkage Pair*	More breastfed, less IMR	High CMR, due to female illiteracy, in spite of sterilization	In spite of female. sterilization, high av child/repro span (not significant)
E.	*Trace Correlation*	**.3193**		
	Wilks Lambda	.7162		
	Chi Square	629.9		
	Significance	.0001		

Socio-Economically and Demographically Underdeveloped States

This cluster of states includes Assam, Orissa, Karnataka, Jammu and Haryana. They are characterized by considerably high female illiteracy, moderate to high level of fertility, and relatively slightly more health services (Mukherji, 2000d, ibid., pp. 100-120). Immunization level is less and so also ANC care. They also represent some common canonical (causal) relations, e.g., (a) more breastfeeding, so less infant mortality rate, (b) ANC care, so higher number of children ever born per mother, and (c) less average number of children over the reproductive span due to urban residence. More details are presented in Tables 28 to 31.

Table 28

Canonical Structure Matrix, Assam

Variables		*Canonical Variate*		
		1	*2*	*3*
A. *Demographic Matrix (Dependent Set)*			*Canonical Weights*	
1. Av child (No. av child/repro. span)		.06	-.10	**-.98**
2. CEB (Children Ever Born)		-.36	**-.94**	.14
3. IMR (Infant Mortality Rate)		**-.93**	.31	-.11
B. *Socio-Economic-Cum-Policy Matrix (Independent Set)*				
4. Residence (Urban residence)		-.10	.08	**.87**
5. Femilliteracy (Prop. female illiterates)		-.12	-.35	-.14
6. Femsterilization (Female sterilization)		-.09	-.57	.26
7. Ancgiven (Antenatal care given)		.48	**.56**	-.37
8. Breastfed (Children breastfed)		**.85**	-.47	.08
C. *Canonical Correlation*		**.41**	**.37**	.11
D. *Meaning of Canonical Linkage Pair*	More breastfed, less IMR	More ANC less CEB		Urban residence and less Av children/ repro. span
E. *Trace Correlation*	**.4020**			
Wilks Lambda	.5750			
Chi Square	607.2			
Significance	.0001			

Table 29

Canonical Structure Matrix, Orissa

	Variables		*Canonical Variate*	
		1	*2*	*3*
A.	*Demographic Matrix (Dependent Set)*		*Canonical Weights*	
1.	Av child (No. av child/repro. span)	.03	.19	**.98**
2.	CEB (Children Ever Born)	**-.86**	**-.51**	-.01
3.	IMR (Infant Mortality Rate)	.49	**-.83**	-.16
B.	*Socio-Economic-Cum-Policy Matrix (Independent Set)*			
4.	Residence (Urban residence)	-.20	.06	-.02
5.	Femilliteracy (Prop. female illiterates)	-.14	-.05	.36
6.	Femsterilization (Female sterilization)	**-.71**	-.31	**-.66**
7.	Ancgiven (Antenatal care given)	**.38**	**.57**	-.53
8.	Breastfed (Children breastfed)	-.53	**.75**	.37
C.	*Canonical Correlation*	**.39**	**.37**	.03
D.	*Meaning of Canonical Linkage Pair*	More ANC, less CEB though little sterilization	More breastfed, less IMR. also more ANC, less CEB.	Not significant
E.	*Trace Correlation*	**.3134**		
	Wilks Lambda	.7270		
	Chi Square	394.4		
	Significance	.0001		

Table 30

Canonical Structure Matrix, Karnataka

	Variables		*Canonical Variate*	
		1	*2*	*3*
A.	*Demographic Matrix (Dependent Set)*		*Canonical Weights*	
1.	Av child (No. av child/repro. span)	-.01	-.05	**-.99**
2.	CEB (Children Ever Born)	-.06	**.99**	.01
3.	IMR (Infant Mortality Rate)	**.99**	.03	.02
B.	*Socio-Economic-Cum-Policy Matrix (Independent Set)*			
4.	Residence (Urban residence)	-.02	-.03	**.84**
5.	Femilliteracy (Prop. female illiterates)	.06	.29	-.32

Contd...

Contd...

6.	Femsterilization (Female sterilization)	-.06	**.75**	.34
7.	Ancgiven (Antenatal care given)	.02	**-.57**	-.25
8.	Breastfed (Children breastfed)	**-.99**	-.03	-.02
C.	*Canonical Correlation*	**.65**	**.42**	.05
D.	*Meaning of Canonical Linkage Pair* Less breast-fed, more IMR		Less ANC more CEB, in spite of sterilization	Urban resi less av child/repro. span.
E.	*Trace Correlation* **.4526**			
	Wilks Lambda .4644			
	Chi Square 879.2			
	Significance .0001			

Table 31

Canonical Structure Matrix, Jammu

	Variables	*Canonical Variate*		
		1	*2*	*3*
A.	*Demographic Matrix (Dependent Set)*		*Canonical Weights*	
1.	Av child (No. av child/repro. span)	-.02	.03	**.99**
2.	CEB (Children Ever Born)	**-.96**	-.29	.01
3.	IMR (Infant Mortality Rate)	-.27	**.95**	-.03
B.	*Socio-Economic-Cum-Policy Matrix (Independent Set)*			
4.	Residence (Urban residence)	.19	-.04	**-.54**
5.	Femilliteracy (Prop. female illiterates)	.38	.04	**.51**
6.	Femsterilization (Female sterilization)	-.46	-.21	-.13
7.	Ancgiven (Antenatal care given)	**.70**	.19	**.64**
8.	Breastfed (Children breastfed)	.31	**-.95**	.07
C.	*Canonical Correlation*	**.50**	**.39**	.05
D.	*Meaning of Canonical Linkage Pair* More ANC, less CEB		Less breastfed, more IMR	More female illiterates, more av child per repro. span among rural people in spite of ANC
E.	*Trace Correlation* **.368**			
	Wilks Lambda .6327			
	Chi Square 360.0			
	Significance .0001			

States in Transition: Economically and Demographically Slightly More Developed States

This cluster of states includes Gujarat, West Bengal, Punjab, Andhra Pradesh and Maharashtra. They are characterized by moderate female illiteracy, moderately high level of fertility, and relatively slightly more health services than the previous groups of states (Mukherji, 2000d, ibid.). They reflect some common canonical (causal) relationships, such as: (a) more ANC care, so less number of children ever born, (b) more breastfeeding, so less infant mortality, and so forth. Often, the third canonical relationships of these states is not statistically significant. Details are shown from Table 32 to Table 36.

Table 32

Canonical Structure Matrix, Gujarat

	Variables		*Canonical Variate*	
		1	*2*	*3*
A.	*Demographic Matrix (Dependent Set)*		*Cnonical Weights*	
1.	AVchild (No. av child/repro. span)	.12	-.01	**.99**
2.	CEB (Children Ever Born)	**-.99**	-.02	.10
3.	IMR (Infant Mortality Rate)	.02	**-.99**	-.03
B.	*Socio-Economic-Cum-Policy Matrix (Independent Set)*			
4.	Residence (Urban residence)	-.01	-.11	-.45
5.	Femilliteracy (Prop. female illiterates)	-.49	-.16	**-.61**
6.	Femsterilization (Female sterilization)	-.78	.07	.57
7.	Ancgiven (Antenatal care given)	**.36**	.08	.18
8.	Breastfed (Children breastfed)	-.03	**.97**	-.20
C.	*Canonical Correlation*	**.50**	**.46**	.04
D.	*Meaning of Canonical Linkage Pair*	More ANC given, less CEB	More breastfed, less IMR	Not significant
E.	*Trace Correlation*	**.3970**		
	Wilks Lambda	.5827		
	Chi Square	512.6		
	Significance	.0001		

Table 33

Canonical Structure Matrix, West Bengal

	Variables		*Canonical Variate*	
		1	*2*	*3*
A.	*Demographic Matrix (Dependent Set)*		*Canonical Weights*	
1.	Av child (No. av child/repro. span)	.08	-.08	**.99**
2.	CEB (Children Ever Born)	-.09	**.98**	-.03
3.	IMR (Infant Mortality Rate)	**-.99**	-.16	.07
B.	*Socio-Economic-Cum-Policy Matrix (Independent Set)*			
4.	Residence (Urban residence)	. 09	.13	**-.72**
5.	Femilliteracy (Prop. female illiterates)	-.13	.30	-.62
6.	Femsterilization (Female sterilization)	-.01	**.44**	.20
7.	Ancgiven (Antenatal care given)	.07	**-.81**	-.21
8.	Breastfed (Children breastfed)	**.98**	.16	.02
C.	*Canonical Correlation*	**.49**	**.45**	.05
D.	*Meaning of Canonical Linkage Pair*	More breastfed, less IMR	Less ANC, More CEB in spite of female sterilization	Rural residents have high Av child reprod. span
E.	*Trace Correlation*	**.3869**		
	Wilks Lambda	.6014		
	Chi Square	659.1		
	Significance	.0001		

Table 34

Canonical Structure Matrix, Andhra Pradesh

	Variables		*Canonical Variate*	
		1	*2*	*3*
A.	*Demographic Matrix (Dependent Set)*		*Canonical Weights*	
1.	Av child (No. av child/repro. span)	.10	-.02	**-.99**
2.	CEB (Children Ever Born)	**-.93**	-.31	.01
3.	IMR (Infant Mortality Rate)	.32	**-.94**	.03
B.	*Socio-Economic-Cum-Policy Matrix (Independent Set)*			
4.	Residence (Urban residence)	-.18	-.03	-.01
5.	Femilliteracy (Prop. female illiterates)	-.31	-.21	**.86**

Contd...

Contd...

6. Femsterilization (Female sterilization)	-.75	-.25	-.23
7. Ancgiven (Antenatal care given)	**.37**	.23	**.43**
8. Breastfed (Children breastfed)	-.39	**.91**	.06
C. *Canonical Correlation*	**.50**	**.46**	.12
D. *Meaning of Canonical Linkage Pair*	More ANC, less CEB	More breastfed, less IMR	Female illiterates, some ANC available, less Av children per repro.span
E. *Trace Correlation*	**.4010**		
Wilks Lambda	.5759		
Chi Square	607.2		
Significance	.0001		

Table 35

Canonical Structure Matrix, Maharashtra

Variables	*Canonical Variate*		
	1	*2*	*3*
A. *Demographic Matrix (Dependent Set)*		*Canonical Weights*	
1. Av child (No. av child/repro. span)	-.01	.14	**.99**
2. CEB (Children Ever Born)	.15	**-.95**	.11
3. IMR (Infant Mortality Rate)	**-.98**	-.24	-.02
B. *Socio-Economic-Cum-Policy Matrix (Independent Set)*			
4. Residence (Urban residence)	.13	-.15	-.01
5. Femilliteracy (Prop. female illiterates)	.01	-.27	-.90
6. Femsterilization (Female sterilization)	.18	**-.86**	**.34**
7. Ancgiven (Antenatal care given)	-.05	**.30**	-.24
8. Breastfed (Children breastfed)	**.97**	.23	-.10
C. *Canonical Correlation*	**.61**	**.54**	.08
D. *Meaning of Canonical Linkage Pair*	More breastfed, less IMR	More ANC, less CEB	In spite of female sterilization, av child span is high
E. *Trace Correlation*	**.4752**		
Wilks Lambda	.4373		
Chi Square	838.1		
Significance	.0001		

Table 36
Canonical Structure Matrix, Punjab

	Variables	*Canonical Variate*		
		1	*2*	*3*
A.	*Demographic Matrix (Dependent Set) Canonical Weights*			
1.	Av child (No. av child/repro. span)	-.02	-.19	**-.98**
2.	CEB (Children Ever Born)	**-.99**	-.03	-.05
3.	IMR (Infant Mortality Rate)	.04	**-.97**	.17
B.	*Socio-Economic-Cum-Policy Matrix (Independent Set)*			
4.	Residence (Urban residence)	-.08	.21	**.80**
5.	Femilliteracy (Prop. female illiterates)	-.31	**-.41**	-.14
6.	Femsterilization (Female sterilization)	**-.64**	.16	.38
7.	Ancgiven (Antenatal care given)	**.67**	-.05	.10
8.	Breastfed (Children breastfed)	-.15	**.86**	-.41
C.	*Canonical Correlation*	**.44**	**.32**	.07
D.	*Meaning of Canonical Linkage Pair*	More ANC, less CEB, though little sterilization	More breastfed & less illiteracy, so less IMR	In urban areas, less av. No. of children/ repro. span
E.	*Trace Correlation*	**.3231**		
	Wilks Lambda	.7099		
	Chi Square	240.6		
	Significance	.0001		

Socio-Economically and Demographically Relatively More Developed States

This group of demographically developed states includes Kerala, Tamil Nadu, Goa and Himachal Pradesh. They are characterized by low female illiteracy, low fertility, and quite high degree of health services (Mukherji, 2000d, ibid., pp. 110-120). They also reflect some common canonical (causal) relationships, such as: (a) more breast-feeding, and so less infant mortality rate, (b) more ANC care, and consequently less number of children ever born per mother, and (c) less female illiteracy, and hence less average number of children over the reproductive span. They also enjoy better child immunization, female sterilization and contraceptive use (for details, see Tables 37 and 38). The tables are self-explanatory; hence not elaborated. As examples, only Kerala and Tamil Nadu are presented; lack of space does not permit discussion on Goa or Himachal Pradesh.

Table 37

Canonical Structure Matrix, Tamil Nadu

	Variables		*Canonical Variate*		
			1	*2*	*3*
A.	*Demographic matrix (Dependent Set)*			*Canonical Weights*	
1.	Av child (No. av child/repro. span)		.05	-.04	**-.99**
2.	CEB (Children Ever Born)		.08	**.99**	-.07
3.	IMR (Infant Mortality Rate)		**-.99**	.03	-.07
B.	*Socio-Economic-Cum-Policy Matrix (Independent Set)*				
4.	Residence (Urban residence)		-.09	.10	-.47
5.	Femilliteracy (Prop. female illiterates)		-.12	.27	**.73**
6.	Femsterilization (Female sterilization)		.06	**.85**	**-.46**
7.	Ancgiven (Antenatal care given)		01	**-.42**	. 07
8.	Breastfed (Children breastfed)		**.98**	-.01	.11
C.	*Canonical Correlation*		**.58**	**.53**	.05
D.	*Meaning of Canonical Linkage Pair*	More Breastfed, Less IMR		Less ANC, high CEB in spite of high Fem. sterilization	Though high illiteracy and low sterilization, still low Av child/span
E.	*Trace Correlation*	**.4605**			
	Wilks Lambda	.4649			
	Chi Square	780.0			
	Significance	.0001			

Table 38

Canonical Structure Matrix, Kerala

	Variables	*Canonical Variate*		
		1	*2*	*3*
A.	Demographic Matrix (Dependent Set)		*Canonical Weights*	
1.	Av child (No. av child/repro. span)	. 01	.13	**.98**
2.	CEB (Children Ever Born)	-.02	**-.98**	.15
3.	IMR (Infant Mortality Rate)	**-.99**	.07	-.06

Contd...

Contd...

B.	*Socio-Economic-Cum-Policy Matrix (Independent Set)*			
4.	Residence (Urban residence)	.10	.04	.37
5.	Femilliteracy (Prop. female illiterates)	.02	-.42	**.80**
6.	Femsterilization (Female sterilization)	-.01	**-.72**	-.36
7.	Ancgiven (Antenatal care given)	.05	**.54**	.26
8.	Breastfed (Children breastfed)	**.99**	-.01	-.02
C.	*Canonical Correlation*	**.51**	**.47**	**01**
D.	*Meaning of Canonical Linkage Pair*	More breast-fed, less IMR	More ANC, less CEB	More female illiterates, more Av child
E.	*Trace Correlation*	**.4038**		
	Wilks Lambda	.5702		
	Chi Square	625.9		
	Significance	.0001		

Conclusion

In sum, the following four groups of states can be identified:

1. Socio-Economically and Demographically Least Developed States: Rajasthan, Bihar, Uttar Pradesh and Madhya Pradesh.
2. Socio-Economically and Demographically Underdeveloped States: Assam, Orissa, Karnataka, Jammu, and Haryana.
3. States in Transition: Economically and Demographically Slightly More Developed States: West Bengal, Gujarat, Punjab, Andhra Pradesh and Maharashtra.
4. Socio-Economically and Demographically Relatively More Developed States: Kerala, Tamil Nadu, Goa and Himachal Pradesh.

8

Poverty Index and Fertility Behaviour in India

"Your work is to serve the poor and miserable, without distinction of caste or colour" (Swami Vivekananda, 1894, Complete Work, Centenary Volume VII, 1963, p. 247).

"Lay down your comforts, your pleasures, your names, fame or position, may even your lives, and make a bridge of human chains over which millions will cross this ocean of life" (Swami Vivekananda, 1894, Complete Work, Centenary Volume IV, 1963, p. 480).

Poverty and Fertility in India

Abject poverty and widespread illiteracy among women and men are ground realities in India, even in the year 2006. This chapter is thus more concerned with the most crucial population and development issue, that is, the causal linkages between abject poverty in India, and consequently, very high levels of fertility and infant mortality in the country, specially in pauperized villages and urban slums. To investigate such a crucial causal linkage between widespread poverty and high fertility seems to be the most fundamental issue for the country now.

Most unfortunately, measurement of poverty is not made in the majority of demographic surveys or investigations. Human Development Index (HDI) is also commonly devised at regional or country level, not at the level of individuals – without which we cannot really understand the underlying socio-economic processes behind such high fertility.

Without the study of people's economic condition or poverty condition, it is most difficult and unscientific to explain India's high fertility or infant mortality levels. Thus, a great need was felt to devise alternative ways to estimate people's poverty condition.

So, this chapter makes a new and novel contribution to this field, by measuring poverty index at the individual level, which is not yet attempted by UN Human Development Reports. An indirect measure of poverty, called Poverty Index, is constructed at the level of the individual woman, as discussed below.

A composite index is thus constructed at the individual level which reflects her poverty score, relative to all others. Based on recent survey data, thus a composite poverty index is computed for each sampled woman respondent of each state of India. Their corresponding fertility and infant mortality levels are also computed. By performing canonical analysis, the links between the demographic data set and socio-economic data set, plus population programmes and policies followed by that individual family are ascertained. A series of such canonical linkage analysis are performed, one for each Indian state, taking every time the data for individual woman as the units of observation (total 91,000 sampled women all over India, in their reproductive ages). Resultant canonical (causal) relations have very clearly proved that unless massive poverty and widespread female illiteracy are not severely and urgently reduced in India, the present-day very high fertility level will not decline. This is the minimum necessary condition for bringing out the desired demographic transition in India. Without the fulfilment of this necessary condition, nothing is going to improve current dismal demographic and development situation in the country.

Policy import of such crucial canonical results is most profound: these indicate that we must very urgently implement very effective programmes for massive employment generation and drastic reduction of dismal poverty situation and for reduction of widespread illiteracy among the masses of women in India, especially in the most neglected states of MP, UP, Bihar, Rajasthan, West Bengal, Orissa, Andhra Pradesh, and so on. These steps are very necessary before the current poverty and illiteracy situation in India lead to catastrophe and great human misery. After independence, 59 years have already been wasted. Lack of planning for the poor, ineffective economic planning, and rudderless family planning programmes have characterized all these years. We must now act on a war-footing to fight out this most crucial battle against widespread poverty and dismal fertility situation in India, before the situation reaches the maximum entropy level and the point of no return.

So, based on surrogate measures, this chapter thus computes Poverty Index at the individual level, and through Canonical model, analyzes its causal effect upon fertility and infant mortality rates for three relatively developed states (viz., Goa, Kerala and Tamil Nadu) and six less developed states (viz., Andhra Pradesh, Bihar, Madhya Pradesh, Rajasthan, Uttar Pradesh and West Bengal). Of course, the condition of poverty and fertility/mortality in 25 Indian states is also analyzed, but in this volume only the findings of three developed states and six problematic states are highlighted.

Method of Computing Poverty Index at State Level

United Nations Human Development Report (1997, Technical Note, Appendix I, pp. 101-7) has devised ways of computing Human Development Index and Poverty Index for different nations. For Poverty Index they have used certain measures like: (a) life expectancy at age 40, (b) female illiteracy rate, (c) per capita Gross National Product (GNP), (d) proportion of people not getting health services, and (e) proportion of people lacking essential drinking water facilities.

Method of Computing Poverty Index at the Individual Level

However, at the individual level, the measure of poverty index is computed here on the basis of following five indicators, because data for their income is not available:

1. female illiteracy,
2. if respondent woman is living in a *kuchcha* house,

3. non-availability of drinking water in the house,
4. non-availability of toilet facility in the house, and
5. non-availability of health facilities to the women respondent and/or her children anytime during four years previous to the survey date.

If answer to anyone of such question is 'yes', then, the woman respondent is given a score of one on each such measure; otherwise she is given a zero score. The sum total of all such "yes" scores marks her poverty index, at the individual level. This index varies between a value of zero (when she is assessed as not poor), and a value of maximum 5 score (when she is in the poorest category). So far, no such attempt of computing individual level of poverty index has been made. This poverty index is computed for all 91,000 women respondents surveyed, for all major states of India (Mukherji, 1997b, pp. 1-25).

Canonical Analysis between Poverty, and Fertility and Mortality Rates

Canonical analysis is performed for each of 25 major states of India. Separate canonical analyses were performed by using data of the poverty index and NFHS data of individual respondent's demographic variables like children ever born, infant mortality index, and population programme variables (e.g., if contraceptives ever used, number of child immunization courses completed, female sterilization done or not, etc). Out of 25 states, findings of only nine states are presented here. All data here refer to individual units. Sample size sometimes exceeds 6,500 or more cases for a state (Mukherji, 1997b, pp. 1-26; 2005g, pp. 1-25).

Canonical analysis is a very high powered statistical analysis between two or more data matrices: and it has unfolded the causal relationships between a set of dependent variables and a set of independent variables. Results of such nine separate canonical analyses showed very many crucial findings, having great practical meaning and statistical power. For technical details see earlier studies by the present author (Mukherji, 1979b, pp. 250-66; 1983b, pp. 1-141; 1989b, pp. 343-73). Many substantive and technical details are also available in Rummel and Mukherji (1981, pp. 10-81).

Canonical Analytic Model

Canonical analysis is a higher form of regression analysis, but instead of a single dependent variable as in regression model, it deals with a matrix of dependent variables, and a matrix of independent variables, and instead of one, yields a set of solutions in a single run of the test, as many as the minimum number of variables in the two sets. In short, canonical analysis can do in a single shot, what hundreds of regression analysis cannot do (Hotelling, 1937, pp. 321-77; Cooley and Lohnes, 1962, 45-65; Mukherji, 1979c, pp. 234-284; Mukherji, 1992, pp. 1-92).

Table 39

Summary of Results of Six Separate Canonical Analysis: AP, Bihar, MP, Rajasthan, UP, and West Bengal (1992-93)

State	*Canonical Linkage Pairs*		
	1	*2*	*3*
Andhra Pradesh: Meaning of canonical linkages	High poverty, high CEB	High IMR, as no ANC, and FP not used, though some sterilization	High CMR in rural areas because less immunization, moderately high poverty, though some ANC available
Bihar: Meaning of canonical linkages	High poverty, high CEB; high IMR as no ANC	High CEB in urban areas where no sterilization, though some immunization	High poverty, high CMR; even in urban areas though some ANC available
Madhya Pradesh: Meaning of canonical linkages	High poverty, high CEB; high CMR as no ANC	Moderately high poverty, high CEB even in urban areas, though less immunization	High CMR in rural areas where FP not used and little immunization, though some ANC available
Rajasthan; Meaning of canonical linkages	High poverty, high CEB; as no ANC	In rural areas, high CMR where little immunization	High IMR in rural areas where no ANC care given, though some immunization available
Uttar Pradesh: Meaning of canonical linkages	High poverty, high CEB; high IMR, as little immunization	Moderate poverty even in urban areas, high CEB, though some FP used	High poverty, high CMR, though some ANC was available
West Bengal: Meaning of Canonical Linkage Pair	High poverty, high CEB, though some ANC available	High IMR in rural areas where some sterilization done, but no ANC, nor FP used	High CMR where FP not used, though ANC available, but low immunization completed

Since here only three variables exist in demographic or dependent matrix, only three pairs of canonical vectors or canonical variates are extracted successively from dependent and independent matrices, with decreasing order of predictability as in principal components analysis. As can be seen from each canonical interrelationship, a specific type of socio-economic-cum-policy variables are *causally linked* with a specific kind of demographic variables, and in each case, the canonical correlations between the pair of vectors is maximized (see Tables 39 to 47).

Table 40

Poverty Index and Canonical Structure Matrix, Bihar (no. of sample cases: 2,909)

	Variables		*Canonical Variates*		
			1	*2*	*3*
A.	*Demographic Matrix (Dependent Set)*			*Canonical Weights*	
1.	CEB (children Ever Born)		**.83**	**.65**	.25
2.	IMR (Infant Mortality Rate)		**.51**	-.45	-.73
3.	CMR (Child Mortality Rate)		.19	-.60	**.62**
B.	*Socio-Economic-Cum-Policy Matrix (Independent Set)*				
4.	Urban residence		.02	**.43**	**.59**
5.	Poverty index		**.84**	.01	**.58**
6.	Female sterilization		-.11	**-.65**	-.06
7.	No ante-natal care		**.47**	.31	**-.50**
8.	Family planning ever used		.01	.31	.16
9.	Number of immunizations		-.20	**.42**	-.10
C.	*Canonical Correlation*		**.23**	**.07**	**.04**
D.	*Meaning of Canonical Linkage Pair*	High poverty, high CEB, high IMR as no ANC		High CEB in urban areas where no sterilization, though some immunization	High poverty, high CMR, even in urban areas though some ANC available
E.	*Trace Correlation*	**.1456**			
	Wilks Lambda	.9367			
	Chi Square	189.6			
	Significance	.0001			

Given a very large sample size of Bihar (2,909), the overall statistical overlap or *trace correlation* is also quite high (0.145), which indicates the extent the independent set has explained the portion of total variance in the dependent set. Besides, there are successively three significant relations that have also emerged in each analysis, with canonical values.

Findings at Canonical Analysis of Individual Level of Data

For example, with reference to Table 40, for the complicated canonical linkage equation for the first pair of variates for the state of Bihar can now be written as follows, based on only high-loadings (usually above 0.40, shown with bold face):

083 *(Children Ever Born, CEB) +* ***0.51*** *(Infant Mortality Rate, IMR)*
= ***0.84*** *(Poverty Index) +* ***0.47*** *(no ANC care given)*

This can easily and meaningfully be interpreted that, for the first largest set of canonical variates, the attribute, "Poverty Index" increases "high level of CEB", especially when female sterilization is absent and when no ANC care given. Canonical correlation between this matched pair of canonical variates is 0.237, indicating that one single factor, alleviation of abject poverty condition among the people/women will greatly reduce fertility rate in backward states of Bihar, and in similar states. This factor has emerged as the strongest determinant of fertility behaviour, amidst a total of nine variables. Conspicuous absence of many other important variables in the first linkage is also noteworthy (like family planning or immunization).

In the like manner, successive canonical correlations, loadings, and corresponding patterns of causal relationships between demographic behaviour set and socio-economic variables-cum-policy set can be easily interpreted. Remaining canonical relationships are briefly stated in the summary Tables 39 and 45, and are detailed in Tables 40 to 47.

A few points need mention. Mostly, interpretations of canonical linkages are easy, and can be done by just linking the highly loaded canonical weights with each variable(s) (shown with bold face). However, often interpretations become complex; when third pair of canonical variate shows bi-polarity or complex relations, then only the clearer polarity is considered (ignoring unclear polarity). Besides, mostly the focus is given on considering the 'positive' canonical weights, ignoring the 'negative' ones, whenever that does not make sense. Furthermore, when a specific variable indicates high canonical weights on two (or more) canonical variate pairs, then, only that specific canonical variate pair is considered with which that variable is loaded highest, ignoring the lower weights.

All these canonical linkage equations are not only statistically significant, but are also practically very meaningful. Each of them has emerged as a separate demographic system, orthogonal and independent of the previous one. Their interpretations and policy implications are very clear. All the three canonical linkages mainly emphasize upon the great need for poverty alleviation programmes and developmental efforts for women, like universal female literacy programmes and their employment, side by side health improvement, nutrition development, and upliftment as required policy instruments, apart from the continuation of the present-day family welfare programmes and spread of contraception. These canonical findings are interpreted as given below (for details see Mukherji, 1997b, pp. 1-25; 2005g, pp. 1-25):

Crucial Findings from Six Less Developed States

The findings are detailed in Tables 40 to 44 and are summarized in Table 39. Only the most important canonical linkage from each state are highlighted as follows:

1. Andhra Pradesh: high poverty, large number of children ever born per mother (CEB)
2. Bihar: high poverty, high CEB
3. Madhya Pradesh: high poverty, high CEB
4. Rajasthan: high poverty, high CEB, also because no ANC care available
5. Uttar Pradesh: high poverty, high IMR, as little immunization given
6. West Bengal: high poverty, though some ANC was available

The results are self-explanatory. State after state repeats the same causal relationship between poverty and high fertility. Further details of other canonical linkages are elaborated in summary Table 45.

Table 41

Poverty Index and Canonical Structure Matrix, Madhya Pradesh (Cases: 2,980)

	Variables		*Canonical Variate*		
			1.	*2.*	*3.*
A.	*Demographic Matrix (Dependent Set)*			*Canonical Weights*	
1.	CEB (children Ever Born)		**.59**	**.63**	-.57
2.	IMR (Infant Mortality Rate)		**.66**	-.76	-.01
3.	CMR (Child Mortality Rate)		.44	.10	**.81**
B.	*Socio-Economic-cum-Policy Matrix (Independent Set)*				
4.	Urban residence		-.01	**.52**	**-.42**
5.	Poverty index		**.77**	**.56**	.08
6.	Female sterilization		-.18	-.34	-.01
7.	No ante-natal care		**.58**	-.39	**-.66**
8.	Family planning ever used		.05	.33	**-.59**
9.	Number of immunizations		.07	**.12**	**-.11**
C.	*Canonical Correlation*		**.23**	**.12**	**.09**
D.	*Meaning of Canonical Linkage Pair*	High poverty, high CEB, high IMR as no ANC		Moderately high poverty, high CEB, even in urban areas though less immunization	High CMR in rural areas where FP not used and little immunization, though some ANC available
E.	*Trace Correlation*	**.1652**			
	Wilks Lambda	0.919			
	Chi Square	249.1			
	Significance	.0001			

Table 42

Poverty Index and Canonical Structure Matrix, Rajasthan (Cases: 2,433)

	Variables	*Canonical Variate*		
		1	*2*	*3*
A.	*Demographic Matrix (Dependent Set)*		*Canonical Weights*	
1.	CEB (Children Ever Born)	**.98**	-.38	-.09
2.	IMR (Infant Mortality Rate)	-.12	.25	**.94**
3.	CMR (Child Mortality Rate)	.07	**.88**	-.31

Contd...

Contd...

B.	*Socio-Economic-cum-Policy Matrix (Independent Set)*			
4.	Urban residence	.13	**-.85**	**-.35**
5.	Poverty index	**.70**	-.34	-.63
6.	Female sterilization	-.25	-.02	-.12
7.	No ante-natal care	**.62**	.05	**.43**
8.	Family planning ever used	.17	-.26	.21
9.	Number of immunizations	-.06	**-.28**	**.47**
C.	*Canonical Correlation*	**.23**	.08	.04
D.	*Meaning of Canonical Linkage Pair*	High poverty, high CEB, as no ANC	In rural areas, high CMR where little immunization	High IMR in rural areas where no ANC care is given, though some immunization available
E.	*Trace Correlation*	**.1480**		
	Wilks Lambda	.9347		
	Chi Square	163.7		
	Significance	.0001		

Table 43

Poverty Index and Canonical Structure Matrix, Uttar Pradesh (Cases: 6,395)

	Variables	*Canonical Variate*		
		1	*2*	*3*
A.	*Demographic Matrix (Dependent set)*		*Canonical Weights*	
1.	CEB (Children Ever Born)	**.77**	**.71**	-.02
2.	IMR (Infant Mortality Rate)	**.60**	-.59	-.47
3.	CMR (Child Mortality Rate)	.14	-.37	**.88**
B.	*Socio-Economic-cum-Policy Matrix (Independent set)*			
4.	Urban residence	-.22	**.68**	.13
5.	Poverty index	**.62**	**.49**	**.72**
6.	Female sterilization	-.16	-.13	.16
7.	No ante-natal care	**.72**	-.02	**-.58**
8.	Family planning ever used	.03	**.46**	-.23
9.	Number of immunizations	.07	.21	-.18
C.	*Canonical Correlation*	**.24**	**.13**	**.03**

Contd...

Contd...

D.	*Meaning of Canonical Linkage Pair*	High poverty, high CEB, high IMR as little immunization and ANC	Moderate poverty even in urban areas, high CEB, though some FP used	High poverty, high CMR, though some ANC was available
E.	*Trace correlation*	**.1642**		
	Wilks Lambda	.9202		
	Chi Square	376. 0		
	Significance	.0001		

Table 44

Poverty Index and Canonical Structure Matrix, West Bengal (Cases: 1,877)

	Variables	*Canonical Variate*		
		1	*2*	*3*
A.	*Demographic Matrix (Dependent Set)*		*Canonical Weights*	
1.	CEB (Children Ever Born)	**.98**	-.56	-.15
2.	IMR (Infant Mortality Rate)	.14	**.73**	**-.45**
3.	CMR (Child Mortality Rate)	.13	.37	**.87**
B.	*Socio-Economic-cum-Policy Matrix (Independent set)*			
4.	Urban residence	.12	**-.44**	.20
5.	Poverty index	**.88**	-.17	.23
6.	Female sterilization	-.25	**.50**	**-.04**
7.	No ante-natal care	**.34**	**.41**	**-.60**
8.	Family planning ever used	.13	**-.56**	**-.69**
9.	Number of immunizations	-.04	-.18	.21
C.	*Canonical Correlation*	**.32**	**.11**	**.03**
D.	*Meaning of Canonical Linkage Pair*	High poverty, high CEB, though some ANC available	High IMR in rural areas where some sterilization done, but no ANC, nor FP used	High CMR where FP not used, though ANC available, but low immunization completed
E.	*Trace Correlation*	**.2010**		
	Wilks Lambda	.8801		
	Chi Square	238.9		
	Significance	.0001		

Crucial Findings from Three More Developed States

The first most important canonical linkage pair that emerged from subsequent canonical analyses of relatively developed states are shown in Tables 46-47, and is summarized in Table 45 (for details see, Mukherji, 1997b, pp. 1-25; 2000d, pp. 85-105; 2005g, pp. 1-25). The first most important canonical linkage pair is shown below:

1. Goa	Little poverty, and much sterilization, so less children ever born (CEB) per mother
2. Kerala	Less poverty, less CEB
3. Tamil Nadu	Less poverty, and high sterilization, so low CEB

Table 45

Summary of Results of Three Separate Canonical Analyses: Goa, Kerala and Tamil Nadu

State	*Canonical Linkage Pairs*		
	1	*2*	*3*
Goa: Meaning of canonical linkages	Little poverty, and much sterilization, so low CEB	High immunization, low IMR, though moderate CMR	Where no ANC and little immunization, quite moderately less IMR
Kerala: Meaning of canonical linkages	Less poverty, less CEB	More sterilization, less CEB, though some IMR also	Moderately high CMR, where immunization less, though ANC given
Tamil Nadu: Meaning of canonical linkages	Less poverty, and high sterilization, so low CEB	Less poverty, low IMR, where some ANC given, but little immunization	Quite high CMR in rural areas even when some immunization and some ANC available

Table 46

Poverty Index and Canonical Structure Matrix, Kerala (Cases: 1,499)

Variables	*Canonical Variate*		
	1	*2*	*3*
A. *Demographic Matrix (Dependent Set)*		*Canonical Weights*	
1. CEB (Children Ever Born)	**-.91**	**-.59**	.05
2. IMR (Infant Mortality Rate)	-.38	**.68**	-.51
3. CMR (Child Mortality Rate)	-.14	.42	**.85**

Contd...

Contd...

B.	*Socio-Economic-cum-Policy Matrix (Independent Set)*			
4.	Urban residence	-.08	.09	-.25
5.	Poverty index	**-.82**	.25	.28
6.	Female sterilization	.28	**.90**	.05
7.	No ante-natal care	-.47	.14	**-.63**
8.	Family planning ever used	.00	-.25	-.37
9.	Number of immunizations	-.03	.90	**-.54**
C.	*Canonical Correlation*	**.37**	**.09**	**.04**
D.	*Meaning of Canonical Linkage Pair*	Little poverty, and so less CEB	More sterilization, less CEB, though some IMR also	Quite high CMR, where immunization less, though ANC given
E.	*Trace Correlation*	**.2422**		
	Wilks Lambda	.82861		
	Chi Square	280.87		
	Significance	.0001		

Table 47
Poverty Index and Canonical Structure Matrix, Tamil Nadu (Cases: 1,427)

	Variables	*Canonical Variate*		
		1	*2*	*3*
A.	*Demographic matrix (Dependent Set)*		*Canonical Weights*	
1.	CEB (Children Ever Born)	**-.99**	**.37**	-.12
2.	IMR (Infant Mortality Rate)	.07	**-.85**	-.34
3.	CMR (Child Mortality Rate)	.10	-.36	**.93**
B.	*Socio-Economic-cum-Policy Matrix (Independent Set)*			
4.	Urban residence	-.03	-.02	**-.66**
5.	Poverty index	**-.42**	**-.56**	-.01
6.	Female sterilization	**.81**	**-.59**	-.04
7.	No antenatal care	-.38	-.43	**-.60**
8.	Family planning ever used	-.05	.27	.10
9.	Number of immunizations	-.08	-.24	.43
C.	*Canonical Correlation*	**.44**	.17	.10

Contd...

Contd...

D.	*Meaning of Canonical Linkage Pair*	Less poverty, and high sterilization, so low CEB	Less poverty, low IMR, where some ANC given, but little immunization	Quite high CMR in rural areas, even when some immunization and some ANC available
E.	*Trace Correlation*	**.28201**		
	Wilks Lambda	.769765		
	Chi Square	372.09		
	Significance	.0001		

In Retrospect

Two noteworthy aspects may be mentioned:

First, the measurements of poverty index at the individual level is a unique contribution in the study of human development index. It provides a simple but meaningful and operational index of deprivation of the individuals. The basic data may be easily collected in common surveys, and this poverty index can be easily computed for the individuals, especially for the females. This will indicate the degree of their deprivation, relative to all others. So, more use of such an effective index will enhance population research and demographic research (Mukherji, 2000d, pp. 85-105).

Second, apart from this poverty index, this chapter has repeatedly demonstrated very many meaningful and causal relations between poverty index and fertility rates and infant mortality rates, both for relatively developed states of Kerala and Tamil Nadu, as well as comparatively less developed states like MP, UP and Bihar. These multitudes of causal findings are great eye-openers and these linkage equations prove the basic fundamental causal relations between widespread poverty and high fertility in India (Mukherji, 1997b, pp. 1-25; 2005g, pp. 1-25). More such meaningful research is henceforth required. Policies are discussed in the next chapter.

9

Policy Implications

"He who wants to serve the father must serve the children first. He who wants to serve Shiva must serve His children – must serve all creatures in this world first" (Swami Vivekananda, 1894, Complete Work, Centenary Volume III, 1963, p. 142).

Policy Import of the Main Findings Emerged So far

These crucial canonical findings have very robust policy import. Female illiteracy is considered in this study as the *proxy* indicator of widespread poverty in the country. Canonical linkages, thus, unravel that it is massive poverty which is singularly responsible for high levels of fertility and infant mortality in India, particularly in neglected states of Bihar, UP, MP, Rajasthan, Orissa, and others. Unjust and iniquitous *syndrome of poverty and high fertility* should be liquidated in India very soon, if we are indeed sincerely committed to onset demographic development in this country.

Important findings, thence, reiterate upon the great requirement of providing universal functional literacy and primary education to all girls and to all adult women of this country, if we are socially committed to actualize fertility reduction in these Indian states, and also to bring down infant mortality levels. This step alone will do the wonder. Without fighting out massive female illiteracy, specially in innumerable villages (of UP, MP. Bihar and Rajasthan where it exceeds 60-70%, even in 2001), nothing can be aspired for India. We will definitely fail to motivate scores of millions of poor and illiterate women and men to accept the family planning programmes, no matter how much we may vainly try to persuade, coerce or allure them. Providing universal female literacy and primary education to them is the requirement of supreme importance now.

Second, there is also the utmost need to vastly improve the family planning programmes, as well as RCH care, child immunization, maternal and child health care, ANC care, and their optimum health delivery system (within existing resources), specially in the villages. There is a great need to revamp all such vital features of primary health services, especially in rural, backward, neglected and remote regions. Thus, both socio-economic development efforts (specially poverty reduction) and programmes for providing RCH services and family planning services should go simultaneously.

Third, the crucial causal relations between illiterate women and very high level of infant and child deaths has manifest again and again. Besides, causal linkages between high TFR and widespread female illiteracy also occur. These evil syndromes between fertility, infant mortality and female illiteracy – which is indeed an index of abject poverty – must be de-linked, before demographic transition will prevail over all parts of India, conclusively and permanently. Without such fundamental socio-economic changes in the Indian society and economy, very little can be hoped for. We must act now. Without any further vacillations. And, we must act with very strong political will and very stringent economic discipline. Both honest political commitment and citizen's active participation are very urgently necessary.

Fourth, regarding findings of Model V (Chapter 6, using three separate factor analyses and their factor score as inputs for canonical model), the meaning of this final canonical interrelationship is crystal clear: very high total fertility and very high level of infant mortality as well as child mortality rate occur in Indian states primarily because of very high female illiteracy, both among the adult women and among young girls, and very widespread poverty among them, as well as due to utter lack of health services and family planning services, specially contraceptives, child immunization and ante-natal care for the mothers. It poignantly tells a story of complete chaos and utter neglect of the poor and downtrodden, particularly in pauperized villages and urban slums.

This finding should be considered as the great eye-opener for all concerned: academicians, policy makers, administrators, and everybody else. We have wasted most valuable 60 years after India's independence in utter complacency and total neglect of the need of the masses of the poor people who are reeling under abject poverty, inequity, and unjust exploitation. The above crucial findings are reiterating the same kind of hard reality time and again.

Fifth, the measurements of poverty index at the individual level is a unique contribution to the study of human development index. It provides a simple but meaningful and operational index of deprivation of the individuals. The basic data may be easily collected in common surveys, and this poverty index can be easily computed for the individuals, especially for the females. This will indicate the degree of their deprivation, relative to all others. So, more use of such an effective index will enhance population research and demographic research.

Sixth, apart from devising the 'poverty index', this study has also amply testified and generated a multitudes of significant causal linkages between poverty index and fertility levels and infant mortality rates, both for less developed states like UP, Bihar, MP, West Bengal, and so forth, as well as for comparatively more developed states of Kerala and Tamil Nadu. Multitudes of causal findings of such states, using the fine-grained individual level data, are great eye-openers and such linkage equations prove the basic causal relations between widespread poverty and high fertility in the country. It is hoped that more such kinds of innovative and meaningful research henceforth will be attempted. Only then relevant policies for each state may be revealed and untangled.

Other Development Policies

Policy relevance of such integrative canonical linkages has been pointed out all through the discussion of results. Below, a few salient points are reiterated:

1. For onsetting fertility decline and for infant mortality reduction in all parts of India, the fundamental requirement is that it should be made mandatory that provision of massive education to all the females and to the general masses (especially adults) be made, and provision of adequate calorie to people, and improving their levels of income and living be urgently made, by enhancing the productivity and through rural industrialization (Mukherji, 1989a, pp. 1-126).
2. Out of multitudes of causal interrelationships, as this study has strongly testified, this is the most fundamental and basic development requirement for ensuring demographic decline and population welfare. Such developmental efforts indeed will provide the necessary improved socio-economic context that will vastly increase the motivation of the people to adopt the small family norm and family planning programmes (Udupa, and Mukherji, 1988, pp. 151-175). Without development efforts for meeting the basic human needs of the people, the adoption of small family norm and use of contraceptives are most difficult to achieve, particularly among the hungry and the illiterate masses.
3. For infant mortality control and child mortality reduction, it is mandatory to provide massive education to all females atleast up to primary school level (Mukherji, 1988a, pp. 10-68).
4. For reduction of maternal mortality, it is mandatory to provide massive education to all females up to at least primary level.

Policies for Improving Health Services in Rural Areas and Inaccessible Tracts

One of the most important recommendations is that more sincere attempts should be made to relieve this syndrome of poverty and to alleviate condition of human living in marginalized villages, if we are really concerned with improving status of health of masses of poverty-stricken rural women and onsetting demographic transition in India.

Second, widespread illiteracy and acute unemployment among women are two basic components of this poverty syndrome. Although Primary Health Centres (PHCs) are not entrusted with the task of relieving poverty, nor with providing general education or employment, but they can at least disseminate more effective health education. Besides, coordination with Block Development Offices or rural development agencies also required to encourage greater dissemination of general education and for work employment among rural women.

Third, it should be mandatory for planners and policy makers, at the district, state and national levels, to recognize the above-mentioned 'causal' interrelationships between syndrome of poverty, poor health, and explosive demographic behaviour, and to frame policies accordingly for providing better welfare condition of human living in the marginalized villages of India.

Thus, well-thought plans and policies and their rigorous implementation are very essential. Situation calls for vast systems transformations. Otherwise, improvements are bound to be transient, and short-lived. Sooner this is realized, the better for our health programmes.

In sum, health and family welfare programmes cannot be treated as isolated. They have to be well-coordinated with economic and social development programmes of state and country. This study has also highlighted the operation of distance-decay phenomenon. It is high time to dive deeply into this phenomenon. Why does it occur? What are the forces underneath?

- In India, most planners believed, and still believe in very illusory concept of 'trickle down effect' – that any plans, programmes, services should be localized, and investment made or facilities set up at a *central place* (say, at PHCs or Community Heath Centres (CHCs); and it is wishfully hoped that its beneficial effects would trickle down and reach over the entire region. But, this concept is illusory, banal, and wrong. Trickle down never occurs in Third World (Mukherji, 1988a, pp. 10-68).
- In reality, the *centre*, where a specific service (say, health) is set up, it usurps all facilities, services, capitals, growth efforts, and resources; and the *peripheries* (vast outlying regions) perpetually remain in the same miserable condition. Trickle down effect never spreads over the space. Even if it ever spreads, the benefits are very marginal. Evidently, this is bound to happen – because the concept itself was wrong, planning faulty, and such design

cannot yield benefits which was beyond its scope and capacity. Some crucial thing was missing from the start, i.e., an utter lack of genuine concern to serve the poor. It was only a lip-service to the socialism. No wonder that results are distance-decay function, polarized distribution, concentrated investment, and neglect of the peripheries (ibid., 1988a, pp. 10-68).

- Then, solution lies, not in further concentrating future capitals, resources, men, money, materials, etc., to a few localized PHCs or Sub-Centres (SCs); rather it lies in maximum decentralization of those afore-mentioned growth efforts/resources over outlying regions, far-flung villages, and backward and hitherto neglected zones. To focus upon those specific zones were health need is so great; and where health services are so lacking!
- Recently, in the mid-1990s, certain SCs are upgraded, certain additional PHCs are set up or renamed, and the former PHCs are now termed Community Health Centres (CHCs). Well, this is a positive endeavour. But, what is emphasized above, regarding the great need for maximum possible decentralization and to do away totally with the faulty 'trickle down principle', is entirely different. It should be understood in the right perspective. Merely renaming some centres, or upgrading some others, will not dispense with present-day polarized (around PHCs) and mal-distributed health services over the national space.

Besides, a few more crucial recommendations are also briefly highlighted (for details, see Mukherji, 1987, pp. 132-138; 1989a, pp. 1-136):

- Infant Mortality Rate (IMR) and Total Fertility Rate (TRF) must be drastically reduced soon. And, control of infant mortality must be given first priority, before fertility transition can be expected to set in. Because, IMR is primal cause, high fertility is effect.
- Health policy-wise and programme-wise, rural health facilities and services must be provided on priority basis specially to hitherto neglected and remote regions, blocks, villages – where need for health services is great and where health services are so insignificant.
- Child immunization, polio vaccination, and child check up services demand much more sincere efforts, since death control of infants/children is a sacred responsibility, and performances achieved are not at all laudable.

- According to General System Theory or Field Theory, any system (here health) cannot be improved without bringing vast system transformation and positive changes in specific socio-economic contexts in which it is imbedded.
- Here, CHCs/PHCs/SCs are imbedded in the socio-economic context of village society which is plagued by *syndrome of poverty* – as manifested in widespread illiteracy, acute unemployment, low occupations, and lower castes. As a result, knowledge and utilization of health services are so poor; IMR and TFR are so high; and such negative demographic behaviour(s) are further regressed due to dismal rates of utilization of existing health services. If we are really concerned with improving health system, then, we cannot ignore those crucial causal relationships in all policies, plans, and implementation – without running risk of getting only repeated failures. These may be beyond the scope of Health Ministry, but certainly not of Planning Departments (e.g., Ministry of Rural Development, Human Resources Development, Education, Labour, Employment, Social Welfare).
- Disseminating health education to women may be task of CHCs/PHCs. On other hand, onus of bringing effective improvements in general education among masses of rural women and providing more employment to unemployed/low-waged women in villages rests on Integrated Rural Development Agencies, Agricultural Extension Agencies, and District and State Planning Departments. These points are highlighted here to draw attention of all concerned to bring better human condition in the country, particularly in villages.

10

Results of Canonical Analysis of 1998-99 Data: Recent Demographic, Socio-Economic and Policy Situation

"Therefore, it is right for you that you should serve millions of brothers rather aggrandise this little self" (Swami Vivekananda, 1894, Complete Work, Centenary Volume III, 1963, p. 446).

National Family and Health Survey (NFHS)-II of India was conducted during 1998-99, and its preliminary data were available in 2000 or later. It is also surmised here to ascertain the recent-most demographic, socio-economic and population policy situation of India, and to assess the broad changes that have occurred. Table 48 provides the detailed data of demographic, socio-economic and population programme variables of Indian states, based on NFHS-II survey (1998-99). Tables 50 and 52 provide the data for rural parts and urban parts, respectively, of various states. In the canonical analysis, the first three variables of Table 48 are treated as dependent variables (dependent matrix), and the next 11 variables as independent variables (socio-economic variables and population programme variables), or two independent matrices. Last two matrices are combined. Thus, these two final data matrices become inputs for final canonical analysis at state level (rural and urban parts taken together). Variable list is given below Table 48.

The same variables are also considered for canonical analysis, separately, of rural parts and urban parts of various states. Thus, three separate canonical analyses were performed, respectively, on data of rural and urban parts of states taken together and the corresponding canonical findings shown in Table 49. Likewise, the canonical linkages for only rural parts are presented in Table 51, whereas canonical relations for urban parts in Table 53.

Demographic and Socio-Economic Situation of India in 1998-99 (Rural and Urban Parts Combined)

Accompanying four maps (Figures 20-23) show the main demographic and socio-economic situation of India during 1998-99, specially in rural and urban parts of all major Indian states. In India, changes do not occur over night. Demographic and socio-economic changes occur very slowly. Thus, the pitiable condition of widespread female illiteracy among adult women in rural India, which had remained very high during 1992-93, has still persisted even in 1998-99 (e.g., in UP, Bihar, MP and Rajasthan) (Figure 20). Consequently, total fertility rate (TFR) also has remained very high in those states (on average 3 to 5 children, even in 1998-99). Thus, although slight reduction in fertility may be noticed in some states during 6-year period (1992-93 to 1998-99), but the fertility decline has not been spectacular in these poor and backward states (Mukherji, 2000C, pp. 10-15). But, they constitute the bulk of India's population and persistently record very high population growth rate. In short, rural socio-economic and demographic scenario virtually remained as untouched by development process, as before (Figures 20-21). Table 50 depicts rural situation very vividly.

In urban India, however, comparatively speaking, slightly more progress is noticed. High female illiteracy still can exist in all northern states (UP, Bihar, MP and Rajasthan), albeit in much reduced form (Mukherji, 2000h, p. 6) (Figure 22). Consequently, total fertility rate (TFR) in urban components of these states has also declined to some extent (Figure 23). It does not exceed 3 children per mother in urban India. Fortunately, TFR is also reaching the replacement level in

Figure 20

India (Rural), Female Illiteracy (age 15-44), 1998-99

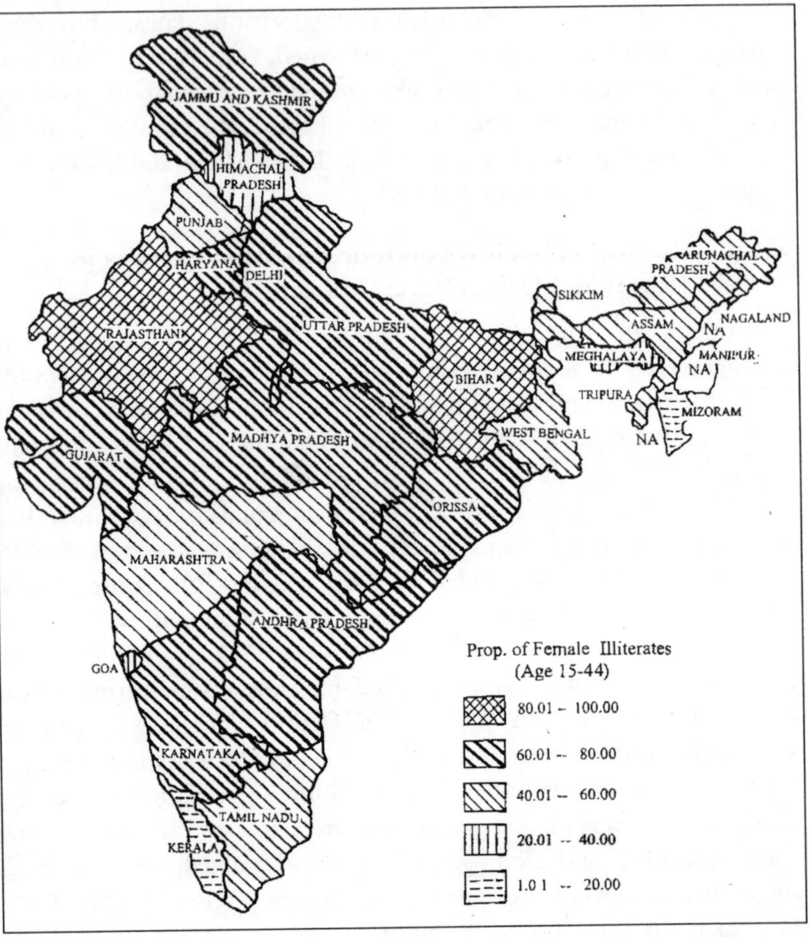

Figure 21

India (Rural), Total Fertility Rate, 1998-99

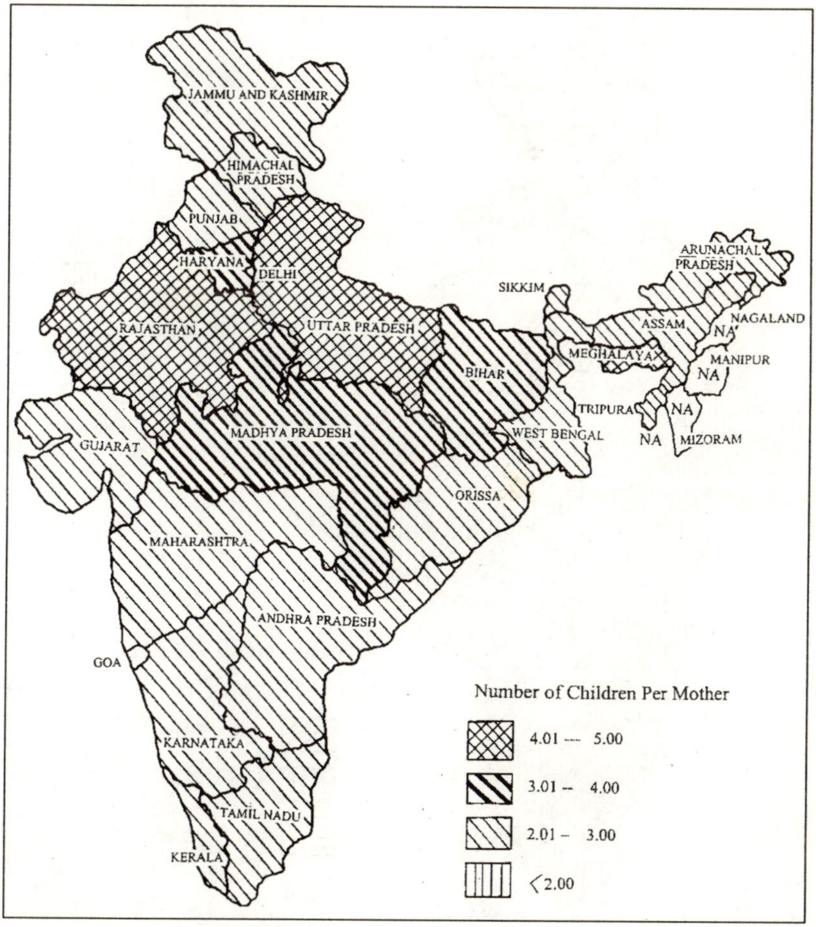

Figure 22

India (Urban), Female Illiteracy (age 15-44), 1998-99

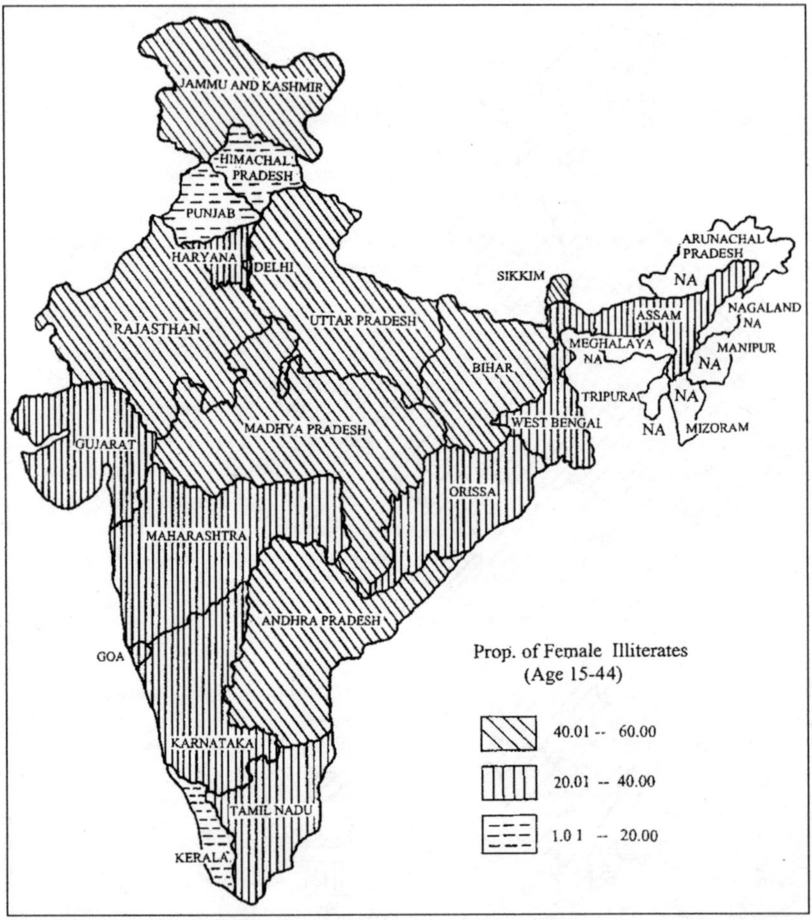

Figure 23
India (Urban), Total Fertility Rate, 1998-99

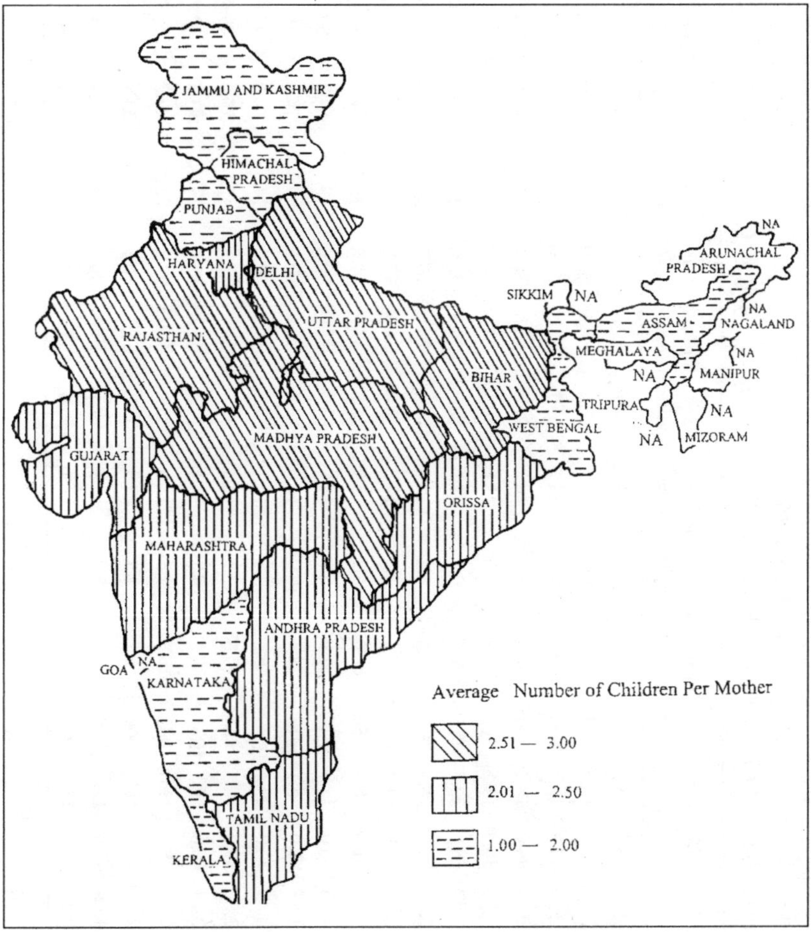

Table 48

NFHS-II Data of Indian States, 1998-99, Rural and Urban Combined, Input for Canonical Analysis

	State	TFR	IMR	GR	Sex ratio	Female illiter	Literate <prim	Primary compl.	Use contra.	Female steril.	Got ANC	Instt. deliv.	Child immun.	Women anaemia	Child anaemia
1.	Andhra Pradesh (R)	2.32	75.0	13.1	990	71.6	5.6	13.3	57.8	52.8	90.5	40.4	48.9	50.7	68.3
2.	Andhra Pradesh (U)	2.07	38.0	15.0	951	40.3	4.0	21.7	62.2	52.4	98.9	78.6	61.0	47.4	66.6
3.	Arunachal (Total)	2.39	44.0	16.4	931	52.7	9.4	14.5	33.7	20.7	61.6	23.9	22.5	62.5	54.4
4.	Assam (R)	2.39	80.0	18.2	941	56.7	12.4	10.2	26.3	15.5	58.1	15.0	14.9	69.2	63.0
5.	Assam (U)	1.50	36.0	14.1	962	23.9	7.3	13.0	30.6	17.9	88.4	59.9	50.1	66.8	50.1
6.	Bihar (R)	3.57	68.0	22.3	953	80.1	2.7	7.6	20.9	18.3	33.0	12.4	9.4	64.0	79.2
7.	Bihar (U)	2.75	51.0	16.6	923	46.2	5.2	12.8	35.4	26.6	67.7	39.9	22.4	59.3	78.4
8.	Delhi (U)	2.42	36.0	14.2	896	29.1	2.7	12.5	55.8	24.9	75.8	59.5	57.8	40.5	69.7
9.	Gujarat (R)	2.98	71.0	18.4	954	64.0	6.2	13.2	53.3	37.8	83.8	33.2	44.9	51.1	74.1
10.	Gujarat (U)	2.33	46.0	15.8	927	31.8	5.9	16.9	53.3	47.0	90.6	69.4	54.3	39.6	64.2
11.	Goa (Total)	1.77	23.0	6.1	1013	28.6	10.9	16.3	34.4	25.6	99.0	90.5	74.9	36.4	51.6
12.	Haryana (R)	3.09	72.0	20.3	869	65.6	2.5	15.1	53.1	43.0	52.0	14.9	58.2	47.6	77.0
13.	Haryana (U)	2.22	59.0	16.3	864	29.5	2.1	12.4	53.4	28.0	77.9	47.1	76.5	45.9	81.3
14.	Himachal Pradesh (R)	2.18	66.0	15.1	1031	38.3	4.5	24.4	60.5	34.1	85.9	25.5	83.7	40.7	67.5
15.	Himachal Pradesh (U)	1.74	38.0	11.6	903	15.8	2.3	15.8	63.9	46.1	97.2	72.2	80.2	38.4	63.9
16.	Jammu & Kashmir (R)	2.98	46.0	15.2	964	75.7	1.5	8.3	36.8	25.3	80.5	28.6	53.4	59.9	69.3
17.	Jammu & Kashmir (U)	1.66	45.0	11.5	889	48.6	1.6	6.4	59.7	37.5	96.2	74.8	73.1	54.3	65.1
18.	Karnataka (R)	2.24	70.0	14.1	996	67.7	4.8	12.7	56.6	53.5	82.6	38.7	60.4	46.0	67.4

Contd...

Contd...

19.	Karnataka (U)	1.89	25.0	13.8	960	31.7	3.7	17.3	56.4	47.1	94.4	78.8	59.0	35.8	62.4
20.	Kerala (R)	2.07	15.0	11.8	1069	13.9	10.0	22.2	55.7	48.6	98.7	91.5	77.9	23.3	43.3
21.	Kerala (U)	1.51	17.0	12.0	1057	8.0	6.8	16.5	57.4	48.5	99.4	99.4	84.9	20.3	47.8
22.	Madhya Pradesh (R)	3.52	104.0	20.2	944	77.8	5.0	10.1	39.3	35.0	55.0	12.3	17.0	57.1	72.4
23.	Madhya Pradesh (U)	2.61	56.0	15.3	904	41.0	6.2	13.7	52.5	37.9	81.8	49.8	41.2	46.1	68.4
24.	Maharashtra (R)	2.74	58.0	14.7	968	55.6	9.7	16.2	62.1	51.9	86.9	34.6	76.8	51.2	73.6
25.	Maharashtra (U)	2.24	32.0	15.0	885	29.0	7.5	20.8	56.7	43.6	94.8	80.9	80.4	44.8	69.9
26.	Meghalaya (Total)	4.49	52.0	20.2	982	38.1	28.4	12.6	15.7	6.4	53.1	17.5	14.3	63.8	67.7
27.	Manipur (T)	2.89	23.0	10.2	1023	10.0	25.7	25.4	56.0	43.8	90.3	57.9	59.6	48.2	55.6
28.	Orissa (R)	2.49	101.0	14.8	963	62.2	9.8	16.0	39.7	34.2	78.5	19.3	42.2	64.1	71.8
29.	Orissa (U)	2.19	66.0	13.3	921	37.9	7.9	20.6	45.2	30.9	86.7	54.7	56.4	54.8	67.4
30.	Punjab (R)	2.42	58.0	15.5	878	48.5	3.1	20.9	53.8	34.3	69.2	32.0	66.3	42.6	75.8
31.	Punjab (U)	1.79	40.0	12.1	938	16.8	2.3	12.5	54.0	17.9	90.3	56.0	86.2	39.1	71.4
32.	Rajasthan (R)	4.01	87.0	23.9	921	85.0	2.0	7.0	35.3	30.1	41.5	15.0	13.1	49.3	77.0
33.	Rajasthan (U)	2.96	60.0	17.8	923	45.9	5.1	13.6	46.9	33.0	69.2	47.2	26.4	46.7	74.1
34.	Sikkim (T)	2.70	52.0	14.8	925	49.4	11.8	15.8	41.6	21.9	70.0	31.7	43.9	61.5	76.7
35.	Tamil Nadu (R)	2.22	59.0	10.4	1024	57.9	4.5	17.5	47.6	44.7	98.1	73.1	76.6	59.1	67.3
36.	Tamil Nadu (U)	2.12	40.0	11.2	996	27.8	4.6	20.8	55.1	46.0	99.0	92.6	81.0	51.6	64.0
37.	Uttar Pradesh (R)	4.27	89.0	22.5	927	77.1	2.6	8.8	18.3	14.1	28.7	11.7	19.2	49.4	70.9
38.	Uttar Pradesh (U)	2.86	65.0	19.1	925	42.5	3.1	10.3	36.6	18.0	63.3	37.3	32.3	46.0	70.1
39.	West Bengal (R)	2.46	56.0	15.7	953	57.4	15.4	14.6	47.5	33.5	88.1	31.5	40.8	64.3	75.1
40.	West Bengal (U)	1.69	41.0	8.2	914	26.1	11.0	15.7	46.4	27.0	96.0	80.1	56.3	57.9	64.3

Contd...

Contd...

Variables (1998-99 sets)

1. TFR = Total Fertility Rate
2 IMR = Infant Mortality Rate
3. GR = Population Growth Rate (SRS data)
4. Sex ratio = No. of females per 1,000 males
5. Female illiteracy = Proportion of women illiterate (age 15-44)
6. Female literate (<primary education) = Proportion of women with less than primary education
7. Female literate (primary completed) = Proportion of women with primary education completed
8. Use contraceptives = Proportion of women (age 15-44) using contraceptives
9. Female sterilization = Proportion of women (age 15-44) undergone female sterilization
10. Got ANC care = Proportion of women who received ante-natal care
11. Institutional delivery of child = Delivery of child in hospital/PHCs, etc.
12. Child immunization = Proportion of children who got complete child immunization course.
13. Women with anaemia
14. Child with anaemia

urban components of Assam and West Bengal and also in urban Karnataka. Considerable decline also occurs in urban parts of Jammu & Kashmir, Punjab and Himachal Pradesh. Nevertheless, the urban components of most northern states still need more rapid fertility decline, in order to initiate a sustained demographic transition (Figure 23). Urban scenario of demographic and socio-economic conditions of various states is presented in Table 51.

NFHS-II (1998-99) survey showed that 36 per cent of ever-married women aged 15-44 were malnourished. It is more pronounced among rural women, illiterate women, and among women having low standard of living index (NFHS, 2000, pp. 141-49).

Canonical Results of States (Rural and Urban Parts Combined): 1998-99 Findings

The first canonical linkage equation can be written as follows, based on only high loadings (for details see Mukherji, 2000d, pp. 1-35) (Table 49):

– 0.65 *(TFR) –* ***0.51*** *(IMR) –* ***0.57*** *(population growth rate)* ***=0.30*** *(contraceptive use) +* ***0.56*** *(got ANC care) +* ***0.41*** *(institutional delivery of child) –* ***0.39*** *(less anaemic children).*

This can be easily and meaningfully interpreted that, for all-India rural-urban combined situation, for the first largest set of canonical variates, the attributes, 'ANC care' and 'contraceptive use' dampen 'IMR' and 'TFR', and also 'growth rate', specially when institutional help for delivery and less anaemic children prevalent. Canonical correlation between this matched pair of canonical variates is 0.96, indicating that 92 per cent (correlation squared times 100) of variance in this set of variate pair is explained by such attribute-bahaviour indicators.

Likewise, successive canonical correlations, loadings, and corresponding patterns of causal relationships between demographic behaviour set and socio-economic attribute-cum-policy set can be easily interpreted (Table 49). The remaining canonical relationships are as hereunder.

The second canonical linkage shows that, one single factor, 'widespread and universal female literacy' would be greatly conducive

Table 49

Canonical Structure Matrix: Canonical Linkage between Demographic Variables and Socio-economic Variables-cum-Population Programme Variables, Indian States, Rural and Urban Combined, 1998-99 Data

Variables	*Canonical Variate Pairs*		
	1	*2*	*3*
A. *Demographic Matrix (Dependent Variables)*		*Canonical Loadings*	
Total Fertility Rate (TFR)	**-.64**	**.79**	.24
Infant Mortality Rate (IMR)	**-.51**	-.29	**.59**
Growth rate of population	**-.56**	-.52	-.76
B. *Socio-Economic–cum-Population Policy Matrix (Independent Variables)*		*Canonical Loadings*	
Sex ratio	-.06	.09	.03
Female illiteracy	-.10	**.37**	**.61**
Literate ≤ primary	-.08	**.50**	.18
Primary complete	.01	.01	.08
Contraceptive use	.30	.10	-.19
Female sterilization	-.37	**-.22**	-.08
Got ante-natal care	**.56**	-.36	**.63**
Institutional delivery of child	**.41**	**.57**	-.16
Child immunization	.23	.14	**.30**
Women with anaemia	.21	-.17	.03
Child with anaemia	**-.39**	.15	.11
C. *Canonical Correlation*	**.95**	**.79**	**.61**
D. *Meaning of Canonical Linkages*	Relatively low TFR, low IMR and low growth rate because of high ANC, high institutional delivery and less children with anaemia	High TFR because moderately high female illiteracy, high proportion of females ≤ primary, and little female sterilization, in spite of high institutional delivery of child	High IMR because of high female illiteracy, and only slight child immuniz- ation, in spite of high ANC
E. *Trace Correlation*	**.8014**		
Wilks Lambda	.0188		
Chi Square	129.0		
Significance	.0001		

to fertility reduction in underdeveloped states. This factor (female illiteracy) alone is manifest as the strongest determinant of fertility, amidst total 11 independent variables (among masses of data, factors, and relationships). Many important population policy or programme variables are also conspicuously absent in this significant canonical linkage.

Such canonical linkages are not only statistically highly significant, but are also practically very meaningful. Each has emerged as a unique demographic field, independent of previous one. Their interpretations and policy imports are very evident. All three canonical linkages mainly highlight the great need for enhancing developmental efforts (like universal female literacy programmes), simultaneously with great need for health improvement, nutrition development, and women's employment, empowerment and development as policy prescriptions, apart from continuing current family welfare programmes and spread of contraceptives. These linkages are now interpreted as follows:

1. Relatively low TFR, low IMR and low population growth rate occur in some states, due to high ANC and some contraceptive use, high institutional child delivery and also due to less children with anaemia (canonical correlation is 0.987).
2. Very high total fertility rate (TFR) occurs in many states, because of moderately high female illiteracy and high proportion of females having less than primary education, and little female sterilization, in spite of high institutional child delivery (canonical correlation is 0.79).
3. High level of infant mortality rate (IMR) occurs due to high female illiteracy, and also due to little child immunization, in spite of some ante-natal care given (canonical correlation is 0.62).

Significance of All-India Findings (Rural-Urban Combined)

Policy imports of such very crucial results are crystal clear. As stated before in this study, female illiteracy is treated as the surrogate indicator of abject widespread poverty in the country. The results based on 1998-99 data set, also, thus, have clearly testified again that widespread and abject poverty or massive female illiteracy is the most crucial determinant of high fertility and high infant mortality in India, specially in wretchedly backward states of Bihar, UP, MP, and Rajasthan, and elsewhere. Very urgently, this evil syndrome of poverty and high fertility must be liquidated, if we are really committed to onsetting fertility decline in this country, everywhere. We cannot afford to be complacent that fertility decline has already set in some southern states (like Kerala, Tamil Nadu or Goa), because fertility level is still perilously very high in most populous and high growth states of UP, Bihar, MP and Rajasthan. Unless and until fertility decline sets in permanently in these large and populous states, there is nothing to rejoice in India.

Findings then highlight on the great requirement of catering universal education to all young girls and all adult women of India, if we are sincerely concerned with bringing in drastic fertility decline in those backward states, and also reducing infant mortality. This remedy is absolutely necessary. Without eradicating massive illiteracy among the Indian females, specially in rural UP, MP, Bihar and Rajasthan – most unfortunately where it still exceeds 75 to 85 per cent – no socio-economic improvement can ever be achieved, notwithstanding how much vain attempts are made to motivate hundreds of millions of illiterate and hungry Indian women to embrace contraceptives and family planning. Sheer impossible! This is the supreme requirement! (Mukherji, 2005g, pp. 1-25)

Precious 60 years have simply vanished since India's independence. We cannot wait more just to reduce such colossal illiteracy among the females. Most unfortunately, and more amazingly, the Indian academia (demographers, population specialists, geographers, social scientists), bureaucrats, planners, policy makers and politicians do not at all appear to be conscious about this great requirement, nor for its rigorous implementation. Sooner this hard reality dawns upon their minds, the better for this country, and for entire world. We cannot continue to behave like the proverbial ostrich with its head buried in the sands; soon dangerous catastrophe will catch us unaware from behind!

Second, as canonical linkages have amply demonstrated, even with 1998-99 data, there is a great urgency to vastly improve family welfare programmes, as well as AN care, MCH care, child immunization, and all components of RCH services. There is a great need to revamp all these crucial aspects of primary health services, specially in the villages, backward states, and hitherto neglected and remote zones. Top priority must be given to such essential health services and family welfare services among the poor, the downtrodden, slum dwellers, the Scheduled Castes, Scheduled Tribes, and very poor and hapless women, specially in most backward and neglected states of UP, MP, Bihar, West Bengal, Orissa, Andhra Pradesh, Rajasthan, and elsewhere. These are zones where benefits of development have not reached the millions of the poor. Thus, the socio-economic development efforts and programmes for providing safe motherhood-cum-child survival programmes and reproductive health should go simultaneously, not in exclusion.

Third, the crucial causal relations between illiterate mothers and very high infant mortality have emerged again with recent 1998-99 data. Moreover, the causal linkages between high fertility and rampant poverty and female illiteracy have also emerged very distinctly, even with recent data. These evil syndrome between poverty and female illiteracy (indeed index of poverty) on the one hand, and high fertility and high infant mortality on the other, must be liquidated, before demographic development will occur permanently over entire India. Without such very fundamental transformations, very little can be expected in India. We must not ever forget the great reality that the hungry and illiterate masses of Indian women cannot go for contraceptives.

This basic social and economic upliftment and this basic and necessary condition for adopting the small family norm must be provided first. Otherwise, all our efforts will be in vain. Precious 60 years are already wasted. Unfortunately, NFHS team and its various reports have not attempted such threadbare and highly powerful analyses. These results, discussed above, are again confirmed mathematically by very high powered canonical findings, and analyzing the latest available 1998-99 data (see Tables 49, 51 and 53). Thus, the truth has emerged, and there is now need for urgent and soulful actions!

Poverty and Female Illiteracy Still Emerged as Most Crucial Determinants of Fertility, even in 1998-99

The Demographic Field Theory is applied by performing canonical analyses upon the three data matrices (D, S, and P), mentioned above.

Table 50

NFHS-II data of Indian States, 1998-99, Rural, Input for Canonical Analysis for 1998-99 Canonical Model

No.	State	TFR	IMR	GR	Sex ratio	Female illiter	Literate <prim	Prim. compl.	Use contra.	Female steril.	Got ANC	Instt. deliv.	Child immun.	Women anaemia	Child anaemia
1.	Andhra Pradesh (R)	2.32	75.0	13.1	990	71.6	5.6	13.3	57.8	52.8	90.5	40.4	48.9	50.7	68.3
2.	Arunachal (R)	2.39	44.0	16.4	931	52.7	9.4	14.5	33.7	20.7	61.6	23.9	22.5	62.5	54.4
3.	Assam (R)	2.39	80.0	18.2	941	56.7	12.4	10.2	26.3	15.5	58.1	15.0	14.9	69.2	63.0
4.	Bihar (R)	3.57	68.0	22.3	953	80.1	2.7	7.6	20.9	18.3	33.0	12.4	9.4	64.0	79.2
5.	Gujarat (R)	2.98	71.0	18.4	954	64.0	6.2	13.2	53.3	37.8	83.8	33.2	44.9	51.1	74.1
6.	Haryana (R)	3.09	72.0	20.3	869	65.6	2.5	15.1	53.1	43.0	52.0	14.9	58.2	47.6	77.0
7.	Himachal Pradesh (R)	2.18	66.0	15.1	1031	38.3	4.5	24.4	60.5	34.1	85.9	25.5	83.7	40.7	67.5
8.	Jammu-Kashmir (R)	2.98	46.0	15.2	964	75.7	1.5	8.3	36.8	25.3	80.5	28.6	53.4	59.9	69.3
9.	Karnataka (R)	2.24	70.0	14.1	996	67.7	4.8	12.7	56.6	53.5	82.6	38.7	60.4	46.0	67.4
10.	Kerala (R)	2.07	15.0	11.8	1069	13.9	10.0	22.2	55.7	48.6	98.7	91.5	77.9	23.3	43.3
11.	Madhya Pradesh (R)	3.52	104.0	20.2	944	77.8	5.0	10.1	39.3	35.0	55.0	12.3	17.0	57.1	72.4
12.	Maharashtra (R)	2.74	58.0	14.7	968	55.6	9.7	16.2	62.1	51.9	86.9	34.6	76.8	51.2	73.6
13.	Meghalaya (R)	4.49	52.0	20.2	982	38.1	28.4	12.6	15.7	6.4	53.1	17.5	14.3	63.8	67.7
14.	Orissa (R)	2.49	101.0	14.8	963	62.2	9.8	16.0	39.7	34.2	78.5	19.3	42.2	64.1	71.8
15.	Punjab (R)	2.42	58.0	15.5	878	48.5	3.1	20.9	53.8	34.3	69.2	32.0	66.3	42.6	75.8
16.	Rajasthan (R)	4.01	87.0	23.9	921	85.0	2.0	7.0	35.3	30.1	41.5	15.0	13.1	49.3	77.0
17.	Sikkim (R)	2.70	52.0	14.8	925	49.4	11.8	15.8	41.6	21.9	70.0	31.7	43.9	61.5	76.7
18.	Tamil Nadu (R)	2.22	59.0	10.4	1024	57.9	4.5	17.5	47.6	44.7	98.1	73.1	76.6	59.1	67.3
19.	Uttar Pradesh (R)	4.27	89.0	22.5	927	77.1	2.6	8.8	18.3	14.1	28.7	11.7	19.2	49.4	70.9
20.	West Bengal (R)	2.46	56.0	15.7	953	57.4	15.4	14.6	47.5	33.5	88.1	31.5	40.8	64.3	75.1

List of variables as in Table 48

Recent NFHS-II data of major states are used, considering rural and urban components separately. Two separate canonical analyses are thus made, separately for rural and urban parts of various states. The variables considered are indicated in Tables 50 and 52. The canonical findings are presented in Tables 51 and 53. Numerous notable canonical equations are generated. These findings are not only statistically very highly significant, but also practically very meaningful, having great policy implications. Most noteworthy fact is that, even with the recent 1998-99 data sets, poverty and female illiteracy have still emerged as the most crucial determinants of fertility and infant mortality in India. This greatly testifies not only the new and novel theoretical contribution of the Demographic Field Theory to population research, but also uphold the central tenet that, first, poverty and female illiteracy must be universally alleviated, before fertility decline and demographic transition set in!

Findings of Rural India (1998-99)

Table 51 presents main findings of canonical analyses performed on data on rural parts of all major states. Here only rural components of states are considered (rural Delhi excluded). Four canonical equations are generated, every time causally coupling only those variables from both the dependent and the independent sets that are causally linked. That is, only those variables are identified in each cycle which belong to that particular *demographic system* or *demographic field*, while reducing others to near zero, and which do not belong to that specific system (field). Important canonical loadings are shown in bold face (Mukherji, 2000d, pp. 5-141; 2000b, pp. 1-35).

The technical details of canonical model are available in Cooley and Lohnes (1962, pp. 45-65); and the way it is integrally used in Demographic Field Theory is given in earlier studies (Mukherji, 1983b, pp. 1-65; 1989b, pp. 342-73).

Following three canonical linkage pairs have emerged, and all of them are statistically of very high value. The general statistical overlap or *trace correlation* is also remarkably high, i.e., 0.91; which means that 82 per cent of total variance in the dependent set is explained by the independent set. Besides, successively three very highly significant canonical linkages also emerged, with canonical values as high as 0.97, 0.89, or, 0.85. It is remarkably rare to find either in physical or social sciences successively such high canonical correlations, specially in a single test. Such canonical linkages are not only statistically very powerful, but also practically considerably meaningful. Most such findings are self-explanatory (see Table 51). Obviously, such crucial canonical equations have great policy implications.

Table 51

Canonical Structure Matrix: Canonical Linkage Relations between Demographic Variables and Socio-economic Variables-cum-Population Programme Variables, Indian States, Rural Parts Only, 1998-99 Data

	Variables	*Canonical Variate Pairs*		
		1	*2*	*3*
A.	*Demographic Matrix (Dependent Variables)*		*Canonical Loadings*	
	Total Fertility Rate (TFR)	.29	**.78**	**.50**
	Infant Mortality Rate (IMR)	.17	-.27	**.46**
	Population growth rate	**.94**	-.54	-.72
B.	*Socio-economic Variables and Population Programme Matrix (Independent Variables)*		*Canonical Loadings*	
	Sex ratio	.13	-.01	-.01
	Female illiteracy	.19	**.52**	**.49**
	Literate < primary	.23	**.45**	.18
	Primary completed	-.14	-.03	.38
	Contraceptive use	**-.03**	.08	**-.60**
	Female sterilization	-.05	**-.39**	**.26**
	Got ante-natal care	**-.53**	-.19	.30
	Institutional delivery	**-.29**	.32	-.12
	Child immunization	-.30	.41	.05
	Women with anaemia	-.54	-.19	-.15
	Child with anaemia	.31	-.04	.03
C.	*Canonical Correlations*	**.97**	**.89**	**.84**
D.	*Meaning of Canonical Linkages Pair*	High growth rate as no ANC, little institutional delivery, little contraceptive use	High TFR because high female illiteracy, large proportion of females with<primary education, little sterilization	Moderately high TFR, moderately high IMR because high female illiteracy and little contraceptive use and little female sterilization
E.	*Trace Correlation*	**.9069**		
	Wilk's Lambda	.0031		
	Chi Square	71.97		
	Significance	.0001		

These canonical findings are identified as follows:

1. High population growth rate occur, because very little ante-natal care is available, little institutional delivery of children is prevalent, and little use of contraceptives recorded (canonical correlation is 0.97).
2. High total fertility rate occurs, because of high female illiteracy and high proportion of females with less than primary education, and very little female sterilization (canonical correlation is 0.89).
3. Moderately high total fertility rate and moderately high infant mortality rate occur, because high female illiteracy prevail, with little contraceptive use and little female sterilization (canonical correlation is 0.85).

Most noteworthy reality is that even with recent 1998-99 data sets, these three canonical linkages have again highlighted the basic truth and 'cause and effect relationships' between high poverty (i.e., high female illiteracy) and high level of fertility and infant mortality in rural parts of all Indian states, which earlier emerged with 1992-93 sets. This basic truth did appear time and again, and has emerged very vigorously and very unambiguously all over rural India, than in urban India, as well as in rural-urban India combined. Note that over 70 per cent of population still lives in rural India, as such, this finding has great policy import for entire India.

Second, Table 51 also emphasizes on the truth that greater use of ANC care, more contraceptive use, and greater institutional facility for safe motherhood and child survival is also absolutely necessary for reduction of high population growth rates in most populous and high growth states (viz., UP, Bihar, MP, Rajasthan and other). This fact must also be equally emphasized. Because, high level of female illiteracy and poverty and great lacuna of health services, together, energizes the most evil syndrome of poverty and high fertility, where high infant mortality and high fertility become almost self reinforcing. It becomes much harder to break the syndrome of poverty and high fertility in those backward states.

Findings of Urban India (1998-99)

Table 53 presents the results of urban parts of major states of India (including urban Delhi). Variables remained the same as earlier. Here

Table 52

NFHS-II Data of Indian States, 1998-99, Urban Parts, Input for Canonical Analysis

No. State	TFR	IMR	GR	Sex ratio	Female illiteracy	Literate <prim	Prim. compl.	Use contra.	Female steril.	Got ANC	Instt. deliv.	Child immun.	Women anaemia	Child anaemia
1. Andhra Pradesh (U)	2.07	38.0	15.0	951	40.3	4.0	21.7	62.2	52.4	98.9	78.6	61.0	47.4	66.6
2. Assam (U)	1.50	36.0	14.1	962	23.9	7.3	13.0	30.6	17.9	88.4	59.9	50.1	66.8	50.1
3. Bihar (U)	2.75	51.0	16.6	923	46.2	5.2	12.8	35.4	26.6	67.7	39.9	22.4	59.3	78.4
4. Delhi (U)	2.42	36.0	14.2	896	29.1	2.7	12.5	55.8	24.9	75.8	59.5	57.8	40.5	69.7
5. Gujarat (U)	2.33	46.0	15.8	927	31.8	5.9	16.9	53.3	47.0	90.6	69.4	54.3	39.6	64.2
6. Haryana (U)	2.22	59.0	16.3	864	29.5	2.1	12.4	53.4	28.0	77.9	47.1	76.5	45.9	81.3
7. Himachal Pradesh (U)	1.74	38.0	11.6	903	15.8	2.3	15.8	63.9	46.1	97.2	72.2	80.2	38.4	63.9
8. Jammu-Kashmir (U)	1.66	45.0	11.5	889	48.6	1.6	6.4	59.7	37.5	96.2	74.8	73.1	54.3	65.1
9. Karnataka (U)	1.89	25.0	13.8	960	31.7	3.7	17.3	56.4	47.1	94.4	78.8	59.0	35.8	62.4
10. Kerala (U)	1.51	17.0	12.0	1057	8.0	6.8	16.5	57.4	48.5	99.4	99.4	84.9	20.3	47.8
11. Madhya Pradesh (U)	2.61	56.0	15.3	904	41.0	6.2	13.7	52.5	37.9	81.8	49.8	41.2	46.1	68.4
12. Maharashtra (U)	2.24	32.0	15.0	885	29.0	29.0	20.8	56.7	43.6	94.8	80.9	80.4	44.8	69.9
13. Orissa (U)	2.19	66.0	13.3	921	37.9	7.9	20.6	45.2	30.9	86.7	54.7	56.4	54.8	67.4
14. Punjab (U)	1.79	40.0	12.1	938	16.8	2.3	12.5	54.0	17.9	90.3	56.0	86.2	39.1	71.4
15. Rajasthan (U)	2.96	60.0	17.8	923	45.9	5.1	13.6	46.9	33.0	69.2	47.2	26.4	46.7	74.1
16. Tamil Nadu (U)	2.12	40.0	11.2	996	27.8	4.6	20.8	55.1	46.0	99.0	92.6	81.0	51.6	64.0
17. Uttar Pradesh (U)	2.86	65.0	19.1	925	42.5	3.1	10.3	36.6	18.0	63.3	37.3	32.3	46.0	70.1
18. West Bengal (U)	1.69	41.0	8.2	914	26.1	11.0	15.7	46.4	27.0	96.0	80.1	56.3	57.9	64.3

List of variables as in Table 48.

also, the following three pairs of canonical causal relations are extracted by canonical analysis, and all are statistically of very high value. Overall statistical mapping or *trace correlation* is also remarkably high, i.e., 0.87; in other words, 76 per cent of total variance in demographic set is explained by the combined set of socio-economic-cum-policy set. Moreover, in successive iterative cycles, three very highly significant canonical equations are also generated, having canonical values as high as 0.98, 0.87, or 0.75. It is extremely rare to obtain successively such a series of high values of canonical correlations in demography or social sciences. These also appeal very much to common sense. Obviously, such canonical findings have great policy implications (Mukherji, 2000d, pp. 125-141). These three findings are:

1. Less total fertility rate, less infant mortality rate, and less population growth rate prevail in urban India, because less female illiteracy occurs, adequate ante-natal care is available, and considerable proportion of women also received institutional assistance in child delivery services (canonical correlation is 0.97).
2. Relatively less total fertility rate occurs in urban India, but moderately high infant mortality and moderately high population growth rate also occur, because less contraceptive used and little institutional delivery is available, in spite of relatively high child immunization services (canonical correlation is 0.89).
3. Less population growth rate occur in urban India, because of little female illiteracy and more literate females with less than primary education, with high contraceptive use, in spite of some women with anaemia (Canonical correlation is 0.75)

Evidently, in urban India, even 1998-99 data clearly demonstrate that wherever female illiteracy is less, fertility rate is also less. Additionally, wherever ante-natal care is more available and institutional delivery of child is more, IMR is also less. This is a very notable finding. This also highlights the great policy implications of simultaneously emphasizing both upon reduction of female illiteracy and also RCH services. Wherever both these 'necessary' condition and 'sufficient' condition are met, as in many urban components of Indian states, fertility decline and infant mortality decline have already set in.

Table 53

Canonical Structure Matrix: Canonical Linkage Results between Demographic Variables and Socio-economic Variables-cum-Population Programme Variables, Indian States, Urban Parts, 1998-99 Data

Variables	*Canonical Variate Pairs*		
	1	*2*	*3*
A *Demographic Matrix (Dependent Variables)*		*Canonical Loadings*	
Total Fertility Rate (TFR)	**-.71**	**-.77**	.35
Infant Mortality Rate (IMR)	**-.37**	**.47**	**.48**
Population Growth Rate (GR)	-.59	**.41**	**-.79**
B. *Socio-economic and Programme Variables Matrix (Independent Variables)*		*Canonical Loadings*	
Sex ratio	.02	-.03	.29
Female illiteracy	**.31**	**.19**	-.01
Literate < primary	-.04	.01	**.38**
Primary complete	-.20	-.06	-.14
Contraceptive use	.08	**-.30**	**.68**
Female sterilization	-.31	.20	-.16
Got ante-natal care	**.73**	.28	-.07
Institutional delivery	**.34**	**-.67**	-.24
Child immunization	-.28	**.47**	**.06**
Women with anaemia	.07	-.02	**.38**
Child with anaemia	.07	-.24	.16
C. *Canonical Correlations*	**.97**	**.86**	**.74**
D. *Meaning of Canonical Linkage Pair*	Less TFR, less IMR, less GR, because less female illiteracy, got high ANC, institutional delivery	Less TFR, moderate IMR and GR, less contraceptive use, little institutional delivery, quite good immunization, also due to less illiteracy	Less GR, more literate<primary, high contraceptive use, but women with anaemia, also IMR, as little immunization
E. *Trace Correlation*	**0.870**		
Wilk's Lambba	0.004		
Chi Square	56.42		
Significance	.0001		

Second, the great importance of need of more use of contraceptives for fertility reduction is also highlighted in the second canonical equation. Thus, more family welfare and greater use of contraceptives is very much required for sustaining fertility reduction and infant mortality reduction. This set of canonical findings has obvious policy import, which can be hardly overemphasized.

One Caveat: Income Poverty and Other Deprivation

NFHS-II (1998-99) survey reveals that 47 per cent of children are malnourished and 74 per cent are anaemic; 36 per cent of ever married women aged 15-49 years have chronic energy deficiency; 54 per cent of women aged 15-49 in rural areas have no education; about 50 per cent of the pregnant women suffer from iron deficiency; 71 per cent of rural households do not have any toilet facility and 19 per cent of villages do not have any health facility (NFHS, 2000, various tables). Such data reveal true situation in rural India, even in recent times.

However, some demographers and social scientists frequently present and utilize such data to show indices of 'multiple deprivations', and argue that it is such multiple deprivations that are more crucial among the poor, and need to be fought out first, and not 'income poverty' *per se*; as if all such deprivations are not the 'consequences' of the crucial causal and fundamental deprivation of income poverty?

As if, when income poverty is to be drastically reduced in rural areas, even then, such multiple deprivations will permanently persist! And, their arguments are – since reduction of all such multiple deprivations is difficult to achieve, so nothing can be done to reduce income poverty. Arguing in these ways, they belittle the whole issue of poverty reduction, misdirect the entire task, and shirk from the entire responsibility of poverty alleviation. These are clearly evidenced in numerous studies and surveys. Thus, NFHS survey never collected 'income poverty' data, nor its various reports analyzed poverty data, even from other sources, and never emphasized in its various reports upon the great need for poverty alleviation among the poor masses.

The same is true with most conventional studies and surveys. Even, recent Reproductive and Child Health (RCH) surveys, (Round I and II), also did not collect income poverty data, and did not relate demographic and health data with income poverty data, as if in such a massive poverty-stricken country like India, this approach is at all scientific and truth-revealing? It seems, these are indeed, conscious or unconscious, hidden strategies of the educated classes to maintain poverty in India perpetually. And, to keep in chain three hundred millions poor masses of India under eternal bondages!

Syndrome of Poverty, Little Utilization of Health Services, and High Fertility

Figure 24 presents a schematic diagram, indicating summary of inter-relationships between (Mukherji, 1987, pp. 132-138; 1997e, pp. 1-12):

(a) *The syndrome of poverty:* As reflected in widespread female illiteracy, low status of women, their low occupation or unemployed condition.

(b). *Very low utilization of health services:* As represented by sampled women's very low utilization rates of health services, caused by above syndrome of poverty among them.

(c) *Explosive demographic behaviour:* Very high infant mortality and very high fertility among those rural women – influenced by various factors of the syndrome of poverty. These explosive demographic behaviour is further aggravated by very low knowledge and utilization of existing health services.

This concept of poverty and high fertility in India in also critically examined and testified in many studies elsewhere (Mukherji, 1987, ibid.; Udupa and Mukherji, 1988, pp. 155-170; Mukherji, 1988a, pp. 10-68; 1999a, pp. 1-20).

The above scenario is further complicated in backward districts, neglected regional pockets, hilly and inaccessible tracts, and in many remote villages, where poverty syndrome is much more pronounced. The above conclusion is true for many parts of northern India as well. And, if Uttar Pradesh or Bihar, Madhya Pradesh or Orissa are considered as a microcosm of rural India, then, these observations are very much applicable to entire India. It is hoped that demographers, geographers and social scientists should properly understand these aspects of the syndrome of poverty and high fertility that is operating in India. For, only with proper understanding, correct policy prescriptions will emerge! (Mukherji, 1997c, pp. 1-12; 2005b, pp. 1-37).

Figure 24

Syndrome of Poverty, Less Utilization of Health Services, and High Demographic Explosion

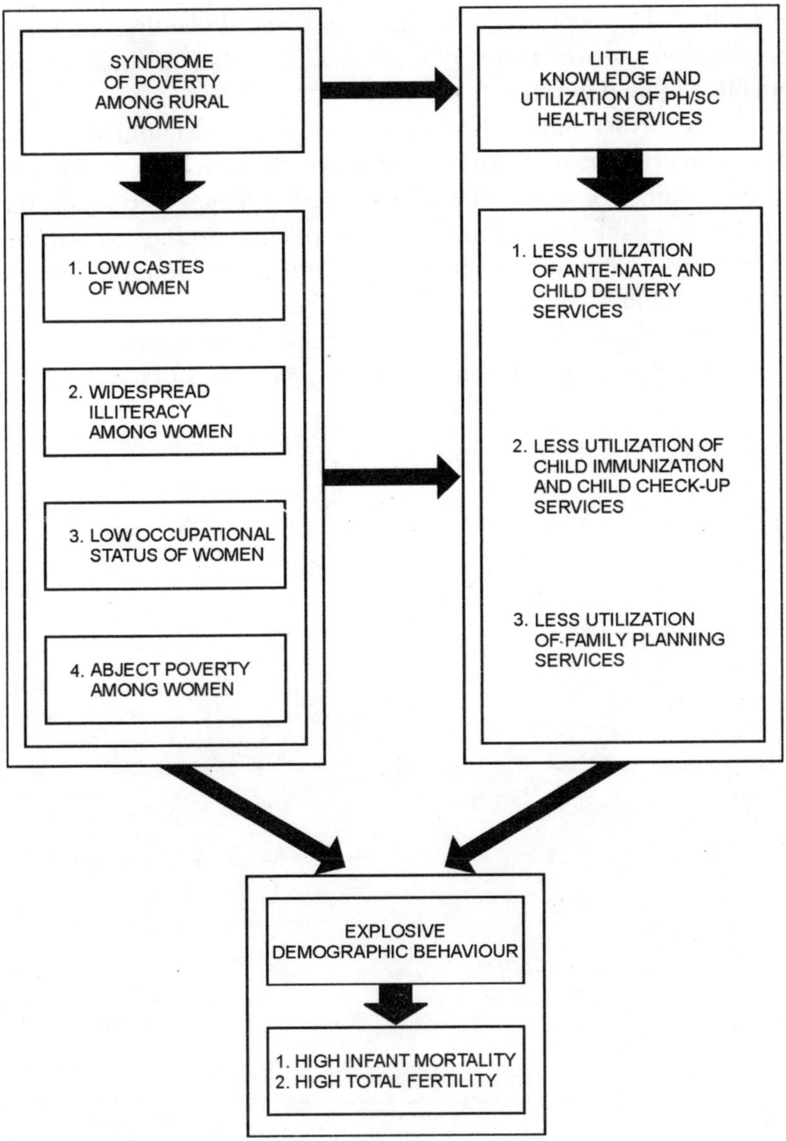

Deprivation, Inequities and Syndrome of Poverty

In Orissa, Haan and Dubey (2006, p. 2328) have found that "the deprivation in terms of lack of access to education, income, markets etc., is compounded by deprivation on the basis of social identity, and social mobilization and articulation of voice to address these inequalities has remained limited in Orissa".

They further argued that "these inequalities are cumulative, and human development disparities reinforce those related to income poverty, and vice versa. They leave out a large section of the population, unable to be economically productive, leading to needs for schemes for social protection, and potentially to political unrest" (Haan and Dubey, ibid.).

In fact, these observations actually indicate the operation of the 'syndrome of poverty and high fertility', which I have discussed above.

11

Most Recent Situation of Poverty and Fertility in India

"Proclaim at the top of thy voice: The Indian is my brother, the Indian is my life. India's gods and goddesses are my God. India's society is the cradle of my infancy, the pleasure garden of my youth, the sacred heaven, the Varanasi of my old age" (Swami Vivekananda, 1894, Complete Work, Centenary Volume IV, 1963, p. 480).

"Let there be dozen such lion-souls in each country, lions who have broken their own bonds, who have touched the Infinite, whose whole soul is gone to the Brahman, who care neither for wealth nor power nor fame, and these will be enough to shake the world" (Swami Vivekananda, 1894, Complete Work, Centenary Volume VIII, 1963, p. 348).

Most Recent Poverty and Fertility Situation (Census 2001 and SRS 2003 Data)

Table 54 provides recent picture of poverty (i.e., female illiteracy) and fertility situation in Indian states, according to Sample Registration Survey (SRS) data of 2003. Proportion of population living below the poverty line is also indicated, according to National Sample Survey Organization (NSSO) data. However, the correspondence between the two indices of poverty (female illiteracy and poverty measure) does

Table 54

Recent Data of Female Illiteracy and Total Fertility Rates, India, (Census of India, 2001 and SRS, 2003) (States arranged according to Female Illiteracy Levels, Total Series)

State	Total		Rural			Urban		
	Female Illiteracy (age 15-44), Census 2001	Total Fertility Rate (TFR), SRS, 2003	Per cent below Poverty Line NSS (1999-2000)	Female Illiteracy (age 15-44), Census, 2001	Total Fertility Rate (TFR), SRS, 2003	Per cent below Poverty Line NSS (1999-2000)	Female Illiteracy (age 15-44), Census, 2001	Total Fertility Rate (TFR), SRS, 2003
India	44.2	3.0	27.4	52.8	3.2	24.7	24.1	2.2
Cluster 1: High Female Illiteracy (High Poverty) and High Fertility States								
Bihar*	68.2	4.2	44.1	72.1	4.4	33.7	35.9	3.1
Uttar Pradesh ***	60.6	4.4	31.4	67.4	4.6	30.6	36.2	3.4
Rajasthan	58.4	3.8	13.4	66.3	4.0	19.5	35.0	2.7
Madhya Pradesh**	49.3	3.8	37.5	58.7	4.1	38.6	27.1	2.4
Cluster 2: Moderately High Female Illiteracy (Moderate Poverty) and Moderately High Fertility States								
Haryana	43.0	3.0	7.4	41.8	3.1	10.2	22.9	2.4
Assam	43.2	2.9	40.4	41.7	3.0	7.6	17.3	1.8
Gujarat	40.0	2.8	12.5	51.0	3.1	14.8	22.9	2.1
Orissa	46.3	2.6	48.3	50.7	2.6	43.8	23.5	2.0
Karnataka	41.1	2.3	16.9	51.4	2.5	24.7	22.9	1.9
West Bengal	38.7	2.3	31.8	45.9	2.5	15.0	21.5	1.6

Contd...

Contd...

Cluster 3: Comparatively Less Female Illiteracy (Poverty) and Slightly less Fertility States								
Andhra Pradesh	49.3	2.2	10.9	57.8	2.3	38.6	28.9	1.9
Punjab	31.2	2.3	6.2	36.5	2.4	5.5	21.4	2.0
Maharashtra	27.9	2.3	23.6	36.2	2.4	26.9	17.7	2.1
Himachal Pradesh.	23.9	2.1	7.6	25.2	2.1	4.6	10.9	1.7
Cluster 4: Low Female illiteracy (Less Poverty) and Low Fertility States								
Tamil Nadu	30.3	1.9	20.6	39.6	2.0	22.7	18.4	1.7
Kerala	5.3	1.8	9.6	5.9	1.8	20.0	3.6	1.7

Sources: 1. *Census of India, 2001, Age and Cultural Tables, India, Series 1,* Various CDs, Registrar General and Census Commissioner's Office, New Delhi, 2001, Various Tables.

2. *Statistical Report of 2003, Report 2 of 2005,* Sample Registration Survey, Census of India, Office of Registrar General and Census Commissioner of India, New Delhi, 2005, pp. 45-49.

3. Regarding Poverty data, National Sample Survey (NSS) data round 55 (1999-2000), and estimated in Popli et al. (2005), pp. 4620-4623.

Note: *Includes Jharkhand. ** includes Chhattishgarh. *** includes Uttaranchal.

clearly exist in some states, but not everywhere; and I seriously consider that 'female illiteracy index' is a much better and more reliable indicator of poverty in India, than others. And, this index also clearly and consistently shows a one-to-one correspondence with fertility levels, irrespective of rural-urban residence, or state variations. Based on Table 54 and Figures 25 to 28, the following four clusters of regions can be delineated.

Cluster 1: High female illiteracy (high poverty) and high fertility states

Includes Bihar, Uttar Pradesh, Rajasthan and Madhya Pradesh. These regions are still plagued by very high female illiteracy (ranging between 50 to 70%), thus very high poverty and very high fertility (TFR 3.8 to 4.2 children per mother). Indeed, the heartland of population explosion in India lies here, even in the 21st century. Unless this belt of abject poverty and high fertility is not specially targeted and maximally served by universal female education programmes, special poverty alleviation actions, and better health services, precious little can be expected for the country, as a whole, in coming decades.

However, it is extremely unjust to label these regions as 'BIMARU' (sick) states, as some population specialists label them with such wrong and derogatory titles, stamping them as sick states, as often we do label and condemn a sickly child to further undescribable neglect, and ultimate death! This is utterly wrong!

A century ago, Swami Vivekananda thundered: "If you call all the time a weak child, 'sick', he will definitely fall sick, and cannot recover. If you call a weak person a sinner, he will definitely fall as a sinner! Rather, we should give such a child our all benedictions, full sympathy, and utmost help; so that he becomes very strong, bold, and brave" (Vivekananda, 1894, Vol. IV, p. 110).

Similarly, maximum developmental help must go to such hitherto historically neglected states of Uttar Pradesh, Bihar, Madhya Pradesh and Rajasthan, which always suffered the onslaught of repeated invasions during last 1,000 years, and also suffered tremendously during the aftermath of India's First War of Independence (1857). These regions are also neglected during post-colonial era. They remain as terribly neglected and extremely backward states.

Figure 25

India (Rural), Female Illiteracy, (age 15-44), Census 2001

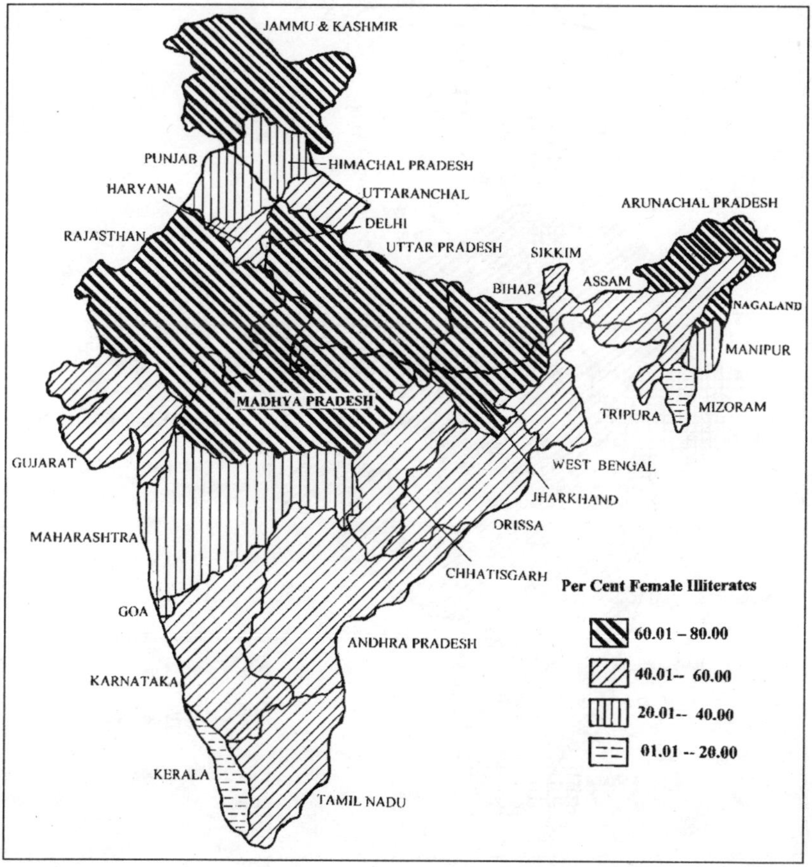

Figure 26

India (Rural), Total Fertility Rate, SRS 2003

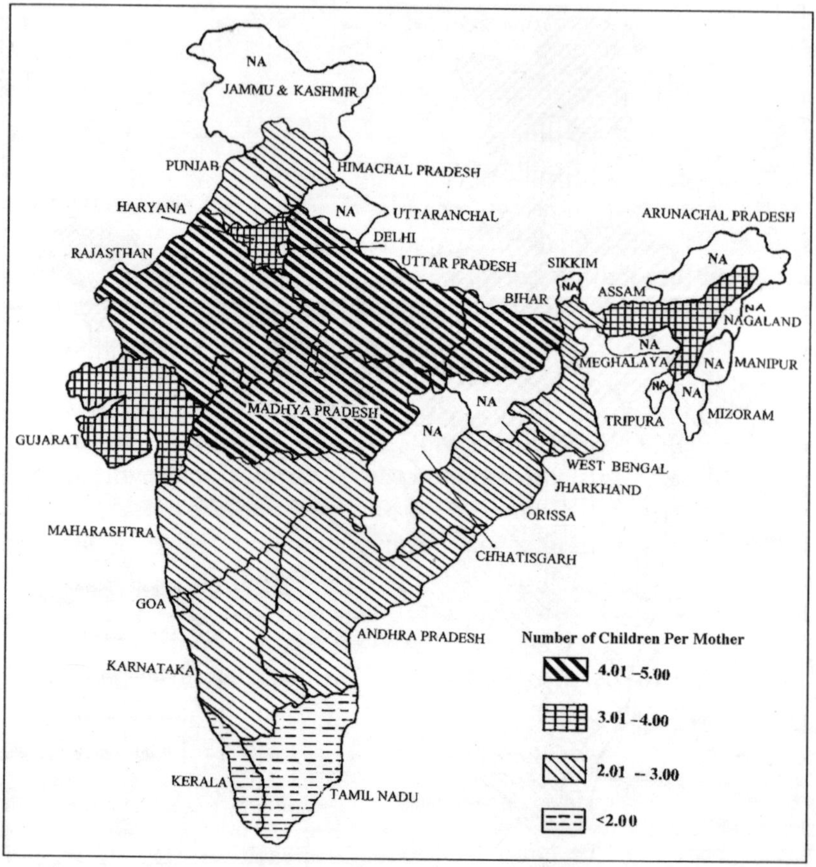

Figure 27

India (Urban), Female Illiteracy (age 15-44), Census 2001

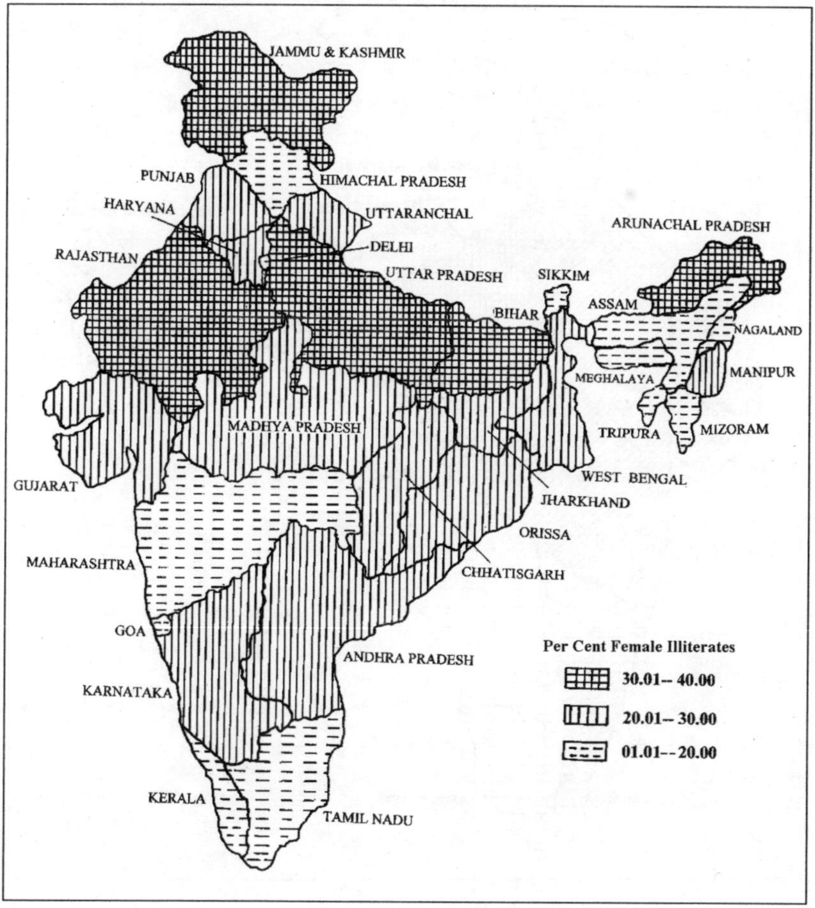

Figure 28

India (Urban), Total Fertility Rate, SRS 2003

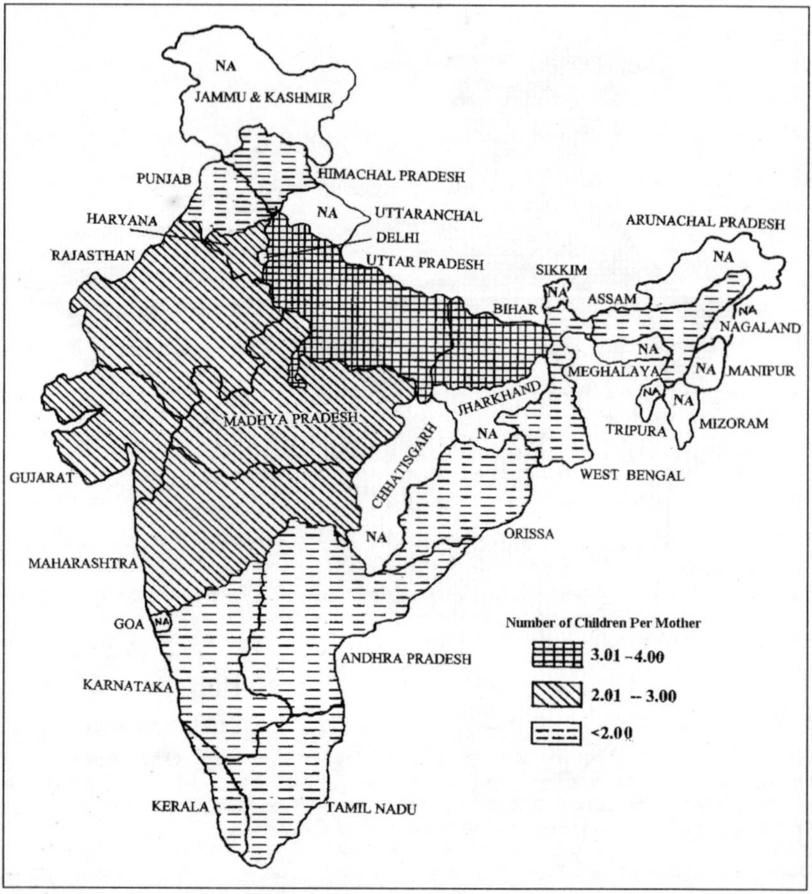

Rather, I shall call them as 'RAMABIRU' states, as Lord Shri Ram was born in Ayodhya in Uttar Pradesh, married Sita in Bihar, made pilgrimage to Pushkar in Rajasthan and were exiled to Dandakaranya forest in Madhya Pradesh. So, these are indeed states of Lord Shri Ram! Call them by that name. And, we must elicit all help from citizens and urge for government's maximum developmental support so that these are soon transformed to higher planes!

Cluster 2: Moderately high female illiteracy (moderate poverty) and moderately high fertility states

This cluster includes Haryana, Assam, Gujarat, Orissa, Karnataka and West Bengal (Table 54), which are characterized by quite high female illiteracy (or poverty), ranging between 38 to 43 per cent, and causing moderately high fertility (between 2.3 to 3 children) (SRS data, 2003). In rural components of these states, female illiteracy is still higher (41% in Haryana to 46% in West Bengal), consequently also higher fertility levels (2.5 to 3.1 children), however not in perfect declining order of relationship. In urban parts, since female illiteracy is much less (21-22%), so fertility is also reduced, e.g., 2.4 children in urban Haryana and only 1.6 in urban West Bengal. This cluster, of course, still needs sustained efforts for further fertility decline.

Cluster 3: Comparatively less female illiteracy (poverty) and slightly less fertility states

This group is represented by Andhra Pradesh, Punjab, Maharashtra and Himachal Pradesh. Even according to SRS data (2003), these states remained in transitory condition, characterized by comparatively less female illiteracy (or less poverty) ranging between 24 per cent in Himachal Pradesh and 49 per cent in Andhra Pradesh, and consequently, slightly still less fertility (2.1 and 2.2 children/mother, respectively). In rural areas of such states, female illiteracy is higher, so also respective fertility levels. For instance, while rural Andhra Pradesh reported 57 per cent female illiterates, corresponding fertility is 2.3 children; whereas rural Himachal Pradesh recorded 25.2 per cent female illiterates, and resultant less fertility (2.1 children). Their poverty levels also correspond with female illiteracy levels, 58 per cent and 25 per cent. However, such correspondence between two indices of poverty is not present everywhere. Indeed, female illiteracy is a much better index of poverty, as it consistently indicates a 'one-to-one correspondence' with fertility levels, irrespective of states, and rural-urban residence.

Cluster 4: Low female illiteracy (less poverty) and low fertility States

Kerala and Tamil Nadu represent this cluster. Such progressive states must serve as the models for demographic decline in India. This cluster has already experienced demographic transition, and is characterized by considerably low female illiteracy (6% in Kerala and 30% in Tamil Nadu), which has substantially dampened fertility levels (ranging between 1.8-1.9 children). Although rural Tamil Nadu still has high female illiteracy, but its fertility is quite low (2 children), while rural Kerala has already achieved almost universal female literacy (94%), whose beneficial effect is reflected in very low fertility in Kerala (1.8 children). Top of all, both urban Tamil Nadu and urban Kerala have achieved a most noteworthy fertility level (1.7 children) that competes with that of Japan (1.55 children) or USA (1.65 children). This is the wonderful effect of female literacy upon fertility transition.

The main argument here is that it is primarily due to very high female illiteracy, which is causing and persisting very high fertility in India. Evidently, given very strong impetus to universal female education, all the first three clusters mentioned above, will soon achieve rapid fertility decline. Thus, the policy prescriptions must be made accordingly.

Just make all women and all girls simply literate, and see this miracle to happen in India! Very soon! It does not require endless NFHS or RCH surveys, nor needs high flying costly conferences, nor high faluting planning debates, nor international meetings, nor even highly sophisticated mathematical models. Neither it needs even Millennium Development Goals (MDGs), nor even expensive PHCs and CHCs. It simply requires only one step, only one positive action, just provide women's universal literacy, and see demographic transition fully arrived in India very soon!

Alas! If Indian politicians, policy makers, and social scientists will ever wake up and do this simple thing!

Who are Poor and Where are they Located?

Measurement of poverty in India is primarily done by National Sample Surveys (NSS, 50th round, 1993-94, and 55th round, 1999-2000). Such surveys usually consider nutritional adequacy and calorie consumption of essential food intakes (2400 or 2100 calories per day per person in rural and urban areas, respectively). NSS have used household consumption expenditure data (1973-74) for estimating expenditure on such goods and services. "Thus, the procedure employed was to calculate the average calorie intake of every expenditure class, identify the lowest expenditure class which consumed the calorie norm, and use the per capita total expenditure of that class as the poverty line" (Sen, 2005, pp. 4611-18). Thus, it has been a quite comprehensive procedure. But, some experts also doubt about its suitability as an index for poverty measurement, or question – can it adequately capture really poor people, or does such a uni-dimensional index do more harm than good for poverty reduction, and so forth (Sen, ibid; Subramanian, 2005, pp. 4625-28; Saith, 2005, pp. 4601-10).

Experts also widely differ regarding the extent of poverty in India and various states (Saith, 2005, pp. 4601-10; Nayyar, 2005, pp. 1631-39; Alderman, 2005, pp. 4837-42). But most usually agree that the proportion of people living below poverty line, even in 2005, ranges at least between 25 to 30 per cent (UNDP, 2005, pp. 19-21). However, in Table 54, NSS data for proportion of people below poverty line are given for rural and urban areas of major states (NSS, 2001; and Popli et al., 2005 pp. 4619-24). Poverty level data may differ, as per estimation techniques adopted by various authors. But, as indicated right from the beginning of this book, I confidently think that data of female illiteracy are much more indicative of poverty situation, and it really manifest considerably greater relevance and significance with the prevailing fertility levels. These become very clearly evident in Tables 54-57.

The nature and extent of poverty condition in India is also reflected in some studies by the present author (Mukherji, 1977a, pp. 1-45; 1979d, pp. 45-65; Mitra and Mukherji, 1979, pp. 32-121; 1981b, pp. 1-255). Recent picture of poverty is also reflected in following investigations (Mukherji, 2000f, p.6; 2000g, p. 6; 2002, pp. 525-559).

Radhakrishna and Roy (2005, pp. 41-58) also recently made a good overview. One very recent study Patodia (2006, p. 10) reveals: "Living conditions in rural India continue to be pathetic with 220 million Indians still living below the poverty line and half of India's children undernourished."

It further states: "The condition of rural infrastructure is far more alarming. Productivity of food grains is very low. Half of our cultivable land is still unirrigated, 30-40 per cent of production of our fruits and vegetables is destroyed for want of adequate transport and storage" (ibid.).

Similarly, according to another study by Radhakrishna and Ray (2005, p. 41), "poverty in India is not merely an economic phenomenon, but also a social one. It is disproportionately high among SCs (Scheduled Castes) and STs (Scheduled Tribes), the share of the STs in poverty had gone up during the 1990s and that of the SCs remained more or less the same". It further says: "It is now widely recognized that while income poverty reduction is relatively easy, elimination of multiple deprivation is more difficult to achieve." Likewise, South Asia Poverty Alleviation Programmes of Mumbai (SAPAP) notes: "Poverty is a product of livelihood systems and the socio-political and economic forces that shape them, and argues that multi-dimensional interventions revolving around land and other property rights, bargaining power for improved wage rates, holistic health care, micro insurance, and physical and social security are needed for accelerating poverty reduction. The key issue is to weaken the strong hold of the rich in the governance of local institutions and facilitate the participation of the poor" (quoted in Radhakrishna and Ray, 2005, p. 42).

"In general, in the developed states, poverty was highly concentrated among the agricultural labour households and, in contrast, in the backward states poverty extended to other occupational groups, including self-employed in agriculture ....In Punjab, Haryana, Maharashtra and Andhra Pradesh agricultural labour households constituted more than 60 per cent of the rural poor in 1999-2000, but they constituted less than 16 per cent in Rajasthan and 28 per cent in Assam" (Radhakrishna and Ray, ibid.).

However, this feature should not surprise us. Actually, this is the effect of labour migration on regional distribution of poverty. Evidently, it is the poor migrant agricultural labourers from backward states moving into developed states of Punjab, Haryana, and others, thus inflating the poor among that landless agricultural labour there, while the remaining other occupational groups continued to stay and remain poor in the backward states of Rajasthan and Assam (Mukherji, 2001, pp. 1-125; Mukherji, 2005, pp. 70-90).

"Among the social groups, SCs, STs, and backward castes accounted for 81 per cent of the rural poor in 1999-2000" (NSS, 2002, various tables).

"The poor among the SCs in rural areas were concentrated in Uttar Pradesh, Bihar and West Bengal. They comprised 58 per cent of the poor among SCs. In urban areas, Madhya Pradesh and Uttar Pradesh accounted for 41 per cent of the poor among the SCs. Incidence of poverty among SCs was high in Bihar, Madhya Pradesh and Uttar Pradesh in both rural and urban areas" (Radhakrishna and Ray, ibid.).

Specifically, poverty reduction programmes need to be focused in these neglected regions, priority-wise. They further noted:

"In terms of income poverty and other indicators of human development also such as education, health, etc., the STs are at the bottom. The increasing concentration of poverty among tribals who suffer from multiple deprivations is a matter of concern.....Bihar, Gujarat, Madhya Pradesh, and Maharashtra together accounted for 75.5 per cent of the poor among STs in 1999-2000. Among STs of these states, rural poverty is highest in Orissa (73%), Bihar (59%), Madhya Pradesh (57%) and West Bengal (50%)" (NSS, 2002, various tables; Radhakrishna and Ray ibid., pp. 46-47).

Thus, poverty alleviation programmes are required to be prioritized in these specific zones. Typically, the zone extending from West Bengal, Orissa, Bihar, Uttar Pradesh to Madhya Pradesh is the heartland of poverty in India, where both SCs and STs predominate among the poor, specially in rural areas.

"Orissa had the highest incidence of the very poor in rural as well as in urban areas in 1999-2000, and presented a different picture in the 1990s in reducing the incidence of the very poor. ...Assam is in league with Orissa in terms of poor performance. Bihar and Madhya Pradesh had a very high incidence of very poor in rural and urban areas. Assam and West Bengal had a high incidence of the very poor in rural areas, as did Maharashtra, Uttar Pradesh, and Pondicherry in urban areas" (Radhakrishna and Ray, ibid., p. 48).

"In rural areas, very poor STs were located mainly in four areas, namely, Madhya Pradesh, Orissa, Bihar and Maharashtra. They comprise 77 per cent of the very poor STs in 1999-2000. In the case of SCs, the very poor were concentrated in Uttar Pradesh, Bihar and West Bengal – they together accounted for 63 per cent of the very poor SCs in 1999-2000. In urban areas, the very poor among SCs and STs were mainly located in these states" (ibid.).

"Clearly, rural-urban disparity widened during the 1990s… The 1990s growth benefited urban areas the most and aggravated the rural-urban divide" (ibid., p. 42).

Regarding malnutrition and poverty among the children and women, the authors found (ibid., pp. 52-54) that "the incidence of undernutrition among children, even though slowly declining, was still alarmingly high during the late 1990s and their incidence is much higher than that of income poverty. About half of the children and slightly over a third of the adults were undernourished in 2000-1".

Further, they (ibid., pp. 55-61) made a good summary of poverty situation in India. A few salient points emerge:

"First, in agriculturally prosperous states, agricultural labour households accounted for the bulk of the rural poor and in the less developed regions rural poverty extended to other occupational groups, including the self-employed in agriculture. In the urban areas, poverty tends to be concentrated more among casual labour households.

Second, Assam, Orissa, Bihar, Madhya Pradesh and Uttar Pradesh have remained laggards in poverty reduction.

Third, the poor are likely to be vulnerable to risks in the labour markets and may increasingly suffer from transient poverty since their dependence on the casual labour market for livelihood is rising both in rural and urban areas.

Fourth, data show that income, and particularly agricultural income growth, is an important channel for alleviating poverty across regions, social groups, economic status, and the occupational groups of the household. Thus, agricultural growth and development is still one of the most important saviours for poverty alleviation in India.

Fifth, agricultural growth is also beneficial to those who are socially excluded in India, such as STs and SCs. Since malnutrition and chronic poverty are closely associated with persistent inadequacy in attaining the minimum income status, income growth, *ceteris paribus*, has a pervasive influence over time on multi-dimensional poverty. This also requires other supportive measures of human development, such as education, health and conducive public interventions, as Kerala and north-eastern states have shown.

Sixth, rural-urban divide is widening.... While urban India is doing better, with even its bottom 30 per cent experiencing growth, there is greater inequality emerging in urban expenditure groups. It is thus easier to escape absolute poverty with a foothold in urban areas and away from the rural abyss, though the relative position of such a household may be quite dismal in comparison".

The authors also noted that, "worsening rural-urban disparity is caused by retarded agricultural growth in last decade, which is itself a matter of concern in employment generation and poverty reduction. ... This also led to slowdown of rural non-farm employment growth" (ibid., p. 56).

Recent Total Fertility Rates Among Illiterates and Literates (SRS, 2003)

Table 55 presents summary of fertility data as per Sample Registration Survey, 2003 (SRS, 2005), classified according to illiterates and literates, and according to rural-urban residence. This table is a great eye-opener, re-confirming what is stated above. Here also, we can visualize four distinct clusters of states, arranged according to female illiteracy and fertility levels. A marvellous sequence of states is manifest, when arranged according to female illiteracy, which perfectly correspond to respective fertility rates. Thus, a 'one-to-one correspondence' between the two emerges out wonderfully. The clusters are:

Cluster 1: High female illiteracy (high poverty) and high fertility states: Serious problematic states: Uttar Pradesh, Bihar, Madhya Pradesh and Rajasthan.

Table 55

Recent Total Fertility Rates among Illiterates and Literates, in Rural and Urban Areas, India, Sample Registration Survey, 2003 (Arranged according to TFR among the Illiterates, Total series)

State	*Total*		*Rural*		*Urban*	
	Total Fertility Rate (TFR), SRS, 2003, among		*Total Fertility Rate (TFR),SRS, 2003, among*		*Total Fertility Rate (TFR),SRS, 2003, among*	
	Illiterate	*Literate*	*Illiterate*	*Literate*	*Illiterate*	*Literate*
India	*4.0*	*2.4*	*4.1*	*2.6*	*3.1*	*2.0*
Cluster 1: High Female Illiteracy (High Poverty) and High Fertility States: Very Seriously Problematic States						
Uttar Pradesh.	5.4	3.1	5.5	3.3	4.5	2.7
Bihar	5.0	3.0	5.0	3.2	4.6	2.4
Madhya Pradesh	4.7	3.2	4.8	3.6	3.1	2.3
Rajasthan	4.5	2.8	4.6	2.9	3.3	2.5
Cluster 2: Moderately High Female Illiteracy (Moderate Poverty) and Moderately High Fertility States: Much Problematic States						
Haryana	4.0	2.5	4.0	2.7	4.2	2.0
Assam	3.9	2.5	4.0	2.6	2.0	1.7
Gujarat	3.8	2.4	4.0	2.7	3.0	2.0
Orissa	3.0	2.3	3.0	2.4	3.1	1.7
Karnataka	2.9	2.1	2.9	2.3	2.6	1.7
West Bengal	2.9	2.1	2.9	2.3	2.4	1.5

Contd...

Contd...

Cluster 3: Comparatively Less Female Illiteracy (Poverty) and Slightly less Fertility States: Transitory States						
Punjab	3.0	2.1	3.1	2.2	2.4	1.9
Himachal Pradesh.	2.9	2.0	3.0	2.0	2.1	1.7
Andhra Pradesh	2.7	1.9	2.8	2.0	2.5	1.7
Maharashtra	2.5	2.2	2.5	2.3	2.6	2.1
Cluster 4: Low Female illiteracy (Less Poverty) and Low Fertility States: Demographic Transition States						
Tamil Nadu	2.5	1.9	2.7	2.0	1.8	1.8
Kerala	1.8	1.4	1.8	1.5	1.7	1.2

Source: Sample Registration System (SRS), Census of India *Statistical Report of 2003, Report 2 of 2005,* Office of Registrar General and Census Commissioner of India, New Delhi, 2005, pp. 45-49.

Cluster 2: Moderately high female illiteracy (moderate poverty) and moderately high fertility states: Much problematic states: Haryana, Assam, Gujarat, Orissa, Karnataka and West Bengal.

Cluster 3: Comparatively less female illiteracy (poverty) and slightly less fertility states: Transitory states: Punjab, Himachal Pradesh, Andhra Pradesh and Maharashtra.

Cluster 4: Low female illiteracy (less poverty) and low fertility states: Demographic transition states: Tamil Nadu and Kerala.

Besides, the following patterns also occur:

1. Fertility levels among the illiterate women are always much higher than that of the literate women, at both all-India and state levels. At all-India level, illiterates have one-and-a half children more (4.0) than that of the literates (2.4), which is a tremendous difference (66%). Such excess burden of fertility is easily preventable, and must be rectified soon.
2. In cluster 1 states, the illiterates have two children more (ranges between 4.5 to 5.4 children) than that among the literates (between 2.8 and 3.1). This difference progressively declines to one-and-a-half children in cluster 2, one children in cluster 3, and, finally, to only-half children in cluster 4. Such differentials indicate tremendously great need for universal female literacy programmes for onsetting fertility reduction. Since in this book, the female illiteracy is considered as an index of poverty, the causal relations between widespread poverty and high fertility is manifest here very loud and clear, even according to 2003 SRS data. Crucial war cry of this study is that poverty must be banished from the surface of India. And, drastic reduction of massive female illiteracy is the first initial step towards this divine goal.
3. Rural-urban differences in fertility are also very prominent. Rural illiterate woman in Uttar Pradesh has very high fertility (5.5 children per mother), which is twice than that of an urban literate woman in the same state (only 2.7 children). Similar differentials exist in all other states also, with decreasing order of differences from cluster 1 to 4. That is, within the same state, an urbanized and literate status of a woman equips her to reduce her fertility to half of that of her illiterate counterparts, living in the villages. That will be a very laudable achievement. Thus, urbanization and

education do have tremendous beneficial effects on fertility decline. Policies and strategies must be taken to promote urbanization and universal literacy. Even a woman's slight transformation from illiterate to literate status, and self-employment, even within the village, can do wonder, without forcibly urbanizing our green villages (into dirty slums).

4. Tremendous spatial variations also exist from cluster 1 to 4, and between backward states like Uttar Pradesh (Cluster 1) on the one hand and developed states like Kerala (cluster 4), on the other. One rural illiterate woman in Uttar Pradesh (with 5.5. children) has 4.6 times higher fertility than an urban literate Keralite woman (1.2 children). Unbelievable! Again, if urban residence and even the literacy status are also ignored, even then, a rural illiterate Uttar Pradeshi woman (with 5.5 children) has three times higher fertility than a rural illiterate Keralite woman (1.8 children). This is again incredible! Here, both the women are illiterate and rural resident, but such a wide difference still occurs due to their respective surrounding social-economic context (i.e., socio-economic component of the demographic field). Unbelievable, that such differences can exist side by side, in the same country! Similar differences also occur between Bihar and Kerala, or between Bihar and Tamil Nadu, and so forth.

A necessary corollary is that, first, the *social or demographic field* concept holds good everywhere, and attempts must be made therefore for positive changes in the socio-economic fields of these women.

Second, fighting poverty and female illiteracy is the first essential step in the war against fertility reduction, which must be supplemented by welfare programmes to make all-round socio-economic development of the females, and also with very strong family planning inputs and health services.

Recent Illiteracy, Poverty, Fertility and Health Situation in 1998-99(RCH Survey)

The present author was the senior-most Research Coordinator of RCH Project during initial 15 months period, and contributed to it much through various papers (Mukherji, 1997f, pp. 1-35; 1998b, pp.

1-30; 1998c, pp. 1-25; 1998b, pp. 1-30; 1998d, pp. 1-16). RCH survey (RCH, 2001) provided detailed data, based on minute analysis of data, the following clusters can be identified:

Cluster 1: Very high female illiteracy, high poverty, high fertility states (with little access to health services): As shown in Table 56, typically, this cluster is represented by highly populous and high growth states of Bihar, Uttar Pradesh, Rajasthan, Madhya Pradesh, Orissa, and also Arunachal Pradesh, where very high female illiteracy or poverty (59 to 73%) causes very high fertility (ranging between 3.6 to 4.5 surviving children). Poverty is also high, if measured by the proportion of *kachcha* houses (32 to 72%). However, female illiteracy is found to be a much better indicator of poverty, as it shows one-to-one correspondence with high fertility. Owing to very high female illiteracy, contraceptive use is also less (ranging between 20 to 30%), so also female sterilization (varying between 13 to 36%). And, only 10 to 20 per cent of all eligible mothers get access to ANC care. Regarding child vaccination, the situation is very precarious, since no vaccination given to 13 to 48 per cent children. Thus, this group of states require very urgent priority and top-most attention. Indeed, they put the greatest hindrance on the path towards demographic transition in India.

Cluster 2: Moderately low female illiteracy, but considerably high poverty and high fertility states (slightly more health services): This cluster is a new one, as small north-eastern states were not considered earlier, due to lack of data. Most of them can also be clubbed with other clusters, based on similarities. But, this cluster includes mainly tribal states like Nagaland, Manipur, Meghalaya, Jammu & Kashmir and Tripura, where incidence of tribal population sometimes reach over 90 per cent. Characteristically, these states have relatively less female illiteracy, but considerably high poverty (reflected by more *kachcha* houses). Besides, they also have relatively better health services than that of cluster 1, for instance, shown by relatively more ANC care (15 to 34%), less proportion of children without vaccination (1 to 21%), and more institutional delivery (13 to 46%). However, use of modern methods of family planning is not high (less than 20%), and female sterilization is not at all high (only 6 to 22%), because of large Muslim (Jammu & Kashmir) or Catholic population. Consequently,

Table 56

Recent Demographic, Socio-economic, Population Programme Variables, and Reproductive and Child Health Services (1998-99) of States, arranged, first, according to Female Illiteracy, and second according to per cent of kuchcha houses (Indirect Poverty Index)

States	*Per cent female illiterate (eligible women) (1998-9)*	*Per cent kachcha houses, (RCH, 1998-99)*	*Per cent kachcha+ semi-pucca house (RCH)*	*Children ever born (CEB) (RCH)*	*Child surviving (CS) (RCH)*	*Per cent SC+ST households*	*Female sterilization*	*Per cent birth-order 3+*	*CPR any modern method*	*Unmet need*	*Per cent full ANC given*	*Per cent institutional delivery*	*Per cent no vaccination given*
India	***56.1***	***39.0***	***70.8***	***4.5***	***3.8***	***27.0***	***33.5***	***45.8***	***42.5***	***25.3***	***31.8***	***34.0***	***18.8***
Cluster 1: High female illiteracy, high poverty and high fertility states													
Bihar	72.9	62.3	83.2	5.5	4.5	25.3	20.5	56.7	23.3	42.0	10.1	14.9	48.8
Uttar Pradesh	70.3	38.9	78.7	5.9	4.6	24.9	13.6	59.9	21.6	38.4	11.2	16.2	28.9
Rajasthan	74.6	31.8	49.9	5.3	4.3	30.3	31.5	51.7	39.0	28.3	16.6	22.5	33.6
Arunachal Pradesh	65.7	71.8	89.3	5.5	4.6	82.4	15.8	56.8	23.8	48.5	19.8	14.9	48.8
Madhya Pradesh	66.4	66.7	82.6	4.8	3.9	38.0	36.3	47.7	43.4	27.1	20.2	21.8	13.2
Orissa	59.5	70.0	89.4	4.5	3.6	41.2	32.5	45.3	39.5	22.0	32.5	23.4	9.7
Cluster 2: Moderately low female illiteracy, but considerably high poverty and high fertility states													
Manipur	41.7	61.7	93.3	4.9	4.5	36.4	9.3	46.3	19.4	36.6	30.9	34.1	20.5
Meghalaya	35.3	44.1	86.2	6.4	5.5	91.3	6.2	57.0	13.2	52.7	30.9	33.4	18.0
Jammu-Kashmir	66.9	33.5	66.9	4.5	4.3	20.4	26.3	25.0	47.0	27.1	23.8	44.4	1.0
Nagaland	34.1	45.8	86.1	5.8	5.4	98.9	12.2	59.9	21.6	40.9	15.6	13.4	8.8
Tripura	29.8	83.1	92.1	4.4	3.8	27.1	22.1	33.4	40.4	12.0	34.8	46.1	16.9

Contd...

Contd...

Cluster 3: Moderately high female illiteracy, moderately high poverty and moderately high fertility states													
Assam	43.5	66.1	86.3	5.0	4.4	24.1	12.4	45.9	28.4	37.6	24.8	23.8	11.6
Sikkim	50.5	37.9	77.6	4.7	4.3	20.7	20.5	43.9	36.7	44.8	31.9	32.3	4.2
West Bengal	48.2	60.9	79.5	4.3	3.7	31.1	30.7	38.5	45.4	12.2	33.4	23.4	10.0
Karnataka	54.0	18.8	79.2	4.2	3.6	25.3	52.4	35.3	57.9	15.3	60.1	50.0	5.7
Cluster 4: Moderate female illiteracy, low poverty and relatively less fertility states													
Haryana	55.6	6.6	52.6	4.5	3.9	23.6	37.7	41.5	52.7	17.5	23.9	25.7	10.4
Gujarat	47.5	21.6	51.8	4.0	3.5	28.7	40.9	37.8	52.0	19.7	42.7	46.1	10.2
Andhra Pradesh	62.8	31.6	66.1	3.8	3.4	27.9	54.0	28.7	58.7	14.0	63.4	50.6	2.4
Maharashtra	40.2	28.7	70.3	3.9	3.5	26.2	47.5	34.6	58.3	19.6	54.8	57.1	1.9
Himachal Pradesh	31.5	26.5	64.1	3.9	3.5	22.3	43.0	31.4	62.4	19.2	52.7	31.7	2.4
Punjab	41.5	5.6	58.0	3.9	3.5	31.5	29.5	35.6	53.6	14.5	25.4	78.8	0.4
Cluster 5: Much less female illiteracy, very low poverty and comparatively still lower fertility states													
Tamil Nadu	41.6	25.4	72.1	3.4	2.9	23.7	45.0	23.6	49.9	21.4	75.3	78.8	0.4
Delhi	21.3	2.1	15.3	3.3	3.1	16.0	26.9	32.2	68.3	12.2	73.1	70.0	2.4
Goa	22.8	3.4	73.2	3.2	2.9	7.0	28.8	22.0	.38.9.	27.0	80.3	93.2	0.0
Kerala	8.5	9.7	43.9	2.9	2.8	12.6	48.5	17.1	57.7	15.2	86.1	97.0	1.8

Source: Reproductive and Child Health Project Surveys, Phase I and II (1998-99), Ministry of Health and Family Welfare, Government of India, New Delhi and International Institute for Population Sciences, Mumbai, 2001, Various Reports and Tables, pp. 1-135 and Various CDs.

List of Variables

1. Per cent female illiterates (among eligible mothers, age 15-44), RCH Survey, 1998-99
2. Per cent *kachcha* houses (non-bricked houses) RCH Survey, 1998-99
3. Per cent *kachcha* and semi-*pucca* houses RCH-I Survey, 1998-99

Contd...

Contd...

4. Children Ever Born (CEB), RCH-I Survey, 1998-99
5. Children Surviving (CS) RCH-I Survey, 1998-99
6. Per cent Scheduled Caste (SC) and scheduled Tribe (ST) households
7. Per cent of birth order 3+ (among all birth orders)
8. Per cent female sterilization (15-44 ages)
9. Contraceptive prevalence rate (CPR) of any modern method, RCH Survey, 1998-99
10. Unmet need for family planning use, RCH Survey, 1998-99
11. Per cent full ANC given to eligible mothers (age 15-44), during pregnancy (atleast 3 visits for ANC, at least one TT injection + 100 or more IFA Tablets), RCH Survey, 1998-99
12. Per cent institutional delivery of child birth, RCH Survey, 1998-99
13. Per cent of children whom no vaccination given to children of 12-23 months, RCH Survey, 1998-99

fertility levels are also high (25 to 60% of birth comprise of 3 + order). Thus, this cluster also requires considerably very high dose of family planning for fertility reduction.

Cluster 3: Moderately high female illiteracy, moderately high poverty and moderately high fertility states (more use of health services): This cluster comprises Assam, Sikkim, West Bengal and Karnataka. This group is coloured by quite high female illiteracy or poverty (43 to 54%), causing moderately high fertility (3.6 to 4.4 surviving children). Due to quite high female illiteracy, the utilization rates of modern family planning methods are still low, ranging between 28 and 58 per cent. Similarly, female sterilization rates also vary widely between 12 and 31 per cent (with exception of Karnataka). Only one-third eligible mothers have access to ANC (25 to 33%), while child immunization situation is slightly better. Overall, this cluster needs much sustained efforts in both family planning and health services for drastic fertility reduction.

Cluster 4: Moderate female illiteracy, low poverty, and relatively less fertility states (with slightly more health services): This group is represented by Haryana, Gujarat, Andhra Pradesh, Maharashtra, Himachal Pradesh and Punjab. Cluster 3 and 4 are very close to each other, and there is no sacrosanct location of any state within a cluster. These are quite flexible. States in cluster 4 are in transitory situation, characterized by moderately high female illiteracy or moderate poverty (31 to 63%), and consequently, moderate fertility (30 to 40% births are of 3+ order). These states also report considerably high utilization rates of health services (no child immunization is only 2 to 10%) and female sterilization (30 to 54%). Unmet need is less than 20 per cent. Although overall performance is quite promising, but still they need sustained efforts as quite high fertility still persists.

Cluster 5: Much less female illiteracy, very low poverty, and comparatively still lower fertility states (quite high use of health services): This cluster is represented by Kerala, Tamil Nadu and Goa (not shown). These states have already enjoyed demographic transition, and are characterized by quite low female illiteracy (9 to 42%) and so considerably dampened fertility (less than one-fifth are of birth of 3+ order). Due to low female illiteracy (or less poverty), the use of modern family planning methods is quite high (ranging between 49 to 58%). Similarly, female sterilization is also high (45 to

49%). Owing to high female literacy, very large segment of eligible mothers do get easy access to ANC (75% to 86%). Similarly, access to child immunization is quite notable (incidence of no vaccination only 2%). This cluster of progressive states must serve as models of demographic decline for India.

Regarding all the above clusters, the main contention here is that it is mainly owing to very high female illiteracy (Uttar Pradesh), that access to health services is also found to be very low, and consequently, fertility rates become very high, and not vice versa. Likewise, due to moderately high level of female illiteracy (Maharashtra), health utilization rates are bound to be also moderate, and consequently, fertility also became moderately high, and not vice versa. Finally, wherever female illiteracy is low (Kerala), access to health services also became easy and utilization rates also increased, and, consequently, fertility levels also declined. So, the keywords are female illiteracy and poverty, which determine the access and utilization rates of health services, and, together, eventually, control fertility and mortality rates. Opposite argument is very naïve and most unscientific. Because, very poor, extremely dispossessed and illiterate women do not have any easy/cheap access to health services, even if PHCs or CHCs are located within 10-20 miles. Who will pay for their transport? Who will buy their medicines (very few PHCs provide freely)? Actual reality is much harsher and cruel, beyond the imagination of conventional demographers, living in ivory towers.

Evidently, given strong impetus for female's literacy, education, female employment, empowerment, and better rural health delivery services, these clusters of states, specially the neglected clusters, will also soon achieve fertility decline. Policies and strategies must be adopted and implemented, accordingly. Top priority must be given to the most backward and hitherto neglected states, districts, and remote tracts.

Recent-Most Poverty, Fertility and Health Situation in 2002-04 (RCH-II Survey)

Very recent picture (2002-04) of these aspects is shown in Table 57, which in fact portrays a slightly modified scene of Table 56 (1998-99). In most cases, little changes have occurred over five years. Following

Table 57

Recent Data of Demographic, Socio-economic, and Reproductive and Child Health Services (RCH Survey, 2002-4), States arranged first according to Female Illiteracy, and second according to per cent of Kuchcha houses (Indirect Poverty Index, 2001)

States	*Per cent female illiterate women, (15-44), Census 2001*	*Per cent kachcha house, Census 2001*	*Total Fertility Rate, TFR (SRS 2003)*	*Per cent birth order 3+*	*CPR any modern family planning method*	*Per cent female sterili-zation*	*Unmet need (limiting and spacing)*	*Per cent no ANC given*	*Per cent full AWC given*	*Per cent institu-tional delivery*	*Per cent full Immuni-zation given*	*Per cent no vaccina-tion given*
India	***44.2***	***40***	***3.0***	***42.1***	***45.7***	***34.3***	***21.2***	***26.5***	***16.4***	***40.5***	***47.8***	***19.0***
Cluster 1: High female illiteracy, high poverty and high fertility states												
Bihar	68.2	57	4.2	54.1	27.3	28.9	36.7	62.1	5.4	23.5	24.4	49.9
Uttar Pradesh	60.6	37	4.4	56.9	26.2	14.4	33.6	42.1	4.4	22.5	28.1	35.5
Rajasthan	58.4	30	3.8	47.1	42.3	31.2	21.8	31.8	5.0	31.4	25.4	29.2
Madhya Pradesh	49.2	54	3.8	49.1	47.3	37.5	21.0	25.8	5.9	28.2	32.5	17.0
Cluster 2: Moderately low female illiteracy, but considerably high poverty and high fertility states												
Nagaland	36.2	61	NA	57.7	35.0	15.2	33.8	44.2	9.5	17.5	14.4	12.3
Manipur	33.8	80	NA	43.1	25.1	8.3	40.1	22.1	10.9	46.3	37.3	11.0
Meghalaya	35.5	53	NA	59.5	14.7	17.1	55.8	45.4	11.7	30.3	14.1	18.7

Contd...

Contd...

Cluster 3: Moderately high female illiteracy, moderately high poverty and moderately high fertility states												
Assam	43.2	74	2.9	40.6	28.7	18.8	22.5	38.2	10.2	26.9	19.3	23.6
Orissa	46.3	62	2.6	42.1	42.9	28.9	19.1	24,1	15.7	34.4	55.1	6.4
Haryana	43.9	7	3.0	38.1	54.4	35.6	14.7	12.8	11.8	35.1	62.9	11.9
Gujarat	40.0	29	2.8	38.1	52.4	35.3	16.3	12.4	25.8	52.2	57.7	6.8
West Bengal	38.7	56	2.3	31.3	55.0	31.6	11.0	9.3	14.0	46.8	54.4	7.5
Karnataka	41.1	31	1.8	29.5	57.7	52.4	15.1	8.5	29.5	58.3	74.1	4.6
Cluster 4: Moderate female illiteracy, low poverty and relatively less fertility states												
Andhra Pradesh	49.3	35	2.2	22.5	62.4	58.1	11.7	5.3	43.9	60.9	62.9	2.8
Maharashtra	27.9	34	2.3	32.1	60.8	48.3	12.1	7.1	23.0	57.9	74.3	2.0
Punjab	31.2	7	2.3	32.1	57.2	30.5	10.1	10.4	16.7	48.9	75.3	9.8
Himachal Pradesh	23.9	29	2.1	24.1	65.4	41.1	11.8	8.7	32.5	45.1	79.4	1.8
Cluster 5: Much less female illiteracy, very low poverty and comparatively still lower fertility states												
Tamil Nadu	30.3	36	1.9	21.3	55.0	49.5	18.1	0.6	23.5	86.1	92.1	0.4
Kerala	6.5	25	1.8	15.5	56.7	45.9	15.2	0.3	69.3	97.8	81.2	0.7

Sources: (1) Ministry of Health and Family Welfare, (2005), Reproductive and Child Health Surveys, Round –II (Phase I and II, 2002-4), Government of India, New Delhi and IIPS, Mumbai, 2005-6, Various Reports and Tables and CDs.

(2) *Census of India, 2001, Population Data series, Social and Cultural Tables,* Registrar General and Census Commissioner, New Delhi, Various Data series(CDs,) 2003-6.

(3) *Statistical Report of 2003, Report 2 of 2005*, Sample Registration System, Census of India, Office of Registrar General and Census Commissioner of India, New Delhi, 2005, pp. 45-49.

Contd...

Contd...

Note: SRS data for Total fertility rates were not available for many states and Union Territories; so also RCH information for them could not be given in Table 57.

List of Variables

1. Per cent female illiterates (among eligible mothers, age 15-44), Census 2001
2. Per cent *kachcha* houses (non-bricked houses), Census 2001
3. Total Fertility Rate (TFR), SRS survey data 2003
4. Per cent of birth order 3+ (among all birth orders), RCH Survey-II, 2002-4
5. Contraceptive Prevalence Rate (CPR) of any modern method, RCH Survey-II, 2002-4
6. Per cent female sterilization
7. Unmet need for family planning use, RCH-II, 2002-4
8. Per cent no ANC given
9. Per cent full ANC given to eligible mothers (age 15-44), during current pregnancy period, RCH-II, 2002-4 (at least 3 visits for ANC + at least one TT injection + 100 or more IFA tablets)
10. Per cent institutional delivery of child birth, RCH-II, 2002-4
11. Per cent full immunization given to children 12-23 months
12. Per cent of children whom no vaccination given to children 12-23 months, RCH-II, 2002-4

five clusters of states can be identified, based on three main criteria (viz., illiteracy or poverty, fertility and health service utilization rates):

1. *Cluster 1. High female illiteracy, high poverty and high fertility states, with very little health services (Bihar, Uttar Pradesh, Rajasthan and Madhya Pradesh):* Over five-year period, slight improvements have occurred in almost all states. For instance, in Bihar, female illiteracy reduced from 72 to 68 per cent, *kachcha* houses (or poverty) changed from 62 to 57 per cent, TFR declined from 4.5 to 4.2, children, CPR slightly increased from 23 to 27 per cent, and unmet need still remained unfulfilled from 42 to 36 per cent, but vaccination not given hovered around at same high level (49%). For Uttar Pradesh, though female illiteracy declined from 70 to 61 per cent, poverty remained virtually stagnant (39 to 37%). TFR only slightly declined from 4.7 to 4.4. children, CPR slightly improved (22 to 26%), but female sterilization remained stagnant (13.6 to 14.6%). Unmet need slightly displaced from 38 to 34 per cent. Although institutional delivery improved from 16 to 28 per cent, but child vaccination was not given to much larger proportion of hapless children (29 to 35%). This is simply unpardonable! Although, there are some progress, but with such snails pace of progress, neither MDG targets can be fulfilled by 2015, nor the 1978 Alma Ata declaration "Health for All" mission by another generation!
2. *Cluster 2. Moderately low female illiteracy, but considerably high poverty and high fertility states, with slightly more health services (Nagaland, Manipur and Meghalaya):* No substantial changes is noticeable in female illiteracy, nor in health service utilization rates. Sometimes deterioration is also recorded, which may be due to better reporting in the latter RCH-II survey in such remote states, than in the former. Situation perhaps has actually degraded in those tribal states. However, institutional delivery and child vaccination have mostly improved in cluster 2.
3. *Cluster 3. Moderately high female illiteracy, moderately high poverty and moderately high fertility states, with moderately more health services (Assam, Orissa, Haryana, Gujarat, West Bengal and Karnataka):* During the five year's period, situation has improved in female literacy and in most health services and so also in most of the

states, but not spectacularly. Noteworthy feature is that Orissa has raised its rank from cluster 1 to cluster 3, while Haryana has slipped down from cluster 4 to cluster 3. Although TFR has also declined below 3 children for most states, but further substantial reduction is very much desirable. CPR has recorded some substantial increase, but unmet need remained sluggish; so also child vaccination. In short, very sustained efforts are further required for onward improvement in such transitory states.

4. *Cluster 4. Moderate female illiteracy, low poverty and relatively less fertility states, with moderately high health services (Andhra Pradesh, Maharashtra, Punjab and Himachal Pradesh):* In these states the female illiteracy has declined, so correspondingly total fertility rates. This is quite commendable. Health services also performed quite well, as reflected in slight decreased levels of unmet need, slightly higher institutional delivery, and less failures in child vaccination. Hence, much future hope can be rested on such improving states, but strict vigilance and sustained urge for reaching the desired goals must also accompany. Then only, such transitory states will achieve the replacement level fertility, universal child immunization and universal ANC care.
5. *Cluster 5. Much less female illiteracy, very low poverty and comparatively still lower fertility states, with considerably high health services (Tamil Nadu and Kerala):* Some further improvements have also occurred in this cluster, though not spectacularly. For Tamil Nadu, female sterilization increased from 45 to 49 per cent, CPR raised from 50 to 55 per cent, unmet need decreased from 21 to 18 per cent, but institutional delivery improved subsequently from 79 to 91 per cent. For Kerala, female illiteracy decreased further from 8.5 to 6.5 per cent, female sterilization slightly declined from 49 to 46 per cent, and CPR also declined from 58 to 57 per cent (may be not properly reported earlier). Unmet need remained stagnant at 15 per cent. However, institutional delivery almost touched the upper limit (99%); so also child immunization (98-99%).

Besides, a few notable features must also be mentioned:

1. *Negative relationships between poverty and fertility rates*: If we notice two columns, viz., female illiteracy and TFR, then we can easily visualize almost a perfect one-to-one relationship between the two.

This is simply remarkable. This appears very clearly in Table 57 for all to see. For example, Bihar has 68 per cent female illiteracy and 4.2 TFR, followed by Uttar Pradesh with 61 female illiteracy and 4.4 TFR, which is, in turn, followed by Rajasthan with corresponding figures of 58 and 3.8, respectively. This, in turn, again, followed by Madhya Pradesh with 49 and 3.8 per cent respectively. Down the column, we can also visualize Haryana (with 44 and 3), Assam (43 and 2.9), Gujarat (40 and 2.8), Andhra Pradesh (49 and 2.2), West Bengal (39 and 2.3), Karnataka (41 and 1.8), Maharashtra (28 and 2.3), Punjab (31 and 2.3), Tamil Nadu (30 and 1.9) and, finally, Kerala (7 and 1.8), in almost perfect sequence and logical order! Of course, the pattern does not present an ideal one, but neither in physical science, nor in social science, even such kind of casual relationship is very rarely achieved. This is simply commendable! And, it must silence conventional critics that such relationships is bi-polar, or opposite causality exists! Only a very naïve person may fail to visualize this basic cause and effect relationship!

On the other hand, if conventional population specialists do really understand this fundamental causal relationship between the two, then, they must not continue to argue the opposite thesis, that "poverty simply arises due to high fertility", as many demographers propagate even today, and undermine the entire issue of poverty alleviation! Rather, all concerned people and policy makers, then, should emphasize upon the supreme importance of poverty alleviation actions, rather than only upon imposing family planning and contraceptives down the throats of poor, hungry, illiterate, and famished Indian women! Poverty elimination actions must now get the topmost priority. Unfortunately, this is not done by population specialists, demographers, geographers and social scientists, nor by planners, policy makers, bureaucrats and politicians. Meantime, very precious 60 years are already wasted!

2. *Inverse relationship between poverty or female illiteracy and health utilization rates:* Second, if we again notice the columns of female illiteracy and any one of the several columns of health services (like female sterilization, CPR, or ANC care, or institutional delivery, or no child vaccination given), we can easily untangle an *inverse relationship* between the two. For instance, Bihar has very high female illiteracy of 68 per cent and CPR only 27, followed by Uttar Pradesh with 61 and 26 respectively, Haryana (44 and 54), Karnataka (41 and 58), Tamil Nadu (30 and 55), and eventually, Kerala (6 and 57). That is, when females become more literate, they get more access to such family planning services, and also more willing to utilize them. Persuasion becomes easier, so also motivation for adopting the small family norm. This is true world-wide. Demographic histories of developed countries world-wide amply testify these. Unless minimum level of education or literacy is given to poor women, and a little bit of hope and aspirations are sown in their abjectly poverty-stricken lives, it is totally wrong to expect them to adopt the small family norm willingly or demand unmet need! This unmet need concept is thrust upon them by demographers. The same is true for low utilization rates for female sterilization, or unmet need, or ANC care or child immunization.

So, if we are really honest to raise the health utilization rates and set in demographic decline among the poor Indian women, first, we urgently need to sit with them, listen to them, look at their moist eyes, and soulfully listen to their untold poignantly sad stories, and try utmost to fill their demands for food, employment, shelter, education, and then only, preach them about contraceptives! If we start to treat them as precious human beings, and give them the minimum means of subsistence and hope, then, they themselves will voluntarily on-set the desired demographic decline! Permanently and securely! Otherwise another century will fly!

Very Little Health Services in Backward States and Remote Areas

Table 58 vividly identifies such backward districts, remote and inaccessible tracts, specially in four most undeveloped states, namely, Uttar Pradesh, Bihar, Rajasthan and Madhya Pradesh. Here, five main aspects of reproductive and child health care are emphasized, like ANC care (check up), safe child delivery, child immunization, utilization rates of modern family planning methods, and female sterilization rate. Table 58 also pinpoints the area of darkness, that is, identifies particular health services, with reference to such five main services, which are not adequately available in such backward and remote tracts. This attempt identifies specific services and particular districts that need immediate attention from District Health

Table 58

Very Little Health Services in Backward, Remote and Inaccessible Areas (RCH-II Survey, 2002-04)

State	Name of few districts where very little health services available, regarding:				
	Ante-natal Care		Child Health	Family Planning	
	No ANC Care to over 50% eligible women(15-44 age)	Less than 30% Safe Child Delivery	No Child Immunization to over 40% children	Less than 30% use Family Planning Methods	Less than 20% Female Sterilization
Uttar Pradesh (Total 70 districts)	26 Districts: Allahabad, Bahraich, Balrampur, Banda, Budaun, Bulandshahar, Chandauli, Chitrakut, Deoria, Etah, Gonda, Hamirpur, Hardoi, Kaushambi, Philibhit, Rampur, Saharanpur, Shahjahanpur, Siddharthnagar, Shrawasthi, Sant Kabir Nagar, Sant Ravi das Nagar, Unnao.	39 Districts: Allahabad, Auraiya, Bahraich, Baghpat, Balrampur, Budaun, Basti, Chandauli, Chitrakut, Etah, Etawah, Farrukhabad, Firozabad, Gautam Buddha Nagar, Gonda, Gorakhpur, Hardoi, Kannauj, Kanpur Dehat, Kannauj, Kaushambi, Kheri, Lalitpur, Maharajganj, Mainpuri, Mirzapur, Moradabad, Muzzafarnagar, Philibhit, Rae Bareily	22 Districts: Agra, Allahabad, Balrampur, Banda, Bareilly, Bijnor, Chitrakut, Deoria, Farrukhabad, Firozabad, Hamirpur Jyotiba Phule Nagar, Kannauj, Kaushambi, Kheri, Mathura, Moradabad, Philibhit, Rampur, Sant Ravidas Nagar, Shahjahanpur, Sonbhadra	49 Districts: Ambedkar Nagar, Auraiya, Azamgarh, Bahraich, Ballia, Balrampur, Banda, Barabanki, Bareilly, Basti, Budaun, Chitrakut, Deoria, Etah, Etawah, Faizabad, Farrukhabad, Firozabad, Fatehpur, Ghazipur, Gonda, Gorakhpur, Hardoi, Hathras, Jaunpur, Jyotiba Phule Nagar, Kannauj, Kanpur Dehat, Kaushambi, Kheri, Lalitpur, Maharajganj, Mainpuri, Mathura, Mau, Moradabad, Pilibhit, Pratapgarh, Rae	22 Districts:Bahraich, Balrampur, Budaun, Etah, Farrukhabad, Firozabad, Gonda, Hardoi, Jyotiba Phule Nagar, Kannauj, Kanpur Dehat, Kheri, Mainpuri, Moradabad, Rae Bareily, Rampur, Sant Kabir Nagar, Shahjahanpur, Shrawasti, Siddharthnagar,

Contd...

Contd...

		Rampur, Saharanpur, Sant Kabir Nagar, Shahjahanpur, Siddharthnagar, Sitapur, Sonbhadra, Shrawasthi, Unnao		Bareily, Rampur, Sant Kabir Nagar, Sant Ravidas Nagar, Shahjahanpur, Shrawasti, Siddharthnagar, Sitapur, Sonbhadra, Sultanpur, Unnao	
Bihar (Total 37 districts)	33 Districts: Araria, Aurangabad, Banka, Begusarai, Bhagalpur, Buxar, Darbhanga, Gaya, Jamui, Jehanabad, Kaimur, Katihar, Khagaria, Kisenganj, Lakhisarai, Madhepura, Madhubani, Munger, Muzaffarpur, Nalanda, Nawada, Paschim Champaran, Purba Champaran, Purnia, Saharsa, Samastipur, Saran, Seikhpura, Sheohar, Sitamarhi,Siwan, Supaul, Vaishali	22 Districts: Araria, Aurangabad, Begusarai, Dharbhanga, Gaya, Jamui, Katihar, Khagaria, Kisenganj, Lakhisarai, Madhepura, Madhubani, Muzaffarpur, Purba Champaran, Purnia, Saharsa, Samastipur, Sheikpura, Sheohar, Sitamarhi, Supaul, Vaishali	22 Districts:Araria, Banka, Begusarai, Buxar, Darbhanga, Gaya, Jehanabad, Kaimur, Katihar, Khagaria, Kisenganj, Lakhisarai, Madhepura,Paschim Champaran, Purba Champaran,Rohtas,Saharsa, Samastipur, Seikhpura, Sheohar, Supaul	30 Districts: Araria, Aurangabad, Banka, Begusarai, Bhagalpur, Buxar, Darbhanga, Gaya, Gopalganj, Jamui, Jehanabad, Kaimur, Katihar, Khagaria, Kisenganj, Lakhisarai, Madhepura, Madhubani, Nalanda, Nawada, Paschim Champaran, Purba Champaran, Purnia, Rohtas, Samastipur, Saran, Seikhpura, Sheohar, Sitamarhi, Siwan	11 Districts: Buxar, Gopalganj, Jamui, Kishenganj, Paschim Champaran, Purnia, Samastipur, Saran, Sheikpura, Sheohar, Siwan

Contd...

Contd...

Rajasthan (Total 32 districts	3 Districts: Barmer, Bikaner, Jaisalmer	2 Districts: Bikaner, Jaisalmer	6 Districts: Banswara, Barmer, Churu, Dhaulpur, Jalore, Sawai Madhopur	2 Districts: Dhaulpur, Jaisalmer	3 Districts: Barmer, Dhaulpur, Jaisalmer
Madhya Pradesh (Total 45 districts)	3 Districts: Chhatarpur, Satna, Sidhi	13 Districts: Bhind, Chhatarpur, Dindori, Jhabua, Katni, Mandla, Rewa, Sagar, Satna, Shahdol, Sidhi, Tikamgarh, West Nimar	31 Districts:Balaghat, Betul, Bhopal, Chhatarpur, Chhindwara, Datia, Dewas, Dhar, Dindori, East Nimar, Hoshangabad, Indore, Jabalpur, Katni, Mandla, Mandsaur, Morena, Narshimhapur, Raisen, Rajgarh, Ratlam,Rewa, Sagar, Satna, Sehore, Seoni, Sahdol, Shajapur, Shivpuri, Sidhi, Ujjain	1 District:Sidhi	No District

Source: Reproductive and Child Health Survey-II, 2002-4, Ministry of Health and Family Welfare and IIPS, Mumbai, 2005, Various Tables and CDs.

Administration, State Health Ministries, and MoHFW. Similar exercises for other states are also done for rest of India, to be shown in another study. As a summary, the following features are highlighted:

Uttar Pradesh: Even in 2002-04, out of total 70 districts, (1) ANC care was unavailable to more than 50 per cent eligible mothers during their current pregnancy in 26 districts; (2) 39 districts showed that less than 30 per cent of total delivery in respective district were safe; (3) 22 districts indicated that child immunization were not given at all to 40 per cent of the children in respective district (age 12-23 months); (4) as many as 49 districts reported that less than 30 per cent eligible women used any kind of modern family planning methods; and (5) female sterilization was less than 20 per cent in 22 districts.

Indeed, Uttar Pradesh *has very poor performance regarding family planning utilization rates, and female sterilization*. Child immunization and ANC care are also very dismal. In sum, there exists worst served 26-30 districts, located both in eastern and western UP, where health services and their utilization rates in all components are very precarious. These most backward and highly neglected districts, specially inaccessible tracts within them, thus, need top-most priority and greatest attention of the District Chief Medical Officers, State Health Ministry, MoHFW, scholars, policy makers, bureaucrats, and all those concerned with India's demographic development. MoHFW must take special notice and care of these most neglected districts of Uttar Pradesh. These tracts are now identified. Trouble shooting must urgently begin. Only then demographic decline in Uttar Pradesh, and in the entire country may set in, vigorously and permanently. Otherwise, the, Alma Ata slogan, "Health for All", would remain a political gimmick for many more decades!

Bihar: According to RCH-II survey, even as recent as 2002-04, out of total 37 districts in Bihar, (1) no ante-natal care (ANC) was given to more than 50 per cent eligible and currently pregnant mothers in as many as 33 districts; (2) 22 districts indicated only less than 30 per cent of total child delivery as safe; (3) almost similar 22 districts also showed that child immunization of any kind was not available to 40 per cent of children (age 12-23 months) in such districts; (4) as many as 30 districts (75%) recorded that less than 30 per cent of eligible women used any modern method of family planning; and (5) female sterilization performed was less than 20 per cent in 11 districts.

In short, 22 districts out of total 37 in Bihar are the heartland of backward zones, where all health services are very dismal, and which need very urgent attention. Such special care and very intensive efforts must be given to them, instead of providing a thin veneer of limited budget allocation and efforts made over entire state. Besides, what is indicated above regarding UP, also holds very true for Bihar. Unless, Bihar and UP are salvaged, specially their most backward and neglected tracts, nothing much can be expected to happen in India, demographically and socio-economically.

These are now well-known facts. But, excessive and corrupt politicking, corrupt political and administrative systems, and laziness and fatalistic attitude of both the governments and the common people in these two most backward and problematic states have left very little hope.

Thus, the only hope lies in what Swami Vivekananda declared a century ago (1893): "First, we very urgently require a character-building and nation-building education for all people, without which nothing can be aspired or sustained" (Vivekananda, 1893, *Complete Work*, 1963, Volume VII, p. 487). This holds true for all aspects of life; for the individuals as well as the nations; for demographic welfare and socio-economic uplift!

Rajasthan: The situation in this state is much hopeful. Out of total 32 districts, (1) fortunately, ANC care was available to more than 50 per cent eligible mothers during current pregnancy in almost all the districts, except only three; (2) only two districts recorded less than 30 per cent safe delivery, the rest of the districts had more safe delivery; (3) only six districts indicated that child immunization were not given to 40 per cent of all children (age 12-23 months) in those respective districts, in the rest it were covered; (4) all the districts reported eligible mothers using more than 30 per cent of modern family planning, except two; and (5) female sterilization was more than 20 per cent in all, but three districts. Thus, compared to other northern states, Rajasthan's performance is much satisfactory. So, health care delivery and utilization situation in Rajasthan is the best in the lot. Recently, it has progressed much faster and to the right direction.

Madhya Pradesh: Out of total 45 districts of Madhya Pradesh, the following five findings emerge: (1) fortunately, ante-natal care was available in most districts, and only three districts showed that no

ANC care was given to over 50 per cent eligible mothers; (2) 13 districts reported less than 30 per cent safe child delivery; (3), unfortunately, 31 districts indicated that no child immunization given at all to 40 per cent of children in the respective districts (age 12-23 months); (4) modern family planning methods were utilized in almost all districts (using more than 30%), except in one; and (5) pleasantly surprising, female sterilization was also over 20 per cent in all districts.

Thus, although Madhya Pradesh has performed satisfactorily in family planning and female sterilization, however, its performance in child immunization is disastrous in 31 districts out of total 45, which indicated that no child immunization was given to over 40 per cent of children in the district. This is simply unpardonable. Consequence is high rates of infant and child mortality in Madhya Pradesh. Such state of affairs is most appalling. To provide maximum sincere efforts for child survival are morally, medically and demographically mandatory.

Summing up, Rajasthan has been progressing considerably well, while Madhya Pradesh's performance is also quite commendable, except in child immunization services (requires tremendous efforts). But, it is Uttar Pradesh and Bihar which are still much lagging behind, and need government's priority attention. These are two states, which need full attention and trouble-shooting on a war-footing. It is not an easy task. Sincere political will, economic discipline, total freedom from corrupt administrative systems, tremendous zeal, and sincere love for common people are the required building blocks for constructing a better and humane health delivery system in these problematic states.

Main Trends

Widespread Poverty in India Even Now

Hunger, acute malnutrition and death among the children are widely prevalent in Maharashtra, Orissa, West Bengal, Bihar, Uttar Pradesh, and many other parts of India, even in 2006. A recent report (*Times of India*, April 19, 2006, p. 30) also mentioned that about 47 per cent of children below the age of three years are still malnourished in India, even in 2005; while their incidence is less than 30 per cent in many African countries. This is mainly caused by rampant corruption in public food distribution system. This is all the more shameful for

India, when millions of tons of foodgrains are rotting in the godowns. "The denial of as little as 200-300 calories in a child's daily diet is what makes the difference between the normal growth and the inevitable decline towards illness and death. Sixty years after national independence, we have yet to free children from hunger" (ibid.). Even in 1998-99, South Asia still had about 40 per cent population below poverty line (percentage of people living below one dollar per day) (Merrick, 2002, pp. 41-46)

Since 1991, India has been more actively following market economy and has also come to the clutches of globalization. Recently, Indian economy has shown much spurt in growth (8% annually), but neither it created much employment for common people, nor reduced poverty in India. It is just limited to a tiny segment of corporate world, and has benefited only a handful of the rich. Rather, economic and social inequalities have widened further. The Human Development Report of India (2004, pp. 25-75) has also indicated that in spite of rapid economic growth, poverty, deprivation and inequities have not declined in India. For instance, even in 2004, 60 per cent of the rural households were denied safe drinking water, 40 per cent did not have access to electricity, 55 per cent did not have sanitary toilets, and over 30 per cent did not have bricked houses.

The recent United Nations Human Development Report (2005, pp. 19-26) has noted that: "Though the incidence of income poverty has fallen from 36 per cent in early 1990s to somewhere between 25 and 30 per cent today. ...But, overall, the evidence suggests that the pick-up in growth has not translated into a commensurate decline in poverty. More worrying, improvements in child and infant mortality are slowing – and India is now off track for those Millennium Development Goals (MDG) targets".

High Fertility and High Infant Mortality Still Persistent

Very high levels of IMR and TFR are still prevailing in India, even in 2005-06, in spite of much hype about the so-called rapid economic growth and development. According to Census of India, 2001 (Census, Provisional Population Total), the overall female illiteracy rate (above age 7) is still 44 per cent, while rural female illiteracy is much higher, i.e., 65 per cent. Infant mortality rate, unfortunately, is still 66 infant deaths (per 1,000 infant born in a year). Indeed, these are not at all signs of development! Rather symptoms of deep-seated poverty, acute deprivation, and utter helplessness! Consequently, TFR is still very high, IMR is also very high, so also under-five child mortality and maternal mortality. Parikh and Radhakrishna (2005, pp. 6-8) thus succinctly noted that, "what is very disquieting is that about 2.2 million children die every-year, and most of these are preventable. Major causes are malnutrition and inadequate supply of vaccines. Preventable and treatable diseases take a huge toll among the poor." Also, "the health gap between the rich and the poor is large" (ibid., p. 6).

Table 59 vividly presents such socio-economic, demographic and health situations in India, during the most recent period, i.e. 1992-93 to 2002-04.

Table 59

Poverty, Demographic, and Health Situations in India, 1992-93 to 2002-04

All-India	*1992-93 (NFHS-I)*	*1998-99 (NFHS-II)*	*1998-99 (RCH-I)*	*2001 (Census)*	*2002-04 (RCH-II)*
Poverty (NSS data)	36.6*	26.9**	26.9**	NA	NA
Female illiteracy (poverty index)	62.0	56.0	56.1	44.2	NA
Per cent kachcha houses (poverty index)	NA	NA	39.0	39.0	NA
Per cent SC/ST	NA	NA	27.0	27.0	NA
No ANC care given	36.8	34.0	35.0	NA	26.5
3 ANC visit made	29.3	27.6	31.8	NA	50.1
Institutional deliveries	25.5	33.6	34.0	NA	40.5
No vaccination to children	NA	NA	18.8	NA	19.0
Full immunization of children	27.5	34.5	54.2	NA	47.8
Use any modern method of FP	36.3	42.8	42.5	NA	45.9
Female sterilization	27.3	34.2	33.4	NA	34.3
Unmet need (spacing and limiting)	19.5	15.8	25.3	NA	21.2
Infant mortality rate	78.5	67.6	NA	66.0	NA
Total fertility rate	3.4	3.2	NA	3.0	NA

Sources: Same as in Tables 1, 48, 54, 55, 56, 57, and 58 for NFHS-I, NFHS-II, RCH-I, Census 2001, RCH-II data, and SRS(2005) Report. Poverty data from NSS data of 50th and 55th round, and Poplin et al. (2005). * NSS 1993–4 data, ** NSS 1999–2000 data.

Low Performance Rates of Most Health Service Indicators

The United Nations Development Programmes (UNDP, 2003; UNMP, 2005) envisaged eight Millennium Development Goals (MDGs), which were split into 18 targets and measured by 48 indicators. Of these, the first five primary goals are (to be fulfilled by 2015): (1) to eradicate extreme poverty by half (measured by proportion of population below poverty line (less than a dollar per day) and prevalence of underweight babies below age five); (2) to achieve universal primary education (measured by net enrolment ratio of children age 6-10, by literacy rate of 15-24 years, and by proportion of children starting at grade one and reaching grade five, age 6-10); (3) to promote gender equity (measured as ratio of girls to boys in primary, secondary and tertiary education); (4) to reduce child mortality by two-third (measured by reduction of IMR rate, by under-five mortality rate, and by proportion of one year old children immunized against measles); and (5) to improve maternal mortality rate (measured by proportion of births attended by health professionals) (ibid., 2003). In reality, these are very basic fundamental human rights. UNDP (2005, pp. 19-26) thus hopes that, "in our highly unequal world, greater equity would provide a powerful catalyst for poverty reduction and progress towards the MDGs." Thus, the Government of India is also a signatory of UN's such MDGs, and expressed its keenness in National Rural Health Mission (GOI, NRHM, 2005) policy document.

But, in India, there are serious gaps between the holy wish and the hard reality. Thus, UN Human Development Report (2005, pp. 19-26) laments that, even when India is considered as a 'software superpower', here "one in every 11 Indian children dies in the first five years of life for lack of low-technology, low-cost interventions" (p. 19)... Malnutrition, which has barely improved over the past decade, affects half of the country's children... About 1 in 4 girls and more than 1 in 10 boys do not attend primary school (ibid., pp. 19-20).

Sadly, as revealed in Table 59, most of these MDGs cannot be reached in India within the specified time schedule (2015), because of very slow progress on these fronts, due to lack of effective health management and absence of a strong political will. For instance, proportion of population below the poverty line (as indirectly measured by female illiteracy) was 62 per cent in 1992-93, which only slightly decreased to 56 per cent in 1998-99, and remained 44.2 per cent even in 2001. That is very little reduction in poverty and female illiteracy have occurred during the decade (1992-2001). Likewise, ante-natal care was not given to 36 per cent of eligible women in 1992-93, which sadly remained unchanged till 1998-99, and only lately recorded 26.5 per cent in 2002-04. Similarly, unmet need was 19.5 per cent in 1992-93, which further declined to 15.8 per cent in 1998-99 and virtually remained unchanged (21.2%) in 2002-04.

TFR, which was 3.4 children in 1992-93, only slightly changed into 3.2 in 1998-99, and still remained as high as 3, according to SRS in 2003 (SRS, 2005). Only 0.4 percentage points over a period of 11 years! Further, IMR changed very sluggishly from 78.5 in 1992-93 to 66 in 2001, whereas performance of even Sri Lanka, Bangladesh and Sub-Saharan Africa is much better (Human Development Report, India, 2004). Female sterilizations were performed on 27.5 per cent of eligible women in 1992-93, which slightly rose to 34 per cent in 1998-99, and got stuck there, even in 2002-04.

Almost similar pictures also emerge with respect to other indicators, like use of any modern methods of family planning (36 to 45%), no vaccination given to children (18 to 19%), full immunization given (27.5 to 47.3%), or institutional delivery (25.5 to 40.5%). Hence, UNDP (2005, pp. 21-22) warns: “If current trends continue, there will be large gaps between MDG targets and outcomes. Those gaps can be expressed in statistics, but behind the statistics are the lives and hopes of ordinary people”... “China and India may seriously fall behind in child mortality MDG targets of 2015” (ibid., p. 21). UNDP (2005, pp. 21-24) continues: “The MDGs themselves are a vital statement of international purpose rooted in a commitment to basic human rights. These rights – to education, to gender equality, to survival in childhood and to a decent standard of living – are universal in nature” (ibid., pp. 23-24).... “The MDGs can be met by 2015 – but only if all involved break with business as usual and dramatically accelerate and scale up action now” (ibid., pp. 21-23).

The report further sternly warns: "To put it bluntly, the world is heading for a heavily-signposted human development disaster, the cost of which will be counted in avoidable deaths, children out of school and lost opportunities for poverty reduction. That disaster is as avoidable as it is predictable" (ibid., pp. 23-24).

Wide State-wise and Spatial Variations in Social and Health Indicators

Apart from afore-mentioned national pictures, very wide state-wise variations exist in health performances, e.g., as regards female sterilization in 2002-04 between Kerala (45.9%) and Tamil Nadu (49.5%) on the one hand, and backward states like Bihar (28.9%) and Uttar Pradesh (14.4%), on the other (see Tables 54-57). Similarly, regarding ante-natal care not given, correspondingly, we have in one extreme Kerala (0.3%) and Tamil Nadu (0.6%); conversely, we have Bihar (62.1%) and Uttar Pradesh (42%), on the other extreme. In a recent paper, Srinivasan (2006, pp. 20-52) has also rightly observed that these backward states lag behind Kerala, roughly 25 to 40 years.

Likewise, there are very wide spatial variations in terms of levels of literacy and income. According to Census 2001, literacy rate (age 7+) is as high as 90.9 per cent in Kerala or 87.5 per cent in Lakshadweep on the one hand, and as low as 39.8 per cent in Bihar or 45.7 per cent in Uttar Pradesh, on the other. Female literacy also ranges from a peak of 87.9 per cent in Kerala or 86.1 per cent in Mizoram to as low as 28.3 per cent in Bihar or 35.8 per cent in Uttar Pradesh. No wonder, as Srinivasan (ibid., pp. 31-32) has indicated that Bihar and Uttar Pradesh would take at least a generation to catch up with Kerala's level of literacy and health indicators. Income-wise also, Punjab is five times richer than Bihar, and Maharashtra four times richer than Orissa. Such large discrepancies adversely affect their demographic performances.

UNDP (2005, pp. 19-21) thus notes:

> "State inequalities interact with gender- and income-based inequalities. Four states account for more than half of child deaths: Bihar, Madhya Pradesh, Rajasthan and Uttar Pradesh. These states are also marked by some of the deepest gender inequalities in India.

> Contrasts with Kerala are striking. Girls born in Kerala are five times more likely to reach their fifth birthday, are twice as likely to become literate, and are likely to live 20 years longer than girls born in Uttar Pradesh."
>
> The Report further pinpoints:
>
> "The differences are linked to the chronic under-provision of health services in high mortality northern states, which is in turn linked to unaccountable state-level governance structures... Translating economic success into human development advances will require public policies aimed explicitly at broadening the distribution of benefits from growth and global integration, increased public investment in rural areas and services and – above all – political leadership to end poor governance and address the underlying causes of gender inequality" (UNDP, 2005, p. 20).
>
> "Gender is one of the world's strongest markers for disadvantage.... Disadvantage starts at birth. In India, the death rate for children ages 1-5 is 50 per cent higher for girls than for boys. Expressed differently, 130,000 young Indian lives are lost each year because of the disadvantage associated with being born with two X chromosomes" (ibid., p. 25).

Besides, as discussed in Table 58, very widespread spatial variations emerge in health performance indicators, over various districts of backward states of Uttar Pradesh, Bihar, Madhya Pradesh, Orissa, West Bengal, Andhra Pradesh, Jharkhand, Uttaranchal, Chhattisgarh, Rajasthan, and even in Maharashtra and Gujarat, specially in villages, remote areas, and tribal zones. Special treatment of these neglected areas is much overdue.

Require Top Priority to Provide Health Services in Backward States, Villages, and Remote Tracts

Very widespread spatial variations occur in health utilization rates, and performance rates, over various districts of backward and neglected states of northern and central India. Such backward districts are listed in Table 58.

These include Uttar Pradesh (specially rural eastern UP, rural south-western UP, Terai districts of UP), Bihar (specially rural parts of northern border districts and eastern districts), West Bengal (specially hilly district, rural north Bengal, rural south Bengal, south-west Bengal), Andhra Pradesh (specially coastal districts, northern and western interior districts), Jharkhand (full tribal belts), Uttaranchal (all hilly districts), Chhattisgarh (all tribal zones), Rajasthan (rural western tracts), even in relatively developed states of Maharashtra (Vidharba region and rural eastern parts) and Gujarat (The Dangs, western parts), and elsewhere, specially in their respective remote, inaccessible, and tribal tracts. Situation in UP is precarious (Mukherji, 1989c, pp. 1-6; 1994a, pp. 1-18).

Hence, health policy-wise, the most important requirement is to identify such zones and urgently provide them with the best possible health services on top priority, along with management information (MIS) system, operational research for optimum health delivery, men, money, and materials, doctors and paramedics, and maximum budget allocation. Then only, some effective dent upon their high fertility and mortality levels can ever be made. Both for such backward states, as well as for entire India.

I have been emphasizing upon these requirements since 1980s (Mukherji, 1983b, pp. 1-141; Mukherji, 1989, pp. 1-121; Udupa and Mukherji, 1988, pp. 1-231, Mukherji 1989b, pp. 325-73), but with not much avail. Only very recently, some researchers are also focusing on this aspect (RCH, 2005; Srinivasan, 2006, pp. 32-52). This is a very heartening change.

One major concern that demands very urgent attention is the health care needs, specially for the poor. Unfortunately, India is rapidly moving towards a market-driven health care system. Towards commercialization of health care services. Parikh and Radhakrishna (2005, pp. 6-8) thus commented:

> "There is a trend towards greater utilization of health care from private providers. Poor access/quality of public facilities may be one reason, but an outcome of this is an excessive use of diagnostic medical services. This may increase cost and also lead to misallocation of scarce resources. It is not only inefficient and iniquitous, but also compromises on the quality of care."

We must rather pursue the goal, what Swami Vivekananda declared 112 years ago (1894):

> "Stretch forth a helping hand, and open the gates of knowledge to one and all, and give the downtrodden masses once more their just and legitimate rights and privileges" (Swami Vivekananda, 1894, Complete Work, 1963, Vol. III, p. 461).

Other Emerging Issues

Differential Fertility between the Hindus and the Muslims

NFHS-I (1992-93) survey showed that total fertility rate (TFR) among the Muslim population was 4.20 children per mother, compared to 2.70 children per mother among the Hindu population, which was 40 per cent higher than that among the Hindus (NFHS, 1995). Still, the report did not add a single more line about such wide fertility differentials; neither explained such phenomena, nor raised the issue about its eventual adverse consequences on India's demographic structure. As if, it was not at all a matter of national concern!

Unfortunately, very few scholars ever took this crucial issue. Some rather argued just the opposite, completely brushing aside the entire issue (see special volume, *Economic and Political Weekly*, September 2004). However, Moulasha and Rama Rao (1999, pp. 3047-51) attempted to draw attention to these phenomena in their study of religion-specific differences in fertility and family planning, with specific reference to Maharashtra, and pinpointed on such high fertility levels among the Muslim population, over the Hindu population. But it did not attract required concern, rather were ridiculed by some demographers.

According to NFHS-II survey (1998-99) (NFHS, 2000) itself, the mean number of children ever born by religion shows that in rural Kerala, on average, the Muslims have 2.70 children per mother (in reproductive ages), compared to 2.05 children among the SCs, 1.93 among Hindu OBCs, and just only 1.70 among other Hindus. Similarly, in rural Uttar Pradesh, the Muslims have on average 4.72 children per mother, compared to 4.13 among the SCs, 4.01 among the Hindu OBCs, and 3.66 among other Hindus. In rural West

Bengal, the Muslims have on average 3.83 children per mother, compared to 2.96 children among the SCs, 2.40 children among Hindu OBCs and 2.60 children among other Hindu castes. Likewise, similar differences can be seen among Muslim fertility and Hindu fertility in urban areas of these states. Quoting such data, a recent study thus also opined: "Hence, it is evident that irrespective of rural and urban stay, Muslims have higher fertility compared to all Hindu segments" (Chattopadhyay, Roy, et al., 2004, pp. 142-43).

In short, on an average, the Muslim fertility is *at least one child higher* than the fertility level of the general Hindu population, in all the states, and in both rural and urban areas. Still, such high fertility among the Indian Muslims did not matter to the researchers, as they concluded that "high Muslim fertility as the resultant of Islamic theology is too naïve, as sometimes believed by Indian scholars in the light of growing evidence of fertility decline among Muslims across world" (ibid., p. 153). However, most such researchers forget that fertility decline among Indian Muslims, if at all occurring, is happening considerably at much slower rate than in other Muslim countries (like Bangladesh, Indonesia, Malaysia, Iran, etc.), because in India they have tremendous demographic and political stake for obtaining majority, staying power, and political votes in India, the factors which are absent in other Islamic Muslim countries, unlike India.

Massive Illegal Immigration from Bangladesh and Its Adverse Consequences

Recently, however, one very important study about India's changing religious demographic structure was made by the Centre of Policy Studies, Chennai (Joshi, Srinivas, and Bajaj, 2003, pp. 87-106). They examined census-based religious population data of all districts of India, over the period 1901-91, specially over 1951-91, and found that religious demographic structure of many bordering districts of India has drastically changed, primarily due to very massive illegal migration of Muslims from Bangladesh.

"The Muslim population is present in large segments and are very much growing in recent decades over a vast continuous stretch of border districts, from Assam, West Bengal, Bihar and Uttar Pradesh. It is a huge belt that starts from Goalpara, Kamrup, Darrang, Nagaon, Dhubri, Barapeta, and Marigaon districts in Assam, continuing on to West Dinajpur, Maldah, Murshidabad, Birbhum, Hooghly, Nadia, and Twenty-Four Paraganas districts in West Bengal, stretching further over to Purnia, Champaran, Muzaffarpur, Darbhanga, Saharsa, and Santhal Parganas districts in Bihar, and over-spreading to Deoria, Gorakhpur, Basti, Bahraich, Bareilly, Rampur, Moradabad, Bijnor, Meerut, Muzzaffarnagar, Haridwar, and as far as Saharanpur districts of Western Uttar Pradesh" (ibid., pp. 100-9).

This belt of illegal Muslim migration stretches over 1,500 miles, from Assam to Western Uttar Pradesh, and widens as far as 300-400 miles, from North to South West Bengal (ibid., pp. 85-87).

The authors have also noted that:

> "In Assam, the proportion of Muslims in total population was 32.42 per cent in 1951, which rapidly increased to 37.15 per cent in 1991. In West Bengal, their comparative proportion rose from 39.89 per cent in 1951 to 47.14 percent in 1991. Most illegal infiltration of Muslims was in West Bengal, because of active political support from Marxist governments in the state. In Bihar, comparative figures are 14.56 per cent (1951) and 21 per cent (1991). In eastern Uttar Pradesh, it rose from 15.40 per cent in 1951 to 20.47 per cent in 1991. Comparative figures in western Uttar Pradesh were much higher, 29.93 and 36.33, respectively" (ibid., pp. 107-8).

Authors have thus noted that:

> "Proportion of Muslims in this belt as a whole is 27.67 per cent: their share has grown by more than 7 percentage points since 1951, when they formed 20.49 per cent of the population of this belt. If we add only the relevant component districts rather than the composite districts, then the proportion of Muslims in this belt turns to be higher at 32.77 per cent in 1991" (ibid.).

The obvious conclusion is that the share of Muslim population has grown from one-fifth in 1951 to one-third of the total population, within this vast northern belt, during a very short span of 40 years (1951-91).

That is the most drastic change and it has already transformed the demographic character of population of these states. If these trends continue unabated, then, very soon, they will constitute the majority of the population in these states, and soon thereafter over entire India (over 50%). This will be the result of comparatively higher fertility levels among the Indian Muslims themselves, but much more compounded by very massive and continuing illegal migration of Muslims from Bangladesh over last 60 years, and very high fertility trends of their progenies, over successive generations.

In spite of comparatively high Muslim fertility in India (evidenced by even recent NFHS-II survey, 1998-99, Census 2001, and other studies), and in spite of clear evidence of very massive infiltration of illegal Bangladeshi Muslims into India, both the print and electronic media totally dismiss such crucial issues as myths of "Saffron Demography of Hindu Communalists" (Rao, *Times of India*, 2006, p. 30). So, the problems not only aggravate, rather become un-surmountable!

Neglect of Basic Primary Health Services and Disease Control

In a recent study, Banerji (2005, pp. 3055-57) discussed the politics in health services in India and indicated that since last two decades the focus is given only upon "Selective Primary Health Care" (SPHC)) (like care for tuberculosis, malaria, fileria, etc.), instead of providing the basic Primary Health Care (PHC) services to the rural poor. And, here lies the root of utter neglect of public health services in the country.

One most important reason for inadequate health systems in India is lack of funds, as Mishra observed (2005, pp. 76-77) that "public expenditure on health as per cent of total government has been declining over the years. There is serious mismatch with allocation biased against rural areas (nearly three-fourths of the population have merely one-tenth of budget allocation)"

He further argues:

> "A major share of allocation is towards family welfare (read as female family planning) and other national programmes. Even within that, more than four-fifths of the expenditure is towards salaries. This leaves hardly any scope for expenditure on infrastructure,

equipment and supplies, and other requirements necessary for providing basic provision for health care" (ibid., p. 76).

Such situations need to be rectified soon.

"There are two straight-forward policy implications – to increase public expenditures in health (to 3.5-4% of GDP in the next 10-15 years) and to ensure maintenance of standards in quality of care" (ibid., p. 81).

In another study, Das Gupta (2005, pp. 5159-65) also pinpointed a few obstacles to effective disease control in India, which need to be dealt with on an urgent basis, like: (1) serious neglect and withering away of government's responsibility for public health (disease control, sanitation, child vaccination, control of food adulteration), as it now follows policies of developed countries and global trends of privatization; (2) neglect of public health regulations and their implementation, due to lack of awareness, vigilance, fund and staffs, and sluggish judicial action against offenders; (3) emphasis given mainly upon clinical or medical services, not upon providing basic public health services and environmental improvement; (4) diversion of funds and personnel from public health services to family planning programmes, strangulating the former; (5) lack of evaluation of performance of public health services and of rectifying policies, vis-à-vis family planning programmes getting all attention; and (6) though impressive administrative or medical capacity exists for intensive campaigns, but their gains are not sustained permanently.

However, recently the government has attempted to improve services through National Rural Health Mission (NRHM) policy document. But Banerji (ibid., p. 3057) indicated that "no focus were given on systematic data collection and operation research for better delivery of health services to the rural population, nor on proper training of different categories of health workers for epidemiological approach to solve community health problems and social orientation. ...Without these, the goals may remain just wishful thinking" (ibid., p. 3057; also see Srinivasan, 2006, pp. 10-21).

Government's Recent Programmes for Rural Development

In order to reduce rural poverty, lately (2005-06), the government is planning to design and implement Rural Employment Guarantee Programme (REGP), under Bharat Nirman Programme, by executing it, first, in 100 districts (out of total 625 districts). It has got mixed responses from the experts, as manifested below:

"Recently, Bharat Nirman Programme is inaugurated. If this is implemented, hopefully, this will create additional 10 million hectares of irrigation facilities, electrify 100,000 villages, construct rural roads and housing and provide drinking water" (Patodia, 2006, p. 10).

"Reforms and policy modifications needed to sustain and accelerate our growth have been recommended and placed before the government from time to time. But decisions are delayed and implementation is too slow. If growth has to accelerate, we have to act and act fast" (ibid.).

Many experts doubt about the government's seriousness of REGP, as Sarkar (2006, p. 5) noted:

> "If document of RGEP is examined, it becomes clear that the government is more interested to appropriate political dividends and votes, rather than really to help the poor. Were it really interested in generating sustainable rural development, then it would not have allocated so meager amount for raw materials and rural infrastructure".

"Given the agrarian distress and problems of low wages and underemployment, the budget (of 2006-07) should have given more focus and higher allocation to agriculture and rural employment" (Dev, 2006, p. 1413).

The crucial problems of deep-seated corruption in India in implementing anti-poverty programmes are very much well known. Some people, however, advice:

> "The delivery systems can be improved with the new approach of participatory development, social mobilisation, right to information, involvement of civil society and panchayati raj institutions" (ibid., pp. 1412-13).

However, most of these ideas of civil society are wishful ideas, because these are not yet operating in India.

> "Promotion of rural non-farm employment is also very important for reduction in poverty... Unless agricultural growth is improved,

one cannot achieve annual GDP growth of 8 per cent and reduction on poverty. Industry and services also may not grow on expected lines without agricultural growth" (ibid., p. 1410).

Gopal (2005, pp. 4523-24) has questioned the euphoria around the National Employment Guarantee Act, 2005-06 by cautioning that unless we learn from past experience of implementation of government programmes and devise corrective measures, there will be few gains for the rural poor. Middlemen must not be allowed to eat away the benefits meant for the real rural poor. Kannan (2005, pp. 4518-22) has also rightly advised that such employment guarantee programmes should be linked with the projects of improving human development, in order to be effective, and more lasting. Thus, such employment guarantee projects must pay the workers adequate wages so that they can come out of poverty line, and must be linked with poverty alleviation programmes, such as, rural housing construction, sanitation, primary health centres, drinking water, etc. (ibid., p. 4522).

Needs Poverty Alleviation and Rural Development

For poverty alleviation, India needs both rapid economic growth with distributive justice, as well as growth that favours pro-poor development and reduces inequality. World Development Bank (1990, pp. 56-79) also advised policies for poverty-reducing growth, through: (a) providing opportunities for the poor, and (b) enabling them to participate in the growth process. The report advocated that these can be achieved by three broad tasks:

- First and foremost, economy-wide and sectoral policies must encourage rural development and urban employment. Experience indicates that this requires moderate taxation of agriculture and relatively undistorted product and factor markets. It also requires public provision of infrastructure and environment that makes technological change accessible to small farmers and the urban poor.
- Second, specific policies are needed to improve the participation of the poor in growth by increasing their access to land, credit, and public infrastructure and services.... Flexible programmes that involve the intended beneficiaries, build institutions, employ

NGOs, and local groups and respond to local needs are the best way of molding infrastructure.

- Third, resource-poor regions, where poverty and environmental degradation are interrelated, require a different approach. Since the potential for growth in these regions is limited and the population is increasing, policies that facilitate out-migration are essential (ibid., pp. 72-73).

Hence, pro-poor growth policies, rural development, urban employment, people's easy access to, and rights over, the basic public infrastructure and services, and out-migration from backward regions may offer some pathways to poverty reduction (Mukherji, 1995b, pp. 1-55; 1997, pp. 1-80). Of them, poverty alleviation through rural development programmes constitute one of the most important components (Mukherji, 1983c, pp. 1-90). However, so far, very limited success has been achieved in India.

The National Institute of Rural Development (NIRD, 1999, pp. 121-22) has reiterated upon the need for revamping the existing schemes for rural development in India, but with greater coordination. It observes:

> "What is needed is 'mainstreaming of poverty concerns' through overhauling the policies of all government departments, under close supervision of the Planning Commission. ... For example, schemes for universal primary education will be successful only when parallel efforts are made for abolition of child labour and vice versa.
>
> Funds for better infrastructure and capital formation, both human and physical, are essential for a decentralised system to function. Thus, investment in roads, irrigation, watersheds and water harvesting structures, electricity, infrastructure for rural industries, village schools and the like, many of which are part of the MNP (Minimum Needs Programme), though never effectively completed, require to be undertaken."

In India, development plans look great, but only on papers! Implementations are very slack and do not reach to the poor. Indeed, never meant to reach to the poor! There are many regions in the country where development has not touched the lives of the people, even after last six decades since independence!

In sum, deep-seated corruption, political bungling, hunger, malnutrition, abject poverty, widespread illiteracy, high fertility, high infant mortality, high child and maternal mortality, and utter lack of government's accountability to do social justice to the poor masses still plague India. The government gives only social lip-service to the poor. Corporate sector and all concerned persons are totally indifferent and unconcerned. India is at the mercy of the terrorists. Rural employment programmes are actually meant to fatten corrupt promoters, constructors and local corrupt political leaders. Social scientists lack social commitments. Terrorists everywhere make life hell and most unsecured at every moment. Massive infiltrations across borders are continuing unabated. And, India sleeps on!

India may now be considered as software superpower, but it fails to wipe out mass poverty among 300 millions Indians!

Amidst these forest of despairs, however, I cannot leave this chapter, without a mission of hope. Let us chant the great message of Swami Vivekananda:

> *"Arise, Awake, great ones! The world is burning with miseries! Can you sleep?"* (Swami Vivekananda, 1894, Complete Work, Centenary Volume VII, p. 501).

> *"Fill the brain, therefore, with high thoughts, highest ideals, place them day and night before you, and out of that will come great work"* (Swami Vivekananda, 1894, Complete Work, Centenary Volume II, 1963, p. 86).

12

Summary and Policy Significance

"I hold all educated people as traitors, who being educated at the expense of the illiterate masses, do nothing for them" (Swami Vivekananda, 1894, Complete Work, Centenary Volume III, 1963).

"Until even a dog remains hungry and unfed in India, we cannot take rest and feel complacent" (Swami Vivekananda, 1896, Complete Work, Centenary Volume VIII, 1963, p. 150).

"Repeat and pray day and night, "O Thou Lord of Gauri, O Thou Mother of the Universe, vouchsafe manliness unto me! O Thou Mother of Strength, take away my weakness, take away my unmanliness, and make me a man!" (Swami Vivekananda, 1894, Complete Work, Centenary Volume IV, 1963, p. 480).

Summary of the Main Findings

Summary I: Findings of Various Canonical Models

This book has performed analyses in following four stages:

- First, this study has further refined and applied the Demographic Field Theory, which was earlier evolved by the present author during 1977-1983, to the data of National Family and Health Survey of India (NFHS-I) of 1992-93, and has performed very many canonical analyses. It has generated a multitude of very useful canonical linkages between three sets of (a) demographic behaviour variables, (b) socio-economic variables, and (c) policy and programme variables.

- Second, the study also repeated the same procedures with recent data of NFHS-II of 1998-99, and performed a new set of three canonical analyses. These exercises yielded many findings having great policy significance.
- Third, most recent demographic and socio-economic situations in India are also critically and minutely examined with Census 2001 and Sample Registration Survey (2003) data.
- Fourth, further, recent-most health service indicators are also thoroughly investigated with data of Reproductive and Child Health Surveys (RCH surveys, Round I, 1998-99 and Round II, 2002-04). Thus, the study is most up-to-date, and portrays the most current demographic and health situations in India (1992 to 2005).

Most pertinent findings of various canonical models (I to IX) are briefly highlighted below:

(a) Canonical Analysis Model I: Crucial Findings of All-India (Total) State-Level Analysis

1. High IMR occurs in India due to high female illiteracy, less immunization and less professionally assisted in child delivery (canonical correlation is 0.987).
2. High total fertility rate and high child mortality occur because of less girls attending schools, less sterilization and less tetanus toxoid given to women (canonical correlation is 0.965).
3. Very high total fertility rate occurs due to high female illiteracy, and due to little ANC, though some sterilization done (canonical correlation is 0.867).
4. Less child mortality occurs due to fewer underweight babies, who were breastfed and also got solid/mushy food. TFR moderately high due to less ANC given (canonical correlation is 0.787).

(b) Canonical Model II: Findings of Rural India, State-Level Analysis

1. Because of high female illiteracy, high total fertility occurs; and also ANC not given, though some Tetanus Toxoid given to mothers (canonical correlation is 0.955).

2. Because less contraceptives used, high crude birth rate occurs, specially when health professionals not available for delivery (canonical correlation is 0.941).
3. Infant mortality is low because female illiteracy low in some states; also contraceptive use moderately high and professional assistance in delivery available (canonical correlation is 0.825).
4. Child mortality rate is low because immunization quite high. Also total fertility rate is high due to less females attending schools (proportion of girls attending school have a definite negative effect on fertility) (canonical correlation is 0.698).

(c) Canonical Model III: Findings of Urban India, State-Level Analysis

1. High TFR occurs because of high female illiteracy, in spite of some contraceptive use. Moderately high child mortality also occurs, because Tetanus Toxoid not given to mothers (i.e., though child surviving in first year, but dies later) (canonical correlation is 0.99).
2. High infant mortality occurs because little immunization is given to children, neither ANC, nor breastfed. Crude birth rate also high (canonical correlation is 0.908).
3. Child mortality rate is high as only partial ANC is given, little breastfeeding, female illiteracy quite high, although some girls attend school (canonical correlation is 0.75).
4. TFR is low, because females attending school (negatively affecting fertility), although female illiteracy is quite high in some states. Contraceptive use also dampen fertility. But, due to high female illiteracy, child mortality high (canonical correlation is 0.60).

(d) Canonical Model IV: All-India Analysis Using State-Level Data (Total Series)

1. High fertility occurs, because of high female illiteracy and also due to very little contraceptives, and high IMR also exists due to little immunization (canonical correlation is 0.88)
2. Less female illiteracy, so less infant mortality occurs, and high total fertility occurs due to less contraceptives used (canonical correlation is 0.66).

(e) Special Factor Analysis Result: Inputs for Model V: Interrelationships between Demographic, Socio-Economic and Population Policy Variables (All-India and States)

1. "High female illiteracy, poverty, high TFR, high IMR, and little health services" dimension (explaining 71.8% of variance).
2. "Prosperity, low TFR, low IMR, more health services and more contraceptive use" dimension (explains another 9.8%).

(f) Canonical Model V: Results of Analysis using Factor Scores as Inputs, taking Rural and Urban Series of States Together

1. Very high TFR, IMR and CMR occur in Indian states, because of poor illiterate females, without minimum sanitation, health and family planning services for them (canonical correlation is 0.904).

(g) Canonical Model VI: Results of Rural India State-Level Series, using Factor Scores and then Canonical Analysis

1. High female illiteracy, poverty, girls not attending school, little health services, nor immunization, nor family planning services; so consequently, high TFR, high IMR, also very high CMR (canonical correlation is 0.91).

(h) Canonical Analysis Model VII: Results of Urban India State-Level Data, using Factor Scores and then Canonical Analysis

1. High IMR, high CMR, high TFR occur even in urban India, because of very high female illiteracy, and virtually no health services, nor family planning services for women and children (Canonical correlation is 0.84).

(i) Canonical Model VIII: Summary Results of Analysis of Individual Level Data of Women and their Demographic Behaviour: Four Types of States emerged according to their Demographic, Socio-economic and Health Positions:

(1) Socio-Economically and Demographically Least Developed States

Four states included in this group are Rajasthan, Bihar, Uttar Pradesh and Madhya Pradesh, and characterized by very high female illiteracy, very high fertility, and very little health services. Also indicate some common canonical links, for instance: (a) more breastfeeding used, so less infant mortality; (b) high female illiteracy and consequently higher number of children ever born(CEB) per mother, in spite of some female sterilization or ANC; and (c) higher average number of children during reproductive span in villages, in spite of some female sterilization or ANC.

(2) Socio-Economically and Demographically Underdeveloped States

This cluster involves Assam, Orissa, Karnataka, Jammu, and Haryana, and is characterized by quite high female illiteracy, moderately high fertility, and slightly more health services. Less immunization and ANC. Represents some common canonical links, viz., (a) more breastfeeding practiced, so less infant mortality, (b) less ANC, so higher CEB, and (c) less average number of children over the reproductive span due to urban residence.

(3) States in Transition: Economically and Demographically Slightly More Developed States

This group includes Gujarat, West Bengal, Punjab, Andhra Pradesh and Maharashtra, and is characterized by moderate female illiteracy, moderately high fertility, and slightly little more health services. Reflects some common canonical-causal equations, such as: (a) more ANC care, so less CEB, (b) more breastfeeding, so less infant mortality, etc. Often, the third canonical relationship is not statistically significant.

(4) Socio-Economically and Demographically Relatively More Developed States

Cluster 4 of demographically developed states includes Goa, Kerala, Tamil Nadu and Himachal Pradesh. These states are characterized by low female illiteracy, low fertility, and quite more health care. Reflect some common causal relationships, e.g., (a) more breastfeeding done, so less infant mortality, (b) more ANC, consequently less CEB, and (c) less female illiteracy, thus less average number of children during reproductive span. They also record more child immunization, female sterilization and contraceptive use.

(j) Canonical Model IX: Findings of Poverty Index and Fertility and Mortality Behaviour (using Individual Level Data)

- First, measuring 'poverty index' at individual level is an unique contribution to study of human development. It gives a simple, meaningful, operational index of deprivation. Basic data can be gathered in usual surveys, and this poverty index can be easily calculated for individual females, showing degree of their deprivation, compared to others. Use of more such useful index will benefit population research.
- Second, apart from devising 'poverty index', this study has also generated a series of useful causal equations between poverty index and fertility/infant mortality, both for less developed states (UP, Bihar, MP, West Bengal, etc.,) and for relatively more developed states of Tamil Nadu and Kerala, with many variations in between. Series of causal findings of such states, using the fine-grained individual level data, are great eye-openers and such linkages prove the main tenet of the study, i.e., basic causal relations between abject poverty and high fertility in India. Application of such innovative research must be encouraged for social research. Then only, relevant policy prescriptions may be untangled, for each state.

Summary II: Serve Underdeveloped and Neglected Regions with Top Priority

One of the most notable findings emphasizes upon the great need for providing development efforts and health services to the most underdeveloped and hitherto neglected regions, on top priority. Based on earlier findings at several levels (Chapters 4 to 11), and considering comprehensively, the following five clusters of Indian states and their (rural/urban) parts can be delineated, which stand at different stages of demographic transition and socio-economic development, and hence require varying degree of actions (Mukherji, 2005b, pp. 1-38). These are not repetition of earlier clusters (of Chapter XI), rather new composite ones, because here rural-urban components of states are also considered (major 18 states, plus minor six north-eastern Indian states and their rural-urban parts, plus Delhi urban, total 49 regional units considered). These are

- ***Cluster I (most underdeveloped regions)**: These underdeveloped regions suffer from very high female illiteracy, high level of poverty, high TFR, high IMR, little health services, and little family planning practices.* Thus, these regions require our greatest attention and very urgent action. They are the most problematic regions, and hold back India's demographic upliftment! This cluster involves four regions, viz., Uttar Pradesh (rural), Bihar (rural), Madhya Pradesh (rural) and Rajasthan (rural).
- ***Cluster II (underdeveloped tribal regions)**: These are special tribal regions, characterized by moderately low female illiteracy, but considerably high poverty and high fertility, with slightly more health services.* This cluster includes Nagaland, Manipur, Meghalaya, Mizoram, Sikkim and Tripura. They include both their rural and urban components. Recently, not much changes are noticed in female illiteracy, nor in health utilization rates. Rather sometimes deterioration can be noticed, perhaps due to their tribal status. However, institutional delivery and child vaccination rates are enhanced lately in most states.
- ***Cluster III (underdeveloped regions)**: These regions also indicate much female illiteracy, widespread poverty, moderately high TFR, moderately high IMR, some health services and family planning practices.* They also need very urgent attention for their transformations. This group includes 12 regions, viz., Uttar Pradesh (urban), Bihar (urban), Rajasthan (urban), Madhya Pradesh (urban), Orissa (rural), Assam (rural), West Bengal (rural), Jammu & Kashmir (rural), Punjab (rural), Gujarat (rural), Haryana (rural) and Maharashtra (rural).
- ***Cluster IV (regions in transition)**: This cluster is characterized by quite low female illiteracy, moderate poverty, quite low TFR, and low IMR, and moderate health services and contraceptive use.* Hence, these regions require further sustained action and efforts for achieving replacement level of fertility. This cluster includes six regions, such as Orissa (urban), Himachal Pradesh (rural), Haryana (urban), Tamil Nadu (rural), Andhra Pradesh (rural) and Karnataka (rural).
- ***Cluster V (relatively more developed regions)**: This cluster of regions depict relatively more prosperity, low TFR, low IMR, relatively little female illiteracy, little poverty, quite good family planning services and*

health services. Thus, they still need persistent efforts for further demographic decline and development This cluster includes 15 regions, namely, Kerala (urban), Goa (urban), Goa (rural), Kerala (rural), Tamil Nadu (urban), Maharashtra (urban), Andhra Pradesh (urban), Karnataka (urban), Gujarat (urban), Himachal Pradesh (urban), Delhi (urban), Punjab (urban), Jammu & Kashmir (urban), West Bengal (urban) and Assam (urban).

Evidently, the first three underdeveloped regions demand and require most urgent action programmes for poverty alleviation and demographic development. Both, poverty reduction programmes and concrete actions for more widespread and better health services to the poor communities, and in inaccessible areas, are very urgently necessary. Unfortunately, neither these are provided so far, nor political will and administrative skill exist. The least developed states and hitherto neglected regions, henceforth, require the greatest actions for poverty liquidation and demographic decline. Only then, India will achieve true and permanent demographic transition.

These are very much neglected and deprived states, not so-called BIMARU states (a great misnomer). They are very wrongly termed as BIMARU states, or sick states, as if their underdeveloped 'stage' is inherent and constitutional, as if these regions did not suffer centuries of much greater neglect and more severe exploitation. By so labelling, conventional scholars, policy makers and government comfortably ignore the stark realities of prolonged historical period of their socio-economic-political deprivation and wrongly put the onus of development upon these deprived regions themselves (as if, likewise, a sick child to be blamed and as if he can automatically recover himself, without outside help). Obviously, such neglected regions require prolonged and utmost care and greater help for their economic and demographic recovery.

Policy Implications

Policy implications of these very crucial findings are very distinct and clear. In this study, female illiteracy is considered as the surrogate or proxy indicator of widespread poverty in India (as none of those surveys ever collected poverty data). The findings thus show that it is the widespread poverty in India, which is most responsible for high levels of fertility and infant mortality, specially in the backward and neglected states of Uttar Pradesh, Bihar, Madhya Pradesh, Rajasthan, Orissa and others. The evil and unjust "syndrome between poverty and high fertility" must be delinked very urgently, if we are really concerned about fertility decline in India.

First, the most fundamental finding that clearly emerges (Chapter V and onwards), separately, for both rural and urban India, is that it is primarily widespread female illiteracy (i.e., poverty) that has caused very high fertility in various states of India. Canonical linkage shows almost a '*one-to-one relationship*' between the two. Unmistakably, this emphasizes that, in India, it is basically very widespread female illiteracy (or abject poverty), which is the fundamental *cause* and high fertility is the resulting *effect*; not vice versa. Compared with female illiteracy factor, other variables contribute much less in determining fertility, often insignificant. These findings therefore reiterate upon the tremendous need for providing general and universal education to all girls and adult women, if we are really sincere about onsetting fertility decline in these Indian states, and also for infant mortality reduction. This step alone will do the miracle! Without combating out massive female illiteracy, specially in innumerable villages in Uttar Pradesh, Bihar, Madhya Pradesh and Rajasthan – where it exceeds 75 to 85 per cent even now – nothing can be changed, no matter how much we may try to motivate scores of millions of poor illiterate women and men to adopt the coveted small family norm! This is the greatest requirement. Now!

Second, and simultaneously, there is also great requirement for enhancing family planning programmes, as well as ANC, child immunization, MCH care, safe motherhood, child nutrition, and all aspects of Reproductive and Child Health (RCH) care services. Canonical findings done at several levels in Chapter V to VII amply testify these. These reiterate that all crucial aspects of primary health services must be activated and strengthened, specially in rural, backward, and hitherto neglected and inaccessible regions. Thus, socio-economic development efforts for poverty alleviation, as well as programmes for providing family planning, safe motherhood-child survival programmes, and catering reproductive health should go, simultaneously, not in isolation! The two must be equally emphasized, not excluding other. Notwithstanding, it must be categorically emphasized that current abysmally low health utilization rates will rise, only, only after, poverty reduction seriously done! Not without that first step!

Third, the crucial causal relationship between illiteracy among the mothers (i.e., poverty) and very high level of infant deaths and child mortality has also emerged time and again (so also between high TFR and female illiteracy) (in many canonical findings of Chapter V to VIII). These evil syndromes between female illiteracy (indeed an index of abject poverty), infant mortality and fertility must be delinked, before demographic decline will set in all parts of India, firmly and securely. Without such very fundamental changes, very little can be expected and achieved. Such causal relationships are repeatedly confirmed by mathematically very highly powerful canonical findings, performed through numerous canonical tests.

Fourth, specifically regarding findings of Model V (Chapter VI) (dealing with total series state-level data), policy import of resultant canonical linkage is very loud and clear: very high fertility and very high infant mortality/child mortality rate prevail in the states, basically due to very high female illiteracy, both among adult women and young girls, and massive poverty among them. Such sordid situations are further compounded by dismal health and family planning services, specially lack of contraceptives, child immunization and ANC. It poignantly tells a very sad story of complete chaos and utter neglect of the poor and downtrodden, specially in pauperized villages and urban slums. Such a finding should be considered as the great eye-opener for all concerned: policy makers, planners, bureaucrats, social scientists, and everybody else. Most precious six decades after India's independence are wasted in foolish complacency and utter neglect about the need of the poor masses – who are reeling under abject poverty, inequity, injustice, and extreme exploitation. The above crucial findings are highlighting the same hard reality, time and again.

Fifth, analyses of data of individuals women respondents and their demographic, socio-economic, and health service utilization rates (Chapter VII) have revealed the following four groups of states, based on their specific characteristics on such dimensions:

- Socio-Economically and Demographically Least Developed States: Rajasthan, Bihar, Uttar Pradesh and Madhya Pradesh.
- Socio-Economically and Demographically Underdeveloped States: Assam, Orissa, Karnataka, Jammu and Haryana.
- States in Transition: Economically and Demographically Slightly More Developed States: West Bengal, Gujarat, Punjab, Andhra Pradesh and Maharashtra.
- Socio-Economically and Demographically Relatively More Developed States: Kerala, Tamil Nadu, Goa and Himachal Pradesh.

As such, they require differential action priorities, that is, top priorities for the most underdeveloped states (Group 1), down to just sustained action for relatively prosperous states (Group 4), with two step-like variations in between.

Sixth, apart from contributing 'poverty index' (which must be encouraged for more use in population research), Chapter VIII has also amply testified numerous meaningful causal equations between 'poverty index' in the one hand and 'fertility' and 'infant mortality' rates, on the other. This was performed, both for less developed states, as well as for relatively more developed states Innumerable causal linkages of such states (that used fine-grained individual-level data) may be treated as findings of supreme importance. Such equations also proved the central notion of this volume, i.e., "causal relations exist between abject poverty and high fertility" in India. When more such meaningful analytical design would be attempted, then, more suitable policies may be generated for each state.

Seventh, moreover, recent NFHS-II survey data (1998-99) are also analyzed in Chapter X, and found that almost similar findings persisted as that of NHFS-I sets of results. So, all major findings remained almost the same, albeit in slight modified form; and such reconfirmation tremendously verified the strength of the Demographic Field Theory and its analytical design, evolved here. Likewise, the crucial policy implications of all main findings are also testified. Nothing changes in India overnight. Levels of fertility and infant mortality, of course, have declined, but not substantially, specially in the most populous and backward states of Uttar Pradesh, Bihar, Madhya Pradesh and Rajasthan. Thus, maximum efforts are now required to eliminate widespread female illiteracy and poverty, and to delink them from high level of fertility and high infant mortality, without any further waste of time and vacillations. This is the main message of this research.

Eighth, Census (2001) and SRS (2003) data also reveal that while fertility and infant mortality rates have improved only very slightly, the poverty and female illiteracy situations have not improved substantially, in spite of tall claims of rapid economic growth in India during the last decade.

Ninth, Reproductive and Child Health (RCH) surveys (Round-I, 1998-99) and (Round-II, 2002-04) data are also minutely examined which unraveled that improvements over the most health service indicators have been quite slow, and these require much more strenuous efforts before Millennium Development Goals (MDGs) can be actualized. Moreover, most of the earlier findings about "syndrome of poverty, fertility and less utilization of health services in India" are also reiterated, even by the recent-most data.

Finally, very wide and very persistent spatial variations do emerge in all demographic indicators (TFR, IMR), also in all socio-economic indicators (poverty, *kachcha* houses, female illiteracy), as well as in health indicators (per cent of child immunization not given, unmet need, or ANC care not provided) over various states. Such variations are very prominent over backward and neglected states and their respective remote and inaccessible zones. Not only spatial variations, but wide variations also occur over time (1992-2004). These are typical backward areas that require top priority attention. Such findings are summed up in Chapter XI. Relevant policies and strategies are also recommended in this chapter.

Various Policies

"Developing countries have continued to grapple with the persistence of mass poverty endemic disease, malnutrition, environmental degradation, and gross income inequality, all of which have caused a degree of human suffering that far exceeds what has been caused by terrorist attacks" (Ramos, 2006, p. 30). India is also plagued by such crucial problems. "The Philippine government has proposed that half of all scheduled debt payments be withheld for a specified period, to be

Figure 29

Required Policies and Strategies for Demographic and Health Improvement

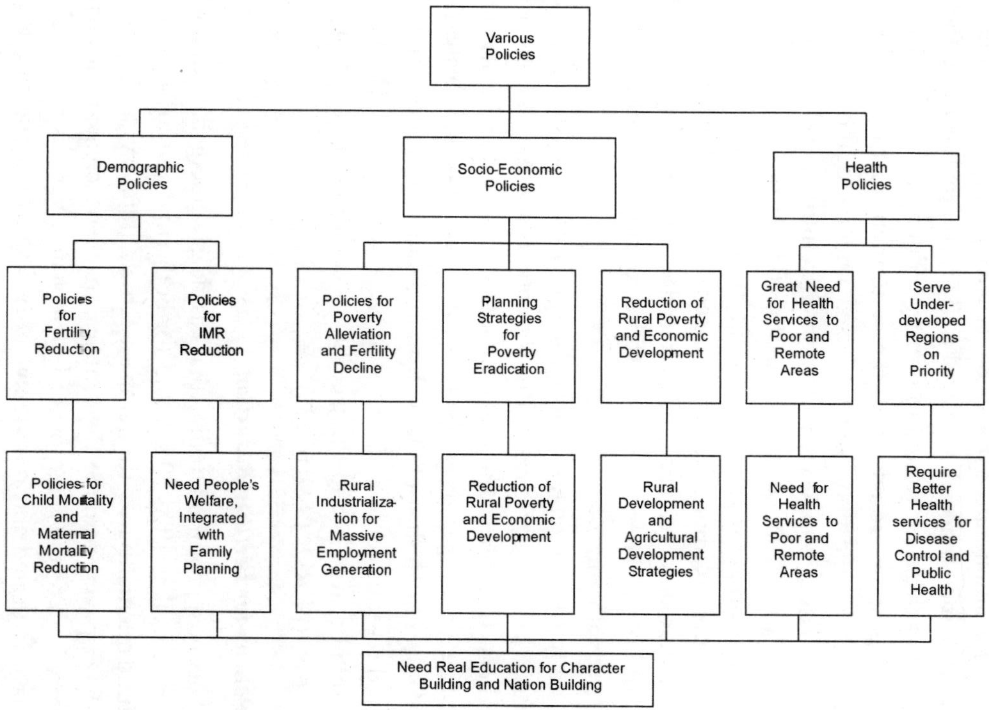

invested in reforestation, clean water, housing, food production, primary health care, sanitation, basic education, farm-to-market roads, ecologically sound tourism, micro-finance, and related projects" (ibid.).

To ameliorate some such crucial problems in India, various policies and strategies are very briefly recommended (see Figure 29). Some of these are related to fertility reduction and mortality control, whereas some are related to the betterment of basic health services, specially to the poor and neglected regions. Some other deal with crucial issues of poverty reduction, agriculture development, massive employment generation and rural reconstruction. Some policies also reiterate upon the great need for integrating rural development actions and family planning strategies. Needless to say that, all such policies and strategies are very much interrelated and need to be very highly coordinated. However, not all strategies could be illustrated, but they are equally important.

In this context, we must also remember that, in India, "there are many lessons: some can learn from others and others can teach to yet others. If full/near full literacy could be reached in Kerala and Tamil Nadu, if cooperatives could work in Gujarat and Maharashtra, if Madhya Pradesh could launch an innovative education programme, if land reforms could be initiated in West Bengal and if green revolution could be sustained in Punjab, there is a lot to learn from such experiences" (NIRD, 1999, p. 121).

Policies for Fertility Reduction

The most profound finding that has clearly emerged, both for 1992-93 set as well as 1998-99 set, and for both rural and urban India, is that fundamentally it is the rampant female illiteracy, and, consequently abject poverty among the females, that have created and maintained very high fertility in most of Indian states. Various canonical linkages have indicated and repeatedly verified almost 'a one-to-one relationship' between the two, between poverty (i.e., female illiteracy) and high fertility. Most persistently, it reiterates that in India widespread female illiteracy has been the 'cause' and high fertility has been the 'effect', not vice-versa. As Tables 52, 54, and 56 have demonstrated, compared with female illiteracy (or poverty) factor, other factors have contributed much less, often insignificant, to determine fertility.

Most conventional demographers and population specialists argue that the relationships between female illiteracy (or poverty) and high fertility is already known, or the relationship is two-way, or that we are yet unsure about which one is the cause and which one is the effect? (Mukherji, 1983c, pp. 75-125). Some researchers even argue: "what is new about it?" So on and so forth. In these ways, they continue to discourage correct and meaningful research to arise, and consequently, always deemphasize the fundamental importance of such a crucial causal relationship. It seems that their hidden objective is – thence, no need arises to take a very serious and soulful concern of this oppressive phenomena, nor to take concrete actions to combat against such agonizing situation! And, then, status quo will be maintained for their own vested interests. I have heard such arguments infinite times, all through my life and in most conferences, both in India and abroad. And, in the meantime, priceless 60 years of Indian demographic time and economic history have vanished, without transforming the fate of millions and millions of the poor and the downtrodden masses, without dampening their high fertility and high mortality levels. Doubtlessly, such conventional attitude and utterly wrong perspective will not solve the burgeoning problems of very rapid population explosion in India!

In this study, both with 1992-93 data and 1998-99 data, very high powered canonical linkages have repeatedly testified and confirmed the great truth, that is, widespread female illiteracy and abject poverty among the masses is the primary cause of high fertility and high infant mortality in India, and that full-fledged war against such evil syndrome must be fought out urgently.

Policy implications of these very fundamental causal relations are crystal clear. It highlights the most urgent need for providing universal functional education to all girls and adult women of India, if we are truly serious about the onsetting fertility decline in hitherto neglected and lagging states, and for infant mortality reduction. Such a massive education programme alone will perform the great miracle. It will definitely bring down fertility and infant and child mortality levels, as various canonical linkages have clearly demonstrated. Without waging a war against the widespread illiteracy among the Indian women, specially in rural areas (Bihar, MP, UP, Rajasthan, where it exceeds even 65-70%), no dent upon the demographic scenario of the country can be made. This is simply impossible, no matter how much we may vainly try to motivate pauperized and illiterate women (and men) to adopt family planning and contraceptives. This is the greatest need of the present time. Sooner this is soulfully understand and acted upon, the better for people and for India (see Figure 29).

Second, as many canonical linkages have testified, both in rural and urban India, there is an urgent need to revamp the family planning programmes, as well as augment ANC care, child immunization programmes, maternal and child health (MCH) care, and all aspects of the reproductive health (RCH), including reproductive tract illnesses (RTI, STI, and HIV/AIDS). Immediate requirement is to activate all such crucial aspects of primary health services, specially in rural, backward, and hitherto neglected regions, and remote and inaccessible tracts. This is almost equally true for urban India, as urban poverty has swelled in many mega cities and large urban centres (Mukherji, 2005e, pp. 25-50; 2005f, p. 1-30; 2006, pp. 1-21). Therefore, both programmes for socio-economic upliftment of the poor and illiterates, and programmes for providing safe motherhood, child survival, and reproductive health should go simultaneously.

Another very important issue concerns with people's lack of access to, and utilization of, health care facilities. As Mishra (2005, pp. 65-81) has also found, wide regional variations exist in people's access to health services, and their utilization rates between the backward states (like UP, MP, Bihar, Rajasthan, Orissa) and the developed states (Karnataka, Gujarat, Tamil Nadu, Goa, Kerala).

NFHS-2 data also indicate that Bihar, Madhya Pradesh, Rajasthan and Uttar Pradesh utilized far less than the low socio-economic group of all-India in ANC care, child delivery, and post-natal care. Conversely, Kerala, Tamil Nadu, Andhra Pradesh, Goa and Karnataka and urban areas of some other states have utilized better than high socio-economic group of all-India (NFHS-II, 2000, various tables).

Thus, the policy prescriptions should be: (1) there is a great need for providing easy access of poor people to the health care facilities in all regions, specially the backward regions; and (2) to make the most efficient management (of men, money and materials) for ensuring the best possible utilization of whatever little health systems exist, particularly for the poor (Udupa and Mukherji, 1988, pp. 120-75; Mukherji, 1989a, pp. 125-35).

These backward areas are: Uttar Pradesh (eastern UP, south-western UP, Terai of UP), Bihar (northern and eastern districts), West Bengal (hilly tracts, north Bengal, Sundarban forests, south-west parts), Andhra Pradesh (coastal, northern and western districts), Jharkhand (tribal belts), Uttaranchal (hilly districts), Chhattisgarh (tribal zones), Rajasthan (western parts), even in Maharashtra (Vidharba region and eastern zones) and Gujarat (Dangs, western semi-arid zones, and elsewhere, especially in their remote, inaccessible, and tribal zones (Table 58, Figures 25-28).

The health policy in India for the next 20 years should, then, be to provide very urgently the best possible health services to such backward regions and states on top priority. This effort must be equipped with the best health management information system (MIS) and operational research for optimizing the health services, even within the available resources. All the requirements for men, money and materials (i.e., doctors and paramedics) should be given on top priority, along with maximum budget allocation. Then, and then only, high levels of fertility and mortality in these backward regions can ever be dampened. That will bring great demographic dividends, both to these backward states, as well as to entire India (see Mukherji, 1983b, pp. 1-141; Mukherji, 1989b, pp. 325-75).

Policies for Infant Mortality Reduction

Third, the causal connection between illiterate mothers and very high infant mortality has occurred time and again; so also the causal links between high TFR and widespread female illiteracy. These evil syndromes between fertility, infant mortality, and female illiteracy – which is indeed an index of abject poverty – must be broken, before demographic development will prevail over entire India, permanently. Without such fundamental changes in the Indian society and economy, very little can be hoped for. We need to take correct actions very urgently, without further directionless thoughts and slipshod planning, without further waste of most precious time (see Figure 29).

Recently, Save The Children (STC) group, a UK-based NGO has revealed in their Global Report on Infant Mortality that India has the highest infant and maternal mortality in the world: about 1.1 million newborns die every year in the country, and nearly 150,000 women perish during childbirth annually (Save The Children, 2006). Every minute an Indian woman dies during child birth, while seven infants die before their first month (ibid., 2006).

UNICEF (2005) also reports that India ranks a dismal 131 out of 193 countries in the under-five mortality ranking (U5MR) – a critical indicator of the well-being of the children. The report cautions that "there cannot be lasting progress if we continue to overlook the children most in need – the poorest and most vulnerable, the exploited and the abused."

India scores low on most basic indicators with 30 per cent of infants born with a low birth weight and 18 per cent of under-fives severely underweight. Primary school enrolment is at 77 per cent and only 61 per cent of school entrants reach grade five. The percentage of central government expenditure allocated to education is a mere 2 per cent in India as compared to 18 per cent in Bangladesh (ibid., 2005).

UNICEF report identifies four key areas in which 'swift and decisive action' needs to take place: poverty and inequality, armed conflict and states which do not take responsibility for their children, HIV/AIDs and discrimination (ibid., 2005).

The report further hopes that "if we can get it right for children – if we can deliver on our commitments and enable every child to enjoy the right of a childhood, to health, education, equality, and protection – we can get it right for people for all ages. I believe we can" (ibid., 2005).

Policies for Child Mortality and Maternal Mortality Reduction

Table 57 has revealed that in India, even as late as 2002-04, one-fourth (26.5%) of all women in reproductive ages did not have access to any kind of ANC care. Only a meagre 16.4 per cent of all eligible women got full ANC care (that includes at least three visits to PHC for ANC check-up, plus one TT injection and 100 IFA tablets during their current pregnancy). Only 40 per cent received institutional delivery and only 46 per cent got safe delivery. The rest were at the mercy of fate and chance survival. No wonder that maternal mortality in India is one of the highest in the world, next only to the poorer sub-Saharan African nations. The situation gets more pathetic in the villages, backward districts and inaccessible areas. The great need is vastly to improve and optimize the ANC services in PHCs and CHCs, specially in remote tracts and neglected states (see Figure 29).

The situation of child immunization and child health care services is neither better. Even in 2002-04, one-fifth (20%) of all children in age 12-23 months never got any kind of child vaccination, only 46 per cent of them got full immunization (Table 57). Only 19 per cent of infants got exclusive breastfeeding during first 4-12 months. Only 19 per cent got Oral Rehydration Solution (ORS) during diarrhoea (2 weeks prior to survey), and 26 per cent of them did not receive treatment for pneumonia (2 weeks prior to survey) (RCH, 2005, Key Indicators Table, pp. 1-6). Consequently, infant mortality in India is pathetically still very high, i.e., 79 infant deaths per 1,000 born annually, even in 2004 (UN, 2004). And child mortality is well above 110, often exceeding to 130 in remote areas of Orissa and Uttar Pradesh. This is simply unpardonable, as happening even 60 years after independence! Infant mortality and child mortality control are morally mandatory and absolutely necessary in a developing country like India. Most such diseases are preventable (as water-borne and air-borne diseases) and must be controlled.

In a recent article, Banerji (2005, pp. 3243-57) has untangled many discrepancies and shortcomings in Government of India rural public health system and policies, as reflected in recent National Rural Health Mission (NRHM) document (GoI, 2004). Such discrepancies are:

> "(1) decline in the organization and management of rural public health system, as only family planning given overriding importance, neglecting primary health care; (2) current focus only upon "Selective Primary Health Care" (SPHC)) (like care for tuberculosis, malaria, fileria, etc.), instead of providing Primary Health Care (PHC) services to the rural poor; (3) serious neglect of rural public

health system and very little growth and expansion of Primary Health Centres (PHCs) and Community Health Centres (CHCs) during last two decades; (4) commodification of the health system, with its increasing focus on privatization and spiraling drug prices beyond the reach of common people; and (5) "Ministry of Health and Family Welfare (MoHFW) and their political masters had never been serious about the plight of deprived sections of the population. Otherwise how can one explain the "advanced stage of decay" of the health services six decades after Independence?"

So, top of all, a paradigm shift is urgently necessary both at central and state levels, from current Specific Public Health Care (SPHC) to old Public Health Care (PHC), and make themselves fully aware of the great need for providing such basic health care services, and rectify such rapid decline over last six decades. India's public heath care systems cannot shirk from its basic duties, leaving poor millions at the mercy of expensive private doctors and merciless private hospitals. It should be made fully responsible to cater to these basic survival needs of millions of hapless children. Top priority must be given to most essential public health needs. The PHCs and CHCs, thus, must be revamped for better health delivery and to optimize health services, within the available resources.

Besides, Mobile Health Vans (MHVs), with child specialists, doctors, paramedics, and all necessary treatment facilities, must make bi-weekly rounds to centrally located villages, and cater to the needs of all surrounding village population, specially in backward districts and inaccessible tracts.

Regarding maternal mortality, the situation needs much care and attention. "According to experts, more than half a million women die from complications in pregnancy or childbirth; this is more than deaths of girls and women by AIDs, hunger, disease or war. And what is shocking is that though the principal causes of these deaths are known and can either be prevented or treated, women still continue to die in large numbers" (Sharma, 2006, p. 32).

"If budgets fail to be sensitive to needs of the poor and women, resources will not be adequately directed to removing gender inequalities and attaining equity goals. Hence, women will keep dying and we will keep continue to make noises regarding skewed sex ratio, which is 922 girls to 1,000 boys (ibid.).

Another recent article pinpoints that "the logistic regression results also show that in both the states (Bihar and Madhya Pradesh) women with high SLI (Standard of Living Index) are experiencing fewer complications. Women with higher birth order are having more complications. Also women who are receiving ante-natal check-up are having significantly less complications" (Jain and Parasuraman, 2004, pp. 196-221). That is, slightly well-off women get more access to ANC care and have less complications; a finding, which has great policy import.

"A sizable proportion of women received no ante-natal care and even those who received ante-natal care are rarely provided with care or advice considered standard components of ante-natal care services" (ibid.).

Given the limitations, still some improvement in child and maternal mortality and morbidity is surely possible, as in north-east Indian states. Rama Rao et al. (2004, pp. 39-55) found that "to minimize and control anemia and morbidity from common disease, the mothers associations, present in almost all villages and involved in socio-religious activities, should be approached to provide education on household hygiene, proper preparation of food and on the practice of effective child breastfeeding as well as the knowledge of right time of solid food supplementation".

Thus, child and maternal mortality reduction is very much required, and possible, specially among the poor segments of the society, particularly in backward states (UP, MP, Bihar, West Bengal, Orissa, Jharkhand, Chhattisgarh, etc.) and their neglected districts, which cannot afford to have expensive health services, nor access to PHCs.

Three Alternative Models for Demographic Decline in India

In India, three distinct models of demographic transition and development have recently emerged: (a) Kerala model, (b) Tamil Nadu model, and very recently, (c) Andhra Pradesh model. Kerala model is now quite famous, which focused on promotion of almost universal general literacy, specially female literacy, its long traditions of social reforms, women's empowerment, women's easy access to education, health services and employment, and also to prosperity through massive emigration to the Middle-East (Zachariah, Rajan, et al., 1994, pp. 20-64; Kodoth and Eapen, 2005, pp. 3278-86; Jeromi, 2005, pp. 3267-77). Thus, in the Kerala model, the cause for rapid fertility reduction was attributed primarily to high female literacy and social reforms, such that demographic decline has occurred there in spite of lack of spectacular economic prosperity. Frequently, the Kerala model is recommended for replication in other states, where poverty is still high, but female illiteracy can be enhanced, rather easily.

In the Tamil Nadu model, the reasons mainly attributed to are a long social tradition of village elders advising to all newly married couples on the critical issue of small family norm (just after wedding ceremony), and efficient health service administrations. So, it is argued that demographic decline has occurred in Tamil Nadu, in spite of slow economic development and prevailing poverty. Of course, this model can also be replicated elsewhere, provided health delivery systems are equally efficient and similar socially-committed advisory elders are also available in experimental states.

In the Andhra Pradesh model, the causal reasons are found to be three: (1) widespread distribution of rice at Rs 2 per kilo; (2) peer group pressures from most village residents upon each male sterilization defaulter, until he is sterilized; and (3) considerably efficient mass male sterilization camps (Mukherji, 2000b, pp. 1-35; IIPS, Hyderabad Conference, 2001, pp. 1-52). Here, the quick success story thus involved much coercion, direct or indirect.

As a concluding comment, it can be said that the Demographic Field Theory perspective, as presented in this book, permits all possible alternative social or policy interventions, without any problems, provided it does not involve any form of coercion upon the human beings, rather encourages them to stand on their own legs and hold their head high! Any kind of models can be adopted, within the demographic field concept, provided it suits the local socio-cultural milieu, and involves people's wilful participation. The ultimate target of the Field Theory is to wipe out all socio-economic-political-cultural barriers from the human fields, and to make humans free from all bondages!

Great Need for Health Services to Poor and Remote Areas

The greatest need of the hour is to cater for the need of health services of the poor and the needy, and the downtrodden people, and to provide the basic health services to the remote and inaccessible areas, over the entire national space (Mukherji, 1989a, pp. 25-125) (see Figure 29). Considerable regional variations are found over national space and among different classes of communities, where proper and adequate health services have not yet reached, specially among the poor and illiterate women, children, the weak, the downtrodden, and the destitute. In spite of 60 years of planning, the development has not reached these poor communities, specially the tribals, Scheduled Castes, hill tribes, landless agricultural labourers, poor peasants, and people living in remote tracts. Development process has not at all touched their lives! Happiness is the most unfortunate lady who has not yet seen the faces of such ocean of helpless humanity!

These communities, as well as these neglected and backward regions, remain perpetually backward and neglected – specially in north-east Indian hill states, Darjeeling and Sikkim hills, eastern UP, northern and southern parts of tribal Bihar, tribal zones of MP, desert tracts of Rajasthan, tribal belts and most undeveloped and poverty-stricken Orissa and West Bengal (Mukherji, 1995a, pp. 1-35). Soon proper and adequate delivery of all health services must be provided to such tracts.

These neglected tracts and backward communities must be provided with Comprehensive Mobile Health Vans (CMHVs), along with all accessories. Only with very sincere and concerted efforts, coupled with a very strong political will, an improved health system can be set and imbedded all over India. Only with such firm and sincere efforts, the war against the 'syndrome of poverty and high fertility' can be won in India! Otherwise, not. This is the distinct lesson emerging from this piece of research.

Need Total Stop to Illegal Migration from Bangladesh

One of the greatest needs of India, now, is to totally stop all illegal migration of Muslims from Bangladesh. Indeed, grave dangers from India's eastern borders are thousand times greater than that from western borders. Because while small infiltrators of terrorists from Pakistan can be fought out with army and ammunitions, but daily, constant and invisible invasion of massive illegal migration from Bangladesh is totally ignored, disregarded and unprotected. In reality, this is almost always welcomed by most political parties for their most mischievous vote-bank politics! And, thus silent invasion is secretly and very gravely changing the entire religious demographic character of India (see Joshi et al., 2002, pp. 10-200). Such daily, non-stop and invasive illegal migration is secretly eating out the very existence of India. Most political parties and the nation act as completely ignorant, totally blind, on this most crucial issue of the country's very existence! Alas! Soon, India will be found only in the Internet! Not in reality!

Not only illegal migrants, but terrorists, ammunitions, explosives, disintegrating forces and militants are also exported from Bangladesh to India, through those routes: West Bengal, Assam and Tripura.

Solution lies in providing very urgent and complete seal of entire 12,000 kms (and over) borders with Bangladesh, heavily fencing with barbed wire and all military installations, and constant army vigilance. Benefit of this step alone will exceed that of endless Five-Year Plans over many millenniums!

Need to Reduce Differential Fertility between Two Communities

Chapter 11 has amply demonstrated that in India, according to NFHS-I (1992-93), the Muslim fertility was 4.2 children, which was 40 per cent higher than that of average Hindu fertility (2.7 children) (NFHS, 1995). Muslim fertility declined slightly later, but not considerably. According to NFHS-II (1998-99) also, Muslim fertility levels are at least one child higher than that of the general category of Hindu fertility; everywhere, irrespective of states, regions, rural or urban residence (NFHS, 2000). Census 2001 also demonstrated this truth glaringly, even when the respective population growth rates are re-calculated (after much hue and cry from pseudo-secularists about comparability, data for Kashmir are excluded from Census 2001, as 1991 Census not done there). It was still found that Muslim population growth in India was 29.9 per cent during 1991-2001 vis-à-vis 19.9 per cent among the Hindus (Census of 2001, Provisional

Population Totals). The fertility differentials between the two communities are too large to ignore. This higher growth may be due to four reasons: (a) their higher fertility rates, (b) massive illegal migration, (c) higher population growth rates among those immigrants and their progenies, and (4) illegal conversions. All such problems must be thoroughly investigated, and counter-veiling policies must be made.

However, most Muslim women and men are very poor, illiterate, unemployed and do not have access to health and family planning services, nor access to RCH services. They also suffer much greater social inequalities and have considerably much less women empowerment. Proportionately, their men-folk also live more below the poverty line. Most are poor, illiterate and unemployed. The society is much more rigid, regarding women's literacy, education, employment and emancipation. It seems that all such factors have adverse effects upon their fertility and infant and child mortality levels. All such reasons must be understood, and relevant policies must be adopted accordingly.

So, the solution lies in providing such socio-economic benefits to them (specially women's education and self-employment opportunities), and their easy and effective access to health and family planning services. When hope and aspirations will be sowed in their lives, naturally, the small family norm will emerge. The demographic benefits, naturally, will be lower levels of fertility, infant and child mortality, as well as lower maternal mortality. Such positive effects will greatly benefit the community's economy, society and health.

Need People's Welfare, Integrated with Family Planning

The solution lies in raising the levels of productivity, employment, wages and incomes among these poor landless agricultural labourers, petty farmers and poverty-stricken rural workers. Rural regeneration efforts are required to be very much integrated with population welfare and family planning programmes, and to be undertaken integrally, not in isolation (Mukherji, 1983c, pp. 1-35) (see Figure 2a and 2b). When their levels of agricultural productivity, income and consumption would rise, then, they would be able to send off their children to school and would begin to look up for hope, aspiration and betterment in future. Then, they will be able to cater for the needs of their children and would cease to expect economic returns from the child labour. Once the seeds for hope and future prospect would be sown, then, these poor peasants and labourers would stop multiplying sheer hands of labour; and consequently, their fertility level would definitely begin to drop; in the same way it has dropped among the educated and the privileged few (see Figure 2a and 2b).

Enhancement of child and maternal health services and other health care of rural primary health centres should consist very important parts of such rural reconstruction programmes. For, control of infant mortality and maternal mortality is both morally mandatory and demographically desirable. For controlling widespread child malnutrition in India, much more than mid-day meals and conventional child nutritional investment programmes will be required; otherwise, India will continue to remain much behind nutrition levels of sub-Saharan Africa (Alderman, 2005, p. 4842).

Require Better Health Services for Disease Control and Public Health

An utter neglect of rural primary health care services emerges in the country. The crucial problem is that now emphasis is mainly given only upon 'Selective Primary Health Care' (tuberculosis, malaria, fileria, etc), instead of providing 'Primary Health Care' to rural poor. And, here lies the roots of dangerous neglect of public health services in India. Concomitantly, health services have gone out of the reach of poor and common people, specially in villages. Privatization of health services is also very rampant. The poor and hapless rural people, and also poor urban dwellers, and the senior citizens, are all put at the mercy of very expensive private doctors, private hospitals, and spiraling drug prices. And, the government is a mute spectator, became a shirker of its essential responsibilities – in a democracy – to provide minimum health services to poor masses. This is a very ominous sign, and soon must be rectified.

Besides, efficient use of Management Information System (MIS) in health and operation research for optimizing health delivery, within given resources and infrastructure, in PHCs/CHCs, is required to be vigorously promoted to maximize rural public health services (Mukherji, 1989a, pp. 25-141). Moreover, the two kinds of lack of motivation, viz., (a) lack of motivation among the PHC's health workers, and (b) lack of motivation among the women users, must also be suitably tackled (Udupa and Mukherji, 1988, pp. 51-171).

Policies for Poverty Alleviation and Fertility Decline

One UN study (1997, pp. 41-120) recommended the following steps for poverty reduction:

1. To empower the individuals, households and communities to gain greater control over their life and resources by:
    - Ensuring their access to assets as a protection against vulnerability: access to credit and other financial services are vital, especially security of tenure, housing and land.
    - Ensuring food security for households and family members.
    - Ensuring education and health for all, along with access to reproductive health care, family planning and safe water and sanitation.
    - Building social safety nets to prevent people from falling into destitution and disaster (UNDP, 1997, pp. 90-121).
2. Strengthen gender equality in order to empower women and to release their vast underused energy and creativity. Poverty eradication without gender equality is impossible.
3. Accelerate pro-poor growth which will:
    - Restore full employment and opportunity expansion as a high priority.
    - Create an enabling environment for small-scale agriculture and the informal sector.
    - Restructure public expenditure and taxation to support poverty reduction.
    - Reverse environmental degradation.
    - Create more employment.
4. To ensure an active state, committed to eradicating poverty and providing an enabling environment for political participation and partnership for pro-poor growth (UNDP, 1997, pp. 105-10).

Gender and Poverty Alleviation

Gender aspect of poverty reduction must also be considered. Many studies found that women and girls in the family suffer disproportionately more, even within the poor families (Mitra and Mukherji, 1977, pp. 32-79); and the women also display more characteristics of poverty and deprivation (Radhakrishna and Ray, 2005, pp. 52-53). Even in 1998-99, 36 per cent of ever-married women (aged 15-49) showed more chronic energy deficiency (CED) (NFHS-II, 2000).

Women are also more vulnerable and face discrimination and marginalization in labour markets (in terms of different wages and other deprivation). They also have less social, legal and political rights and capital resources and thus suffer more poverty and deprivation (World Bank, 1991, pp. 11-23). Widows are more vulnerable and thus suffer doubly. Hence, in poverty reduction programmes and policies, such deprived people and vulnerable gender must be given greater attention and priorities.

Gender inequality is a very serious disadvantage for women and girls. Long ago, in four important studies (Mukherji, 1982b, pp. 12-16; Mukherji, 1982c, p. 4; Mukherji, 1990, pp. 1-25, Mukherji, 1994, pp 1-25), the concept of the 'demographic and economic field of women' was developed, which conceptualized that all the socio-economic-political-cultural components of a woman's life must be treated integrally, not in isolation, linking them with her demographic behaviour and population policy considerations; treated as a whole, as a gestalt. And, as a corollary, they further emphasized that social and economic investment made on women's development will be much more rewarding than that made on men, because such effort will not only liberate her from clutches of poverty, illiteracy and ill-health, but will also benefit her children's education, health and future employment prospects.

Only very recently, UNDP has also echoed similarly: "Poor women are less likely to be educated and less likely to receive ante-natal care when they are pregnant. Their children are less likely to survive and less likely to complete school, perpetuating a cycle of deprivation that is transmitted across generations" (UNDP, 2005, p. 25). Thus, as envisaged above, programmes for poverty reduction, gender inequalities, and health provision for women and their children must be very tightly integrated. The rewards will be many splendoured. Benefits!

Planning Strategies for Poverty Eradication

Widespread illiteracy and pathetic poverty among the masses are two great curses in India. In this context, we must remember the great utterance of Swami Vivekananda, who said 113 years ago (in 1893), that "education itself is a great privilege, which is available only to a handful privileged few, at the expense of the great illiterate masses who are made to pay for the education of the elites" (Swami Vivekananda, 1893, Complete Work, Centenary Volume I, 1963).

This is extracted from the poor classes in the form of indirect taxes. So, it is our bounden duty to repay our great debt to the illiterate masses, at whose expenses the elite and educated classes get this privilege. We should give education to the illiterate masses, specially to hundreds of millions of illiterate women living over entire rural India. This alone will do the wonder, by drastically reducing their fertility, as it has already demonstrated among the privileged and educated classes!

In the same vein, poverty is a great curse. The great majority of people of India, especially in rural parts, are reeling under extreme poverty. Again, according to Swami Vivekananda, "Poverty is man-made; not God-made. It is the educated and privileged elites who deliberately maintain poverty among the poor and the downtrodden, and do nothing to alleviate it." He further thundered: "I hold all educated people as traitors, who being educated at the expense of the illiterate masses, do nothing for them" (Swami Vivekananda, 1894, Complete Work, Centenary Volume I, 1963).

The rural people, thus, denied of education, employment, and any scope for uplift, are bound to remain in the bondage of poverty, fatalism and utter despair (since many centuries). We greatly need real planning for the poor, and its true implementation. The planning, which will directly benefit the poor; not to be usurped by the middlemen and exploiters; not to disappear in the political debacles; not to be camouflaged under illusory ideas of downward-filtration of developmental benefits from the rich to the poor. We need real planning for the poor and employment for the poor, not current jobless growth, entangled with slavery to globalization, which hurts the poor most!

So, our most sacred duty is to uplift the masses of the poor from poverty level, in the same way as handful rich, educated and privileged classes got affluence (see Figures 2a and b and 29). Fertility level of the poor peasants and labourers will automatically decline, as it came down among advantaged groups (Mukherji, 1983c, pp. 10-121). Because scientific explanation states that, under a given condition (i.e., no poverty), if a true event has occurred once (i.e., fertility has declined among non-poor educated families), then, it will definitely recur again, if the same condition is brought forth again. Only the vested interests do not want to face this glaring truth; and ritualistically preach about onsetting fertility decline, without ever changing the most dismal socio-economic context of poverty, within which poor masses are imbedded since many centuries! Such utopian idea will never work. You cannot force to swallow contraceptive down the throats of hungry and impoverished women and people! (Mukherji, 2005c, p. 38-75).

In India, presently utter 'jobless growth' is occurring, under liberalization, privatization and globalization. High-flying movie-multiplexes, shopping malls, scores of fly overs are built, presenting a pseudo-picture of virtual affluence, under psychedelic neo-signs. But, in reality, only a handful of rich and novo-rich get fattened, at the expense of hundreds of millions of impoverished masses – who are relegated to a stature of beggars and destitute (Mukherji, 2006, pp. 160-85). Lands are perched, jobs are very scarce, factories locked out, and farmers forced to commit suicide for non-payment of loans on high interest. Prices of daily commodities soar very high. Corruption is very rampant, everywhere. The academia is bankrupt and soulless! They may lynch you, if you ever dare to talk about poverty in India! Very poor governance is the rule. Political bungling and worst type of corruption have eaten out the very basic root of the Indian society. Criminals rule and move around barechested in the broad day light!

So, economic growth is occurring in India currently, but without any distributive justice. Even 60 years after the independence, abject poverty is very widespread and visible everywhere, specially in rural areas and in urban slums. Their makeshift cheap houses are bulldozed every time, in order to give space for parking lots, shopping malls and flyovers. Jobs are nowhere. The youths are forced to turn to crime, violence, despair, living lives without any hope and aspirations!

Thus, in India, the economic growth has to be fully integrated with distributive justice, and with really effective work programmes for massive employment generation, specially in villages and urban slums. Political gimmicks and lip-service to socialism will not resolve the very dangerous problems of massive unemployment, and overall despair that swaying over the entire country. Shackles need to be unchained. Barriers in the fields need to be demolished.

UNDP (2005, pp. 25-26) has also recently expressed: "The progressive growth approach focuses attention on the structural inequalities that deny poor people and marginalized groups an opportunity to contribute to and participate in growth on more equal terms. It puts distribution, alongside growth, at the centre of the policy agenda for reducing extreme poverty." But, we know globalization hurts the poor most and very strongly reinforces social and economic inequalities between those eating the cake of globalization, and those denied!

Although, the United Nations and other international agencies seem quite serious about reducing poverty and inequalities across developing nations, but neither the UN, World Bank and IMF-led pathways for economic development have yet resolved the crucial issues of underdevelopment, poverty and social injustice in such nations, nor UN and world trade agencies have so far dispensed with their uneven and unjust trade barriers and other bondages imposed on developing countries.

We might thus ponder over what Swami Vivekananda warned long ago (in 1893) that "no sacred work can ever be achieved through conceit means and hypocrisy!" The rich nations have yet to come out as honest and sincere in such action fields!

Reduction of Rural Poverty and Economic Development

Experts differ regarding effectiveness of different strategies for rural poverty reduction, as reflected in many studies. However, most agree that rapid agricultural growth, employment creation and distributive justice in favour of the poor peasants offer the best solutions:.

> "The major poverty alleviation programmes include self-employment programmes, wage employment programmes, PDS (public distribution system of food and essential commodities) and nutrition programmes, and social security programmes. Employment creation through investment in infrastructure development. and pension schemes for the elderly are recent initiatives" (Radhakrishna and Ray, 2005, p. 40).

> "For reducing rural poverty, agricultural growth is important. Low relative food prices are needed for reduction in both rural and urban poverty. Any strategy for reducing poverty has to concentrate both on employment intensity as well as labour productivity. Effective measures are needed for raising agricultural labour productivity without compromising on the employment intensity of agriculture" (Dev, 2000 pp. 823-36).

Some of these ideas are illustrated in Figure 29 and elaborated in various sections:

> "It is recognized that along with growth promoting policies, direct poverty alleviation programs are also needed to raise the incomes and purchasing power of the poor particularly in the short and medium runs. Investments in rural roads and agricultural research and development have the greatest impact, while government spending specifically targeted to poverty reduction such as rural development and employment programs have only modest effects" (ibid., p. 831).

> "Rapid economic growth remains the best bet for reducing India's immense problems of inequality and poverty. Along with rapid economic growth, efforts must be made to see that that the distribution of consumption does not get skewed further" (ibid.).

> "In order to promote economic growth and redress poverty, policy makers will need to promote agricultural intensification for both higher and low potential regions. Striking the right investment balance between irrigated and rain-fed regions, and between high and low potential rain-fed areas will be particularly important" (ibid.).

In a recent article, Nayyar (2005, pp. 1631-39) also unravels that economic growth is a necessary, but is not a sufficient condition for poverty reduction; it needs to be strengthened by initial social conditions of adequate literacy and social protection of the poor.

In short, for effective poverty reduction in India, a votary of inter-related socio-economic-political and institutional policies is very urgently required, namely (Mukherji, 1981c, pp. 150-278; 2002; pp. 525-59; 2006, pp. 280-325):

1. Enhance rapid economic growth, specially in rural areas, and also in small and intermediate towns and metropolitan urban slums.
2. Need primary and middle schools, health dispensary, paved all-weather rural roads, and essential rural infrastructures for rural regeneration.
3. Execute real land reforms in favour of the poor, and easy bank/cooperative credits to small farmers need to be given for seeds, fertilizer, cold storage, and irrigation or water pumps.
4. Implement institutional protection of the poor from their exploitation by village moneylenders, banks, credit societies, marketing agencies, middlemen, panchayat office, and so forth.
5. Provide marketing cooperatives/facilities, so that rural agricultural semi-processed goods get easy and protected markets, free from all exploitations from middlemen/bureaucrats.
6. Promote gender equality and women's empowerment.
7. Demand socio-economic-political accountability of Panchayati Raj and all local public institutions.
8. Ensure total freedom from politicization of village people, rather need their democratization, decentralization and maximum participation in designing and implementation of local projects.

Poverty Alleviation Programmes through Agricultural Growth

Radhakrishna and Ray (2005, pp. 56-57) have made a very good summary of location of the poor and relative success story of poverty alleviation programmes in India. They noted:

> "Data on regional variation of poverty reduction through income growth shows that it has a strong agricultural link. Green revolution mainly occurred in 'irrigated' regions of Punjab, Haryana and Western Uttar Pradesh, and also in delta areas of Andhra Pradesh,

Tamil Nadu and Karnataka. Here, even small farmers were benefited, and poverty was least. In contrast, green revolution bypassed 'rainfed' (and non-irrigated) regions of Telengana in Andhra Pradesh, Maharashtra, Madhya Pradesh, and West Bengal, and arid/semi-arid regions of Gujarat and Rajasthan. In such areas, depth of poverty were in abundance. Endemic poverty persisted, compounded further by abundance of socially excluded groups like SCs and STs."

The authors further argue:

"If it were possible to refocus agricultural growth to extend to the vast geographical areas under the 'rainfed' agro-ecological system areas (AES), considerable progress could be made in poverty reduction even with the existing structure of asset holding and property rights ... These are the major pockets of poverty. It is the map of agricultural growth that could be modified with considerable mileage for poverty reduction. It may be noted that the rainfed AES covers about 54 per cent of land area and 60 per cent of the net-cropped areas (NCA) of the country and support about 44 per cent of the population" (ibid., p. 57).

"It is imperative, therefore, agricultural growth be stepped up and its thrust should be on the hitherto bypassed regions of central and eastern India in order that the resultant poverty reduction be sustained.... So emphasis on irrigation development – which is in some sense difficult but crucial in parts of these regions – agricultural technology – to sustain growth in them – and requisite policy support – to spur growth – would be critical in this quest. Along with agricultural growth, rural non-farm employment and income will also likely to go up" (ibid., pp. 56-58).

As noted elsewhere (Mukherji, 2001a, pp. 1-165; 2001c, pp. 1-24; 2006, pp. 65-121), the majority of urban-ward migrants in India come from the same rural backward regions of Bihar, Uttar Pradesh, Madhya Pradesh, Orissa, Andhra Pradesh, etc., to the metropolitan cities like Kolkata, Mumbai, New Delhi and Chennai and to the regional headquarters like Bangalore, Ahmedabad, Hyderabad, Kanpur, Lucknow, Jaipur, Patna and Pune. They are poor illiterate and unskilled migrants from rural areas, who move out and somehow eke out living in their urban El Dorado. Besides, massive migration of unskilled and illiterate labourers also occurs from agriculturally backward and hitherto neglected states of Bihar, Orissa, Uttar Pradesh and Madhya Pradesh to agriculturally prosperous states of Punjab, Haryana, Western Uttar Pradesh, and also partly to Karnataka and Maharashtra (Mukherji, 2005, pp. 25-50). It is this vast hinterland of poverty where the projects and programmes for poverty alleviation must be directed to.

Besides, massive non-farm employment generation is a must. As Parikh and Radhakrishna (2005, p. 5) noted: "Agricultural productivity improvements and growth of the non-farm sector are essential for long-term poverty eradication. This has been the process of transition from an agrarian economy towards an industrial one – adopted by many East and South East Asian Countries, which resulted in a sharp decline in poverty."

Rural Development and Agricultural Development Strategies

There are innumerable ways for poverty alleviation, if we are soulfully honest and sincere to find the ways and implement them. Rural development programmes are also required to be integrated with family welfare programmes (see Figure 2a and 2b). The two should go hand in hand, not in isolation.

Measures like rural industrialization, the creation of widespread network of surface and underground irrigation, multiple cropping, rural construction work, integrating industries and agricultural products, value-adding process of agricultural goods, etc., will be the greatest generators of rural employment (Mukherji, 1977a, pp. 1-45). Such steps will rise the levels of agricultural productivity, household income, and consumption. Massive generation of employment for rural women and men is a great necessity, which can be actualized by the creation of household industries, village industries, agro-industries, horticulture, food-processing, handicrafts, weaving, oil pressing, and various other cottage industries in the villages. Some UN reports (UN-ESCAP, 1977, pp. 17-18 and 21-27; UN, 1989) and World Bank reports have also emphasized upon similar requirements for rural employment generation (World Bank, 1993, 2003a and b).

World Development Report, 2003a (pp. 83-95) also emphasizes upon the great need for reducing various types of inequalities, as a strong instrument for poverty reduction, by noting:

> "Inequality reduces the participation of poor people in political processes, both directly and indirectly. This in turn reduces the likelihood that poor people have access to education, health care, and other service that would contribute to growth. Inequality can hinder the establishment of independent and impartial institutions and the enforcement of binding rules, because they might reduce the benefits of the privileged."

It further advises:

> "Thus, countries should where still possible, give a high priority to creating egalitarian endowments of land, water, and human capital for its people as they make the transition from rural to urban human settlements" (ibid., pp. 83-86)... "Another strategy is eliminating rural poverty and preparing out-migrants.... And, creating rural non-farm employment" (ibid., pp. 86-88).

Besides, the changes in the iniquitous patterns of land ownership and adequate safeguards against drought, floods and seasonal unemployment are very essential in order to alleviate poverty among the pauperized villagers. Rural cooperative societies for credits, rural banks and marketing cooperatives for village products will be extremely necessary. Many farmers and village workers are forced to commit suicide (e.g., in Andhra Pradesh, Maharashtra, etc.) because of very high interest rates of village moneylenders, and lack of credits facilities for them at reasonable rates. This must immediately stop. And, village credit societies and marketing cooperatives must emerge and operate in every village.

One National Institute of Rural Development (NIRD, 1999, p. 121) study opined that:

> "Land reform is not just distribution of land. Its aims are to break the land-caste based political controls, loosen the interlocking behaviour of factor markets, guarantee access to technology and credit and create conditions for maximum production and marketable surplus,

all so necessary for rural transformation. All its elements need to be addressed in a holistic rather a piecemeal fashion."

Land reforms, cooperative farming, irrigation, innovative measures for agricultural development, rural banks, adequate marketing facilities, multiple cropping, agro-industries, etc., are the only answers to such rural maladies. Decentralization of economic power, more even distribution of development facilities and credits, and lessening of socio-economic inequalities between the owning and non-owning classes, should get priority in order to ameliorate the sad miserable condition of the poor masses in the villages, both men and women. Too much politicking in village societies, political bungling in all political parties, and a very deep-seated corruption among the village panchayats, power-hungry village elites, and village development agencies have usurped all the energies of village regeneration in India. Reforms in such domains indeed require a Herculean task!

On a limited scale, some pathways are however indicated in one World Bank study (World Bank, 1996, pp. 77-95) and again recently reiterated (World Bank, 2003b, pp. 21-22), that:

(1) Put in place a market-based foodgrains policy that protects the poor through safety nets, while mitigating drastic supply shocks through a cost-effective and well-managed stabilization mechanism.
(2) Reduce input subsidies (for food, fertilizers, pump irrigation, electricity, seeds, etc.) that are fiscally unsustainable and distorting input use. Savings thus to be appropriated should be used to fund more productive investments in agricultural research/extension, rural roads and electrification.
(3) Provide decentralization and institutional changes, which would improve the cost effectiveness and sustainability of rural infrastructure development.

However, serious doubts arise whether essential subsidies (food, fertilizers, electricity, irrigation pumps, etc.) should be reduced in India, without hurting the poor most. Rather, such subsidies still need to continue, but only for the poorest, excluding others not so poor. However, suggested better accountability of the institutions and better governance are very much required.

Rural Development Through Decentralization and Panchayati Raj

Decentralization of rural development programmes through people's participation and revamping Panchayati Raj are often found to beneficial. As an important study by National Institute of Rural Development (NIRD, 1999, p. 119) rightly emphasized on the need for people's participation, by observing that "central to the overall failure are excessive reliance on top-down centralised bureaucracy and scarcity of funds". It further elaborates that "an elaborate system of patronage, thriving on disempowerment of the poor and hapless, distributes largesse to a chosen few at the cost of multitudes. As for the funds, rural development, meaning about half the country's population's development, has attracted less than a tenth of the expendable funds at any time. An acute urban bias is all pervasive" (ibid.). It further reiterates:

> "Without a positive trust towards the socio-economic transformation of the marginalized groups, growth may bypass the poor and safety net schemes may only remain short-term palliatives. Thus, economic growth *per se* is not the solution" (ibid., p. 120).

The study further emphasized upon the great need for decentralization and developing the Panchyati Raj Institutions (PRIs) (rural local self-government), and opined:

> "The present constitutional amendment has made the third tier of governance statutory but its span of activities is yet not adequately defined. The need of the hour is to strengthen the localized elected base in contrast to the appointed authorities" (ibid.).

> "Government interventions should not only improve the incomes of the poor but their bargaining power *vis-à-vis* the moneylenders, landlords, and bureaucracy. Such empowering measures need to be distinguished from the popular measures which merely act as doles and do not enable the poor to stand on their own legs or fight for their rights. Empowerment is good in itself, leads to higher incomes, checks corruption and arbitrary use of power" (ibid.).

In sum, NIRD emphasizes upon the two basic requirements for effective rural development in India, by stating that "the ultimate goals should be to achieve rural prosperity through participatory development process…. No such development is possible without bestowing the real decision making power on the community" (ibid., pp. 121-22).

Second, there is no alternative to finding funding resources. This is of course difficult. NIRD observed that "what can still be expected is reduction of excessive expenditures on the bureaucracy, both administrative and political, non-productive budget expenditures, and concealed subsidies, particularly to the non-poor segments of the population. This would release a significant amount of resources for deployment in social sectors" (ibid.).

Hence, people's active participation in designing, implementing and controlling the entire budget and all the processes of rural development work, without the intervention of the bureaucrats and, even powerful elite of the Panchayati Raj, should be activated. Otherwise, the happiness will, again, be an unfortunate lady, who will not be able to see the faces of the rural poor!

Rural Industrialization for Massive Employment Generation

Rural industries can become the greatest generators of rural employment. Creation of massive non-farm rural employment through industrialization of agro-products will create a large number of work opportunities in the villages. However, these need many associated changes also. As one important recent study has opined: "To generate growth the main policy components are ensuring sound macro-economic management and macro-economic stability, boosting domestic demand, adopting fiscal discipline, accelerating industrial production, reforming financial sector institutions and promoting good governance" (HCSI Herald, 2001, pp. 13-18). The study has further observed that "pro-poor growth is needed both for reducing poverty and for making growth a stronger and a more indigenous process… Maximisation of employment and through this maximisation of welfare of individuals shall have to be defined as the goal of economic programme….Speedy expansion of small business seems to be a viable alternative for India" (ibid., pp., 13-14). We need to encourage small scale industries and enterprises because "this sector can promote large scale employment with relatively much less capital requirement, a more equitable distribution of income, effective mobilization of resources and promotion of dispersed growth" (ibid.).

Special Rural Development Programmes and Massive Employment Creation

Recently, in a study, Bhaduri (2005, pp. 1-90)) has opined that market economy is not at all capable of poverty reduction and mass employment generation in India. For these objectives, we need to devise special rural development programmes for generating mass employment among the poor unemployed rural workers, and to create national assets. It needs programmes that will benefit the poor directly. According to Bhaduri,

> "There are roughly 35 million unemployed rural people. If employment is to be provided to these people for 300 days per year, at the rate of Rs 60 per day, that would cost Rs 630,000 million (Rs 63,000 crores). Plus, if cost of essential materials are also added, then, the total cost would be only 4 per cent of the Gross National Product – two and half per cent of GNP for wages, and only one and half per cent for required materials" (ibid.).

Bhaduri (ibid.) further says, the entire work will be executed through Panchayati Raj systems, through government's recent Right to Information Act (in order to curtail corruption and misappropriation of funds). His argument is that:

> "The benefits will work in two ways: (1) first, it will provide money in the hands of the workers, which, in turn, will create demands for consumer goods, which in turn will generate additional mass employment everywhere; thereby starting a wheel of economic prosperity; and (2) second, the project will also create permanent national assets and by raising national productivity, eventually, it will generate national wealth. Additionally, the greatest benefits will be encouraging people's massive and active participation in the national reconstruction" (ibid., pp. 75-90).

Although the above are profound ideas, however, some questions also arose (Sarkar, 2006, pp. 95-96). First, the estimate of only 35 million rural unemployed is untenable, it must be three times more;

second, thus, the cost of wages will be also three times more, i.e., Rs 1,900,000 millions (Rs 190, 000 crores). Plus, the cost of materials will also be three times more to make it meaningful and permanent assets. Thus, the total cost of the project will be 12 per cent of GNP, not just 4 per cent, as author dreamt.

In spite of these limitations, I very strongly think that such Rural Massive Employment Generation Programme (RMEGP) is much more commendable, and should be seriously attempted, rather than government's presently envisaged National Rural Employment Generation Programme (NREGP), which has very limited scope and coverage. NREGP is a half-hearted programme, taken mainly for vote-bank politics, not really to ameliorate widespread poverty and hunger in India. Otherwise, much greater fund would have been allocated and countrywide coverage made.

Rural Infrastructure Improvement and Rural Employment

As discussed earlier, land reforms alone cannot be a panacea; it must be supplemented by seed and fertilizer depots, credit and marketing facilities, as well as good rural infrastructures, like all-weather metal road, electricity, cold storage, warehouses, marketing cooperatives, and related institutions.

> "The poor need a ladder to climb out of poverty, not palliatives that keep them dependent on government handouts. Subsidies for rural power, canal water and fertilizers benefit mainly large farmers. Subsidies for food, education and health overwhelmingly benefit urban folk and richer rural areas. Rural employment schemes are a palliative that help greatly in droughts when agricultural jobs plummet, but they are plagued by corruption and waste. They have failed to create durable assets" (Aiyar, 2005, p. 18).

For poverty eradication and mass rural employment creation, hence, we require alternative strategies that will benefit the poor directly, such as, permanent roads, stable supply of electricity and rural micro-credit societies, and so forth. Recently, one expert has also opined:

> "Many studies have shown that all–weather roads (which need capital-intensive construction) are the best way to reduce rural poverty, while temporary roads built by labour-intensive employment schemes achieve little. Even illiterate Bihari villagers will tell you that if every village has a paved road plus electricity plus telecom, businesses will spring up all over the place and provide millions of new jobs. The talent is in place, even the finance is in place, only the infrastructure is missing. Provide that and rural India will take off" (ibid.).

Policies for Agricultural Development and Security of the Poor

UNDP (1998, pp. 87-88) recommended the following policies for agricultural development in developing countries:

- We need to strengthen agricultural research and extension systems. Need is also to establish clear, long-term property rights over land, and access to credit.
- We need to promote sustainable intensification of agriculture and sound management of natural resources, especially in areas with fragile soils, limited rainfall and widespread poverty.
- We need to develop low-cost markets and transport networks for inputs and outputs.
- We need to expand and improve assistance in food and agricultural development.

Promotion of Agri-Business and Rural Employment

Recently, some experts suggest the likely benefits of agri-business and bio-energy for creating massive rural employment (Firodiya, 2006, p. 30). He advocates to promote agri-business in each village by "focusing on export of a variety of processed food, seafood, herbal products and flowers, with the help of friendly bank loans, and insurance companies for necessary cover" (ibid.). It will create mass of rural employment. Textile export will also provide another opportunity. Agri-business and textiles will generate crores (tens of millions) of new well-paid jobs. It is also suggested that "oil companies should create a bio-energy cluster in each village, which will use local feedstock to produce biogas, bio-diesel, and ethanol. Biogas may be used for electricity, bio-fertilizers, and bio-pesticides; while bio-diesel and ethanol may be further processed and blended with diesel and petrol for energy use" (ibid.). It will generate further crores of rural employment.

For promotion for agri-business management, we also need to enhance value addition and marketing. Some studies also suggest (e.g., Singh and Sharma, 2006, pp. 456-58) such steps as: (1) post-harvest management of agro-products, e.g., pre-processing facilities, washing, packaging, etc.; (2) agro-processing facilities like cold chain, low cost pre-cooling facilities close to production areas to avoid wastage and reduce transportation costs; (3) proper technology for agro-industrial processing; (4) warehouses and infrastructures for storage and transportation of unprocessed products; and (5) integration of small and unorganized processing units and transforming them into national and global players, with incentives for brand building and optimum marketing. Thus, several such important policy initiatives should be promoted for agricultural management.

Although, the ideas are good, but their implementation is quite difficult. Additionally, many crucial questions remain: can the farmers at all afford to produce such crops, in the face of frequent climatic hazards and market uncertainties? Second, if local feedstock would be enough for bio-fertilizers, and ethanol?

Besides, recently, Ghosh (*Ananda Bazaar Patrika*, May 21, 2006, p. 4) pinpointed various dangers of further penetration of capitalism, both Indian and international, into agri-business and commercialization of crops in Indian agriculture. As envisaged now, this will be done mostly in the form of 'contract farming' under the control of multinational companies (MNCs).

"The dangers lies in the fact that, (1) then, MNCs will determine the nature of crop; (2) will determine nature and amount of seeds, water, fertilizers, everything; (3) will give seed money to small and petty farmers on MNC's own high rate of interest; (4) after harvesting, the majority of crops will be purchased by MNCs, but at their own determined low rate; and (5) all risks of agricultural failure or marketing uncertainties will have to be borne by the small and petty farmers, not by MNCs" (ibid., 2006).

MNCs thus have no responsibilities. They entail no risks. They will harvest only the heaps of benefits at the cost of the poor peasants, and the small and petty farmers will be bound by endless bondages! Soon, their land will be mortgaged; harvest confiscated; loan with high interests will tightly engulf their neck. Soon, the land would degenerate into wastelands, and millions of petty farmers, relegated as beggars!

These have repeatedly happened in Latin American and African countries. This has already happened in Andhra Pradesh, Maharashtra and West Bengal, in India, during last 3-4 years, where scores of thousands of commercial crop farmers were forced to commit suicide, because of crop failures, failure to repay loans with high interest, climatic hazards, lack of cold storage, and declining market prices for such crops in Indian or international markets.

Such brute exploitation is going on since many years. So, all these precautions must be taken by the state and central governments and by local cooperatives (both agricultural and marketing), before agri-business and crop commercialization are extended on wider scale. The poor peasants cannot take such high risks. The governments must provide them with all helping hands, instead of remaining as mute, deaf and blind spectators!

Notwithstanding, we also need to explore innovative options for rural employment, albeit with much cautions. Thus, many-sided efforts for poverty alleviation are required now. Details are also presented elsewhere (Mukherji, 2001b, pp. 160-225; 2006, pp. 298-325).

Indeed, we very seriously need to make a frontal attack on abject poverty and hunger in India. And, we must all the time remember the divine declaration of the great monk Swami Vivekananda 113 years ago (1893): "Until even a dog remains hungry and unfed in India, we cannot take rest and feel complacent" (Vivekananda, 1893, Complete Work, Centenary Volume VIII, 1963 p. 150).

Education and Development

Radhakrishna and Ray (2005, pp. 59-60) have rightly indicated that among the tribal states of Mizoram, Meghalaya and Nagaland, the incidence of 'very poor' is absent and the people enjoy inalienable rights on land and assets. So, these people cannot be displaced or dispossessed easily as elsewhere. They also show better indicators of human development. So, education has contributed a lot for their development. Thus, education is an important component of health, nutrition, and material well-being of this people, and this has reduced poverty in the region. "Thus, combined with income growth, human development in the form of education and health contribute to poverty reduction." Hence, as lessons for poverty reduction for other regions, human development components (like education, health, and nutrition) must be given priorities (ibid.).

Implementation of Programmes and Issue of Funding

Often arguments are made that above-mentioned policies are utopian ideas, and they cannot be implemented due to shortage of funds. In reality, these arguments are mischievous designs by vested interests. Well, wherefrom money/resources come for governments' extravaganza? For very expensive perks and wasteful expenditures of all political representatives? Why is money always available for rich 300 universities, but not for village primary schools? Why subsidies, meant for the poor are always usurped by the middle class and the rich? Why Reserve Bank always protect the interests of the super-rich, corporate houses, and business sectors, draining out money from the common people? Why are trillions of bank loans, scattered to defaulting business houses never recovered? Why are vast black money, manifold larger than the governments entire exchequers, never controlled and confiscated? The money and resources for the afore-mentioned development strategies for the poor should come from the same sources! Planning must be made for the poor, and the poor only!

Need Education for Character Building and Nation Building

Swami Vivekananda thundered more than 112 years ago (1893): "A nation-wide real educational effort for character-building of all men, women and children of India, and their transformation for nation building seem to be the only panacea.".. "You should go to the sinking millions of India, and take them by the hand" (Swami Vivekananda, 1893, Complete Work, Centenary Volume III, 1963, p. 433).

Most unfortunately, since independence, this greatest requirement of human-making is entirely missing from India's educational and developmental efforts. Sooner the leaders and common people will understand its great requirement, and will ceaselessly strive for achieving this, the better for India's survival!

Conclusion

In short, three kinds of policies and strategies have been highlighted.

First, policies for fertility reduction, infant mortality reduction, child mortality and maternal mortality reduction are very strongly recommended. The great need for providing basic health services to the poor and remote areas is also tremendously emphasized, as well as policies for poverty alleviation and fertility decline, and gender aspect of poverty alleviation. The need for revamping family planning and RCH care services is also candidly reiterated.

Second, focus is also given upon the need for people's socio-economic welfare programmes to be integrated with family planning programmes, and also upon the requirement for better health services for disease control and basic public health. Besides, the great need to reduce differential fertility between the Hindus and the Muslims is also emphasized, and also highlighted utter need to make total stop to illegal migration from Bangladesh.

Third, an entire battery of economic development policies and strategies is also recommended, which include steps for poverty eradication, reduction of rural poverty and economic development, poverty alleviation programmes through agricultural growth, rural development through agricultural development, rural industrialization through decentralization and Panchayati Raj, rural industrialization for massive employment generation, special rural development programmes for employment creation, rural infrastructure improvement, policies for security of the poor, promotion of agri-business for rural employment, social development through education, and top of all, the greatest need for education for character-building and nation-building.

In sum, much more emphasis has been placed upon the need for effective socio-economic development and poverty eradication programmes for delinking the evil syndrome of poverty and fertility, rather than only upon sterilization and usual family planning programmes.

Of course, the family planning programmes are also very essential, and should be enhanced more rigorously. Specially, contraceptives must reach to the poor and downtrodden women and men, who are always denied access to such services. Everyone of us definitely has seen very emaciated faces and looks of many beggar women in the villages, railway stations, urban slums, or road junctions, trailed by three, four or more children and infants. Indeed! It is they who need to be given contraceptives on top priority, and such facilities must be provided at their doorstep. And, provided, first you have also given them one plate of warm rice!

At the same time, it is always worthwhile to remember that these family planning programmes will be much more effective, only when, proper motivation is created in the minds of the poor rural masses in favour of the small family size. Unless poverty is alleviated, such motivation is very hard to emerge and persist.

Thus, I end this book, quoting the divine utterances of the Great Saviour, Swami Vivekananda:

> *"Be fearless, the Lord is with you, and He will yet raise the starving and ignorant millions of India"* (Swami Vivekananda, 1894, Complete Work, Centenary Vol V, 1963, pp. 23-24)

> *"Vow, then, to devote your whole lives to the cause of the redemption of these three hundred millions, going down and down every day" (now 1.12 billion on June 10, 2006)* (Swami Vivekananda, 1894, Complete Work, Centenary Volume V, 1963, p. 17).

References

Abler, A., Adams, B. and Gould P. (1971), *Spatial Organization*, New York.

Aiyar, Swaminathan S. Anklesaria (2005), "Globalising Rural India", *Times of India*, December 18, Edit Page Article, p. 18.

Alderman, Harold (2005), "Linkages between Poverty Reduction Strategies and Child Nutrition: An Asian Perspective", *Economic and Political Weekly*, November 12, pp. 4837-4842.

Banerji, Debabar (2005), "Politics of Rural Health in India", *Economic and Political Weekly*, July 23, pp. 3253-3257.

Berelson, B. (1969), "Beyond Family Planning", *Science*, 169, pp. 533-543.

Berry, B.J.L. (1966), *Essays on Commodity Flows and the Spatial Structure of the Indian Economy*, Department of Geography, University of Chicago, Research paper No. 111, Chicago, University of Chicago Press, pp. 6-151.

Berry, B.J.L. (1969), "Interdependency of Spatial Structure and Spatial Behaviour: A General Field Theory Formulations", *Regional Science Association*, Vol. 19, pp. 10-20.

Bhaduri, Amit (2005), *Development with Dignity: A Cass for Full Employment*, National Book Trust, New Delhi, pp. 1-90.

Caldwell, J.C. (1982), *Theory of Fertility Decline*, Academic Press, London.

Caldwell, J.C. (1988), "Family Change and Demographic Changes: The Reversal of the Generation Flow" in Srinivasan, K and Mukerji S. (eds.), *Dynamics of Population and Family Welfare*, Himalaya Publishing House, Mumbai, pp. 71-96.

Census of India, 2001, *Population Tables, Series I, India*, Various Data Series (CDs), 2003-6.

Census of India, 2001, *Social and Cultural Tables, Series I, India*, Various Data Series (CDs), 2003-6.

Census of India, 2001, *Types of Household Tables, Series I, India*, Various Data Series (CDs), 2003-5.

Chandrasekar, S. (1972), *Infant Mortality and Fertility in India*, Allen and Unwin, London.

Chattopadhyay, Aparajita, Roy, T.K. et al. (2004), "Hindu-Muslim Fertility Differential: Study of Selected States of India", in *Population, Health and Development in India* by Roy, T.K., Guruswamy, M. and Arokiswamy P. (eds.), Rawat Publications, Jaipur and New Delhi, pp. 137-156.

Coale, Ansley J. and Hoover, Edgar (1958), *Population and Economic Growth in Low Income Countries: India and Mexico*. Princeton.

Cooley, W.W. and Lohnes, P.R. (1962), *Multivariate Procedure in the Behavioural Sciences*. Wiley, New York, pp. 45-65.

Das Gupta, Monica (2005), "Public Health in India; Dangerous Neglect" *Economic and Political Weekly,* December 3, pp. 5150-5165.

Demeny, Paul (1972), *The Economics of Population Growth*. East-West Population Institute's Reprint Series, Honolulu, Hawaii, pp. 1-20.

Dev, Mahendra S. (2000), "Economic Reforms, Poverty, Income Distribution, and Employment", *Economic and Political Weekly*, Vol. 35, No. 10, pp. 823-836.

Dev, Mahendra S. (2005), "Agriculture and Rural Employment in the Budget", *Economic and Political Weekly,* April 2, pp. 1410-1413.

Firodiya, Arun (2006), "Back to Roots: Agribusiness and Bio-energy can create 27 Crore Jobs", *Times of India*, January 4, Edit Page Article, p. 30.

Ghosh, Shankar (2006), "Dangers of Contract Farming in West Bengal", *Ananda Bazaar Patrika* (in Bengali), May 21, 2006, p. 4.

Gillespie, D.G. (2004), "Whatever Happened to Family Planning and for that Matter, Reproductive Health?", *International Family Planning Perspective*, New York, Vol. 30 (1), pp. 34-38.

Gopal, K.S. (2005), "Is the Euphoria Justified?", *Economic and Political Weekly,* October 15, pp. 4523-4524.

Government of India (2001), *Nutritional Intake in India, 1999-2000,* National Sample Survey Organisation, Ministry of Statistics and Programme Implementation, New Delhi.

Government of India (2004), *Human Development Report of India, 2004*, Planning Commission, New Delhi.

Government of India (2005), *National Rural Health Mission 2005*, Ministry of Health and Family Welfare, New Delhi.

Haan, Arjan De and Dubey, Amaresh (2005), "Poverty, Disparities, or the Development of Underdevelopment in Orissa", *Economic and Political Weekly,* May 28-June 4, 2005, pp. 2321.-2329.

Harman, H.H. (1967), *Modern Factor Analysis*, Chicago University Press, Chicago, pp. 11-67.

HCSI Herald (2000), "Memorandum to the Planning Commission", Herald of Small Scale Industries, New Delhi.

Hotelling, Harold (1936), "Relations Between Two Sets of Variate", *Biometrika,* 28, pp. 321-377.

International Institute for Population Sciences (2000), Summary of Proceedings of Seminar on Population and Development in Andhra Pradesh, IIPS and State Ministry of Health and Family Welfare, Hyderabad/Mumbai.

Jain, Ruchi and Parasuraman, Sulbha (2004), "Maternal Morbidity and Utlilization of ANC Services: A Study of Bihar and Madhya Pradesh", in *Population, Health and Development in India* by Roy, T.K., Guruswamy, M. and Arokiswamy P. (eds.), Rawat Publications, Jaipur and New Delhi, pp. 196-221.

Jeromi, P.D. (2005), "Economic Reforms in Kerala", *Economic and Political Weekly,* July 23, pp. 3267-3277.

Joshi, A. P., Srinivas, M.D. and Bajaj, J.K. (2003), *Religious Demography of India*, Centre for Policy Studies, Chennai, pp. 40-85, 87-106, and 107-133.

Kannan, K.P. (2005), "Linking Guarantee to Human Development", *Economic and Political Weekly,* October 15, pp. 4518-4522.

Kodoth, P. and Eapan, M. (2005), "Looking Beyond Gender Parity: Gender Inequities of Some Dimensions of Well-Being in Kerala", *Economic and Political Weekly,* July 23, pp. 3278-3286.

Lewin, Kurt (1951), *Field Theories in Social Sciences*, Harper, New York, pp. 1-297.

Merrick, Thomas W. (2002), "Population and Poverty: New Views on an Old Controversy", *International Family Planning Perspectives*, New York, Vol. 28(1), pp. 41-46.

Ministry of Health and Family Welfare, Government of India (1994), *National Population Policy 1994 (NPP, 1994),* National Commission on Population, Government of India (GoI), New Delhi, pp. 1-40.

Ministry of Health and Family Welfare, Government of India (2000), *National Population Policy 2000 (NPP, 2000),* National Commission on Population, Government of India (GoI), New Delhi, pp. 1-55.

Ministry of Health and Family Welfare, Government of India (2001), *Reproductive and Child Health Surveys, Phase I and II (1998-99),* Ministry of Health and Family Welfare, New Delhi and International Institute for Population Sciences, Mumbai, 2001, Various Reports and Tables, pp. 1-135 and various CDs.

Ministry of Health and Family Welfare, Government of India (2004), *National Rural Health Mission (NRHM*), Government of India (GoI), New Delhi.

Ministry of Health and Family Welfare, Government of India (2005), *Reproductive and Child Health Project Surveys, Round –II (Phase I and II, 2002-4*), Ministry of Health and Family Welfare, Government of India, New Delhi and International Institute for Population Sciences, Mumbai, 2005-6, Various Reports and Tables. and CDs.

Mishra, Srijit (2005), "Public Health Scenario in India", in *India Development Report, 2004-05,* by Parikh and Radhakrishna (eds.), Ibid., pp. 62-83.

Mitra, A. and Mukherji, Shekhar (1979*), Population, Food, and Land Inequality: The Geography of Hunger and Insecurity in India*, Indian Council of Social Science Research, and Allied Publishers, New Delhi, pp. 32-121.

Mitra, A., Mukherji, Shekhar and Bose, R.N. (1980*), Indian Cities,: Their Industrial Structure, In-migration, and Capital Investments,* Indian Council of Social Science Research (ICSSR) and Abhinav Publishers, New Delhi, pp. 1-190.

Moulasha, K. and Rama Rao, G. (1999), "Religion Specific Differences in Fertility and Family Planning", *Economic and Political Weekly*, October 16-23, pp. 3047-3051.

Mukherji, Shekhar (1971), "A Field Theory Formulation of Migration Flows Through a System of Indian Cities", Seminar Paper, Department of Geography, University of Hawaii, Honolulu, Hawaii, pp. 1-40.

Mukherji, Shekhar (1972a), "Inter-State Migration and State-Income Inequalities in India", Paper, presented to The East-West Center, Honolulu, pp. 1-25.

Mukherji, Shekhar (1972b), "A Spatio-Temporal Model of Mobility Patterns in a Multi-ethnic Population in Hawaii", Paper, 22nd International Geographical Congress, Edmonton, Canada, pp. 1-35.

Mukherji, Shekhar (1974), "A Spatio-Temporal Model of Mobility Patterns in a Multi-Ethnic Population, Hawaii", in *People on the Move: Studies in Internal Migration* by L.A. Kosinski and R. Mansell Prothero (eds.), Methuen, London, pp. 325-346.

Mukherji, Shekhar (1975), The Mobility Field Theory of Human Spatial Behavior: A Spatial Behavioural Approach to the Study of Migration and

Circulation in Indian Situation. Doctoral Dissertation, Department of Geography, University of Hawaii, Honolulu (Xerox University Microfilms, Ann Arbor), pp. 20-65.

Mukherji, Shekhar (1976a) "A General Field Theory of Migration Behaviour", 47th Australia and New Zealand Association of Scientists (ANZAAS), Hobart, 1976, pp. 1-25.

Mukherji, Shekhar (1976b),"A General Field Theory of Movement Behaviour: Pathway to Migration Planning for Underdeveloped Countries", 23rd International Geographical Congress, Minsk, 1976 (in Russian), pp. 21-32.

Mukherji, Shekhar (1977a), "Spatial Disorganization and Internal Migration in India: Alternative Strategies for Restructuring the Space Economy and Development", Paper, Expert Working Group Meeting on Population Growth and Economic Development in Sub-national Areas, UN-ESCAP, Bangkok, September-October, 1977, 1-45.

Mukherji, Shekhar (1977b), "Assessing Interrelationships between Population Policies, Social Systems, and Demographic Behaviour in India: An Analytical Framework", *Demography India*. 6, Nos. 1-2. pp. 250-266

Mukherji, Shekhar (1979a), "The Mobility Field Theory: A Spatial Behavioural Foundation to Movement Dynamics, with Application to Indian Situation", IGU Working Group on Transformation of Rural Habitat and National Geographical Society of India, Research Monograph No. 25, Banaras Hindu University, Varanasi, pp. 1-80.

Mukherji, Shekhar (1979b), "General Field Theory of Movement Dynamics: Pathway to Migration Planning for Underdeveloped Countries", *Geografiska Annaler, Human Geog (Sweden)*, 1980, Series B, Vol. 62B, pp. 18-32.

Mukherji, Shekhar (1979c), "Understanding Canonical Analysis through Human Mobility Research", *Geographical Review of India*, Kolkata, September, 1979 (b), pp. 234-249.

Mukherji, Shekhar (1979d), "Spatial Disorganization and Internal Migration in India: Strategies for Restructuring Space Economy and Development", *Canadian Studies in Population*, 6, 1979, pp. 45-61.

Mukherji, Shekhar (1980), "Understanding Mobility Field Theory", *Demography India*, Vol. 8, No. 4-6, 1980, pp. 254-284.

Mukherji, Shekhar (1981a), "The Demographic Field Theory", Occasional Paper No. 1, Department of Geography, Visva Bharati University, Santiniketan, West Bengal, pp. 1-56.

Mukherji, Shekhar (1981b), "Demographic Field Theory: Interrelationships between Socio-economic System, Population Policy and Demographic behaviour in India", International Union for the Scientific Study of Population (IUSSP), Manila, 1981, pp. 1-55.

Mukherji, Shekhar (1981c), *Mechanisms of Underdevelopment, Labour Migration and Planning Strategies in India,* Prajna Pub, Kolkata, 1981, pp. 1-278.

Mukherji, Shekhar (1982a), *Poverty and Mobility in India: A Field Theoretic Perspective*. Prajna, Kolkata, pp. 1-248.

Mukherji, Shekhar (1982b), "The Value of Women in India" (Bharate Narir Mulya) (in Bengali), *Desh*: A Bengali Weekly, October, 1982, Kolkata, pp. 12-16.

Mukherji, Shekhar (1982c), "The Concept of the Demographic Field of Women: Demographic and Economic Value of Women", (Narir Jana-sankhik O Arthanaitik Mulya) (in Bengali), *Aaaj-Kaal:* A Bengali Daily, Kolkata, p. 4.

Mukherji, Shekhar (1982d), "Demographic Field Theory: Theoretical and Empirical Example of Geo-Demography", International Geographical Congress, Symposium on Population Geography, Sao Paulo, August 1982, Proceedings, pp. 1-30.

Mukherji, Shekhar (1983a), "Poverty and Fertility in Birbhum District, West Bengal", Chapter 7, in *Essays on Rural Development*, Utsargo Publications, Varanasi, pp. 161-177.

Mukherji, Shekhar (1983b), *The Demographic Field Theory: Population Policies and Demographic Behaviour in India*. Thinkers Library, Allahabad, pp. 1-141.

Mukherji, Shekhar (1983c), *Essays on Rural Development*, Utsargo Publications, Varanasi, 1983, pp. 1-225.

Mukherji, Shekhar (1985a), "Process of Wage Labour Circulation in Northern India", in *Labour Process and Labour Policies, International Labour Organisation (ILO),* by Guy Standing (ed.), Croom Helm, London, 1985, Chapter 9, pp. 252-279.

Mukherji, Shekhar (1985b), "Syndrome of Poverty and Wage Labour Circulation: Indian Scene", in R. Mansell Prothero and Murray Chapman (eds.), *Circulation in the Third World*, London, Routledge and Kegan Paul (1978), published in 1985, Chapter 10. pp. 280-299.

Mukherji, Shekhar (1985c), "A Canonical Model of Migration to Cities", 24th International Geographical Congress, Rouen, France, 1984, in Espace, Movements and Settlements: Proceedings, Rouen, 1985, pp. 45-52.

Mukherji, Shekhar (1985d), "Multi-variate Linkages between Demographic Behaviour, Social Systems and Population Policies in India", International Union for the Scientific Study of Population (IUSSP), Mathematical Demography Section, Florence, Italy, July-August, 1985, pp. 1-20.

Mukherji, Shekhar (1985e), "Demographic Field Theory: Integrative Model of Fertility and Mortality Behaviour in India", International Symposium on Population Mapping, National Atlas Organization and Thematic Mapping, Calcutta, pp. 1-12.

Mukherji, Shekhar (1986a), "Interrelationships between Economic Structure of Indian Cities, Migration and Capital", Special Monograph, Economic Geographical Society of India, Utkal University, Bhubaneshwar, pp. 1-20.

Mukherji, Shekhar (1986b), "Canonical Model of Population Displacement from Rural to Urban Poverty," Proceedings, Seminar on Urban and Regional Development, Department of Applied Geography, University of North Bengal, District Darjeeling, 1987, pp. 169-85.

Mukherji, Shekhar (1987), "Findings of Survey on Primary Health Services to Rural Women in Varanasi District, Uttar Pradesh", *Journal of Health,* Indian Council of Medical Research Project, Institute of Medical Science, Banaras Hindu University, Varanasi, 1987, pp. 132-138.

Mukherji, Shekhar (1988a), Operation Research on Delivery of Rural Health Services in Varanasi *District,* Indian Council of Medical Research Project, Institute of Medical Sciences, Banaras Hindu University, Varanasi, pp. 10-68.

Mukherji, Shekhar (1989a), Systems Analysis of PHCs of Varanasi District. ICMR Health Project, Institute of Medical Sciences, Banaras Hindu University, Varanasi, pp. 1-126.

Mukherji, Shekhar (1989b), "Application of the Demographic Field Theory to Study Demographic Behaviour, Socio-economic Systems, and Population Policies in India", in *Dynamics of Population and Family Welfare 1989* by K. Srinivasan and K.B. Pathak (eds.), Himalaya Publishing House, Mumbai, pp. 343-373.

Mukherji, Shekhar (1989c), "Utilization of Rural Health Services of Varanasi District", *Journal of Health Services,* Indian Council of Medical Research (ICMR) Project, College of Medical Sciences, Banaras Hindu University 1989, pp. 1-6.

Mukherji, Shekhar (1990), "Field Theory Perspective of Women's Demographic and Socio-Economic Situations", Seminar on Population, Gender and Development in India, International Institute for Population Sciences, Mumbai, March 4-6, 1990, pp. 1-24.

Mukherji, Shekhar (1992), "Application of the Demographic Field Theory to Developing and Developed Countries", International Institute for Population Science Research Monograph, Mumbai, pp. 10-92.

Mukherji, Shekhar (1993), "A Canonical Model Linking Spatial Structure and Spatial Behaviour in India: Linking Difference in Socio-Economic

Structure of States and Inter-State Migration", in *Dynamics of Population and Family Welfare 1993* by K.B. Pathak, et al. (eds.) Himalaya Publishing House, Mumbai, Chapter 8, pp. 245-275.

Mukherji, Shekhar (1994a), "Poverty and Fertility in Uttar Pradesh: Strategies for Poverty Alleviation and Better Health Services", Background paper for the Session on Poverty, Employment, and Population Change in Uttar Pradesh. Seminar on Population and Development in Uttar Pradesh, Institute of Medical Sciences, Lucknow, December 4-6, 1994, pp. 1-18, B.R. Publishers, New Delhi (1996).

Mukherji, Shekhar (1994b), "Demographic and Economic Field of Women", Symposium on Space, Gender, and Development in Developing Countries, International Geographic Congress, Department of Geography, University of Dhaka, Bangladesh, November 1994, Proceedings, pp. 1-25.

Mukherji, Shekhar (1995a), "The Syndrome of Poverty and High Fertility in India and The Third World: Strategies Required for Fertility Decline and Better Health Deliveries", Paper presented to International Seminar on Population, Development and Health in Developing Countries, Department of Geography, Banaras Hindu University, 1995, pp. 1-36.

Mukherji, Shekhar (1995b), "Poverty-Induced Migration and Urban Involution in ESCAP Region," Background paper for UN-ESCAP Expert Meeting on Population and Poverty, Bangkok, Sept 1995 (Summary and Recommendations appeared in UN-ESCAP Expert Group Meeting's proceedings volume, May/June, 1996).

Mukherji, Shekhar (1996), "Poverty-Induced Migration and Urban Involution in ESCAP Region: and Urban and Regional Planning Lessons from Japan." IDE/VRF Monograph No 300, Institute of Developing Economies, Tokyo, Dec 1996 (published March, 1997), pp. 1-81.

Mukherji, Shekhar (1997a), "Poverty and Fertility in India: Results of Findings of the Demographic Field Theory – Linking Demographic Behaviour, Socio-economic System, and Population Policies in India", *IIPS Newsletter*, Mumbai, 1997, January, Nos. 4-6, pp. 1-6.

Mukherji, Shekhar (1997b), "Poverty Index and Its Linkages to Fertility Behaviour in India", presented to the 21st Indian Social Science Congress, Session: Population Studies, Tamil University, Thanjavur, pp. 1-26.

Mukherji, Shekhar (1997c), "Poverty and Fertility in India and Required Research Priorities", Presidential Address, Population Science Section, 21st Indian Social Science Congress, Tamil University, Thanjavur, Tamil Nadu, pp. 1-45.

Mukherji, Shekhar (1997d) "Causal Linkages between Syndrome of Poverty and High Fertility in India: A Very Neglected Aspect of Population Studies in India", Presented in International Seminar on Environment, Energy and Technology: Regional and Global Perspectives, Banaras Hindu University, Dept of Geography, Dec 1997. (Published in Professor R.N. Dubey Memorial Lecturers 2004, *Poverty and Population in India*, R.N. Dubey Foundation, Allahabad, pp. 38-74.

Mukherji, Shekhar (1997e) "The Syndrome of Poverty and Fertility in India", Paper, IGU Seminar on Gender, Environment, and Health, Dept of Geography, Chiang Mai University, Thailand, January 1997, pp. 1-12.

Mukherji, Shekhar (1997f), "Basic Research Proposal and Research Design for Rapid Household Survey of District Level Reproductive and Child Health Services in India", International Institute for Population Sciences, Mumbai, pp. 1-35 (During first 15 months of organizing, designing and training for survey, June 1997–Sept 1998, the present author was the Senior-most Coordinator of this All-India survey, taken up at the request of World Bank and Ministry of Health, Government of India).

Mukherji, Shekhar (1998a) "Poverty and Fertility in India: Required Policy Changes", IGU Symposium on Changing Health Problems in Developing Countries, MS University of Baroda, Proceeding Volume, March 1998, pp. 250-270.

Mukherji, Shekhar (1998b), "Training Guidelines for RCH Project: Rapid Survey". *Manual Prepared for Training for the Trainers*, International Institute for Population Sciences (IIPS), Mumbai, May, 1998, pp. 1-30

Mukherji, Shekhar (1998c), "Methodology of Rapid Survey: Reproductive and Child Health Project (RCH Project)", Background Paper for Training for the Trainers, International Institute for Population Sciences (IIPS), Mumbai, May 1998, pp. 1-25.

Mukherji, Shekhar (1998d), "Research Design and Methodology of Rapid Household Survey: Reproductive and Child Health Project (RCH Project)", Background Paper presented in Reproductive and Child Health (RCH Seminar), International Institute for Population Sciences (IIPS), July 1998, Mumbai, pp. 1-16.

Mukherji, Shekhar (1999a), "The Syndrome of Poverty and Fertility in India", Paper presented to United Nations funded Symposium on Nihon University Seminar in Population and Socio-Economic Transformations. in Asia, United Nations Population Project, Nihon University, Tokyo, March 3, 1999, pp. 1-20.

Mukherji, Shekhar (1999b), "Demographic and Socio-Economic Conditions in India", Paper, Presented to Japan Women's University, Department of Study of Contemporary Societies, Kawasaki, Japan, July 1999, pp. 1-15.

Mukherji, Shekhar (2000a), "Poverty Index and Its Linkages to Demographic Behaviour in India", presented to National Seminar on Land-use, Rural Development and Transfer of Technology, Department of Geography, Banaras Hindu University, February 2000, pp. 1-25.

Mukherji, Shekhar (2000b) "Poverty and Fertility in India and Andhra Pradesh: A Demographic Field Theoretic Perspective", presented in Seminar on Rapid Fertility Decline in Andhra Pradesh, Hyderabad (Brief summary in Proceeding Volume), March 2002, pp. 1-35.

Mukherji, Shekhar (2000c) "The Syndrome of Poverty and Fertility in India", *Yojana,* Ministry of Information and Braodcasting, New Delhi, May 2000, pp. 1-5.

Mukherji, Shekhar (2000d), "Application of Demographic Field Theory: Causal Linkages between Demographic Behaviour, Socioeconomic Systems, and Population Policies in India." International Institute for Population Sciences, IIPS Research Monograph 27, December 2000, Mumbai, pp. 1-145.

Mukherji, Shekhar (2000e), "Poverty and Rapid Population Explosion in India", *Yojana (Journal*), Ministry of Information and Broadcasting, Government of India, New Delhi, August 2000, pp 10-15.

Mukherji, Shekhar (2000f), "Poverty-Induced Migration and Acute Urban Decay in India", *Free Press Journal,* Mumbai, July 2000, Edit Page Article, p. 6.

Mukherji, Shekhar (2000g), "Metropolitan Explosion and Urban Degradation in India", *Free Press Journal,* June 2000. Mumbai, Edit Page Article, p. 6.

Mukherji, Shekhar (2000h), "Population Explosion and Its Consequences", *Free Press Journal*, Sept 2000, Edit Page Article. p. 4.

Mukherji, Shekhar (2001a), "Poverty-Induced Migration and Urban Involution in ESCAP Region: Required Planning Strategies." Research Monograph No 25, International Institute for Population Sciences, Mumbai, March 2001, pp. 1-165.

Mukherji, Shekhar (2001b), "Causal Linkages between Migration, Urbanization and Regional Disparities in India: Planning Strategies Required," International Institute for Population Sciences (IIPS). Research Monograph No. 28, Mumbai, March 2001, pp. 1-225.

Mukherji, Shekhar (2001c), "Causal Linkages between Migration to Cities and Regional Disparities in India: Processes and Planning Strategies", IUSSP Population Conference, Salvadore, Bahia, Brazil, August 18-24, pp. 1-24.

Mukherji, Shekhar (2002), "Urbanization and Migration in India: A Different Scene", in *International Handbook of Urban Systems*, by H.S. Geyer (ed.), Edward Elgar, Cheltenham, U.K., 2002, Chapter 20, pp. 525-559.

Mukherji, Shekhar (2005a), *Poverty and Population in India,* Professor R.N. Dubey Memorial Lectures, 2004, Professor R.N. Dubey Foundation, Allahabad, pp. 1-95.

Mukherji, Shekhar (2005b), "The Syndrome of Poverty and High Fertility in India: Programmes for Poverty Eradication and Health Services", in *Poverty and Population in India* by Shekhar Mukherji, Professor R.N. Dubey Memorial Lectures, 2004, Professor R.N. Dubey Foundation, Allahabad, pp. 1-38.

Mukherji, Shekhar (2005c), "Syndrome of Poverty and High Fertility in India", in *Poverty and Population in India,* by Shekhar Mukherji, Professor R.N. Dubey Memorial Lectures, 2004, Professor R.N. Dubey Foundation, Allahabad, pp. 38-75.

Mukherji, Shekhar (2005d), "Distressed Migration and Urban Decay in India", in *Poverty and Population in India,* by Shekhar Mukherji, Professor R.N. Dubey Memorial Lectures, 2004, Professor R.N. Dubey Foundation, Allahabad, pp. 76-95.

Mukherji, Shekhar (2005e), "Distressed Migration and Urban Involution in India", *Oriental Geographer, Golden Jubilee Volume*, December 2005, Department of Geography, University of Dhaka, Dhaka, Chapter 2, pp. 25-50.

Mukherji, Shekhar (2005f), "Distressed Migration and Urban Decay in Some Asian Metropolises: Phenomena, Processes, and Planning", in Felicitation Volume of Prof L.R. Singh, Department of Urban and Regional Planning, University of Akron, USA, 2006 (forthcoming), pp. 1-30.

Mukherji, Shekhar (2005g), "Poverty Index and High Fertility in India", Paper, International Conference on Geography and Environment, Department of Geography, University of Dhaka, Dhaka, December 6-12, 2005, pp. 1-25 (forthcoming in a journal).

Mukherji, Shekhar (2006), *Migration and Urban Decay: Asian Experiences*, Rawat Publications, Jaipur and New Delhi, pp. 298-325.

National Institute of Rural Development (NIRD) (1999), "Rural Development Programmes", in *India: Rural Development Report, 1999, Regional Disparities in Development and Poverty*, NIRD, Hyderabad, Chapter 6, pp. 99-122.

National Family and Health Survey (NFHS) (1994), *Report of the National Family and Health Survey of Uttar Pradesh*. Population Research Centre, Lucknow, and International Institute for Population Sciences (IIPS), Mumbai, Chapters 6, 8, and 9, pp. 1-112.

National Family and Health Survey (NFHS-I) (1994), *India: Introductory Report, NFHS-I Survey*, IIPS, Mumbai.

NFHS (1995), *National Health and Family Survey-I, India (1992-93),* Mumbai, IIPS, 1995 (data sources and reports).

NFHS (2000), *National Health and Family Survey-II, India (1998-99),* Mumbai, IIPS, 2000 (data sources and reports).

Nayyar, Gaurav (2005), "Growth and Poverty in Rural India: An Analysis of Inter-State Differences", *Economic and Political Weekly,* April 16, pp. 1631-1639.

Parasuraman, Sulbha, Roy, T.K., Radha Devi, D. et al. (1999), *Role of Women's Education in Shaping Fertility in India: Evidences from NFHS*, Himalayan Publishing House, pp. 134-136.

Parikh, Kirit S. and Radhakrishna R. (eds.) (2005), "Overview: Ten years of Reforms, What Next?", in *India Development Report, 2004-05,* by Parikh, Kirit S. and Radhakrishna R. (eds.), Indira Gandhi Institute of Development Research, Oxford University Press, New Delhi, pp. 1-20.

Patodia, D.N. (2006), "Catch an Elephant by its Ears: India Must Act Fast if it Wants to Take Advantage of Economic Reforms", *Hindustan Times,* Edit Page Article, p. 10.

Phillips, Warren (1972), "Understanding Canonical Analysis", Department of Political Science, The Ohio State University, Columbus, Ohio, (mimeo), pp. 1-21.

Popli, G., Parikh, A. and Palmer-Jones, R. (2005), "Are the 2000 Poverty Estimates for India a Myth, Artefact or Real?", *Economic and Political Weekly,* October 22, pp. 4619-4624.

Pyle, Gerald F. (1974), *The Spatial Dynamics of Crime*, University of Chicago, Department of Geography, Research Paper No. 159, Chicago, pp. 21-101, and 107-141.

Radhakrishna, R. and Ray, Shovan (2005), "Poverty in India: Dimensions and Character", in *India Development Report, 2004-05,* by Parikh and Radhakrishna (eds.), ibid., pp. 40-61.

Rama Rao, G. Ladusingh, L. and Pritamjit, Rajkumar (2004), "Nutritional Status of Children in North-East India", *Asia-Pacific Population Journal,* September 2004, pp. 39-55.

Ramos, Fidel (2006), "Beneath the Embers: Forgotten Side of War on Terrorism", *Times of India,* February 3, Edit Page Article and Project Syndicate, 2006, p. 30.

Rao, Mohan (2006), "Saffron Demography: Hindu Communalists Spread Population Myths", *Times of India,* Edit Page article, April 20, 2006, p. 30.

Rummel, R.J. (1965), "A Field Theory of Social Action with Application to Conflict within Nations", *General Systems*, Vol. 10, (1965), pp. 183-197.

Rummel, R.J. (1970), *Applied Factor Analysis*, Northwestern University Press, Evanston, pp. 17, 121-123, 343-345.

Rummel, R.J. (1974), "Population Policies and Demographic Change: Dimensions, Projections, and Linkages", Paper, PATH Institute, Honolulu, Hawaii, USA pp. 1-18.

Rummel, R.J. (1975), "Analysing Population Policy and Demographic Change", A Research Proposal for National Science Foundation (USA), Dimensionality of Nation's Project, Department of Political Science, University of Hawaii, Honolulu, Hawaii, pp. 1-46 (mimeographed).

Rummel, R.J. (1975), *Dynamic Psychological Field: A Psycho-Philosophical Prolegomenon to the Dynamics of Conflict and War*, Sage Publishers Los Angeles.

Rummel, R.J. and Mukherji, Shekhar (1981), *Analysing Population Policy and Demographic Change*, Prajna Publishers, Kolkata, pp. 1-81.

Rummel, R.J. (1979), *Field Theory Evolving*, Sage Publishers, Los Angeles.

Saith, Ashwani (2005), "Poverty Lines versus the Poor: Method versus Meaning", *Economic and Political Weekly*, October 22, pp. 4601-4510.

Sarkar, Avhirup (2006), "Lessons from the History of America's Recession in the Thirties: For India's Rural Employment Guarantee Programmes", *Ananda Bazar Patrika* (in Bengali), February 8, Edit Page Article, p. 5.

Sarkar, Avirup (2006), "Exceptional and Straightforward: A Critique of the Book on Development with Dignity" by Amit Bhaduri (in Bengali), *Desh:* A Bengali Fortnightly, April 12, 2006, pp. 95-96.

Sample Registration Survey, Census of India (2005), *Statistical Report of 2003, Report 2 of 2005,* Sample Registration Survey Unit, Office of Registrar General and Census Commissioner of India, New Delhi, 2005, pp. 45-49.

Save The Children (STC) (2006), *Global Report on Infant Mortality,* Save The Children Committee, London, U.K.

Schwind, Paul J. (1975), "A General Field Theory of Migration", *Economic Geography*, Vol. 51, No. 1, January 1975, pp. 1-18.

Sen, Pranab (2005), "Of Calories and Things: Reflections on Nutritional Norms, Poverty Lines, and Consumption Behaviour in India", *Economic and Political Weekly,* October 22, pp. 4611-4618.

Sharma, Benita (2006), "Budgets, and the Invisible Woman", *Times of India*, February 28, Edit Page Article, p. 32.

Singh, Amarendra P. and Sharma, J.K. (2006), "Management Strategies for Promotion of Agriculture", *Journal of Rural Development*, Vol. 24 (4), pp. 445-458.

Srinivasan, K. (1988), "Modernisation, Contraception and Fertility Change in India", *International Family Planning Perspectives,* Vol. 14, No. 3, pp. 94-101.

Srinivasan, K. (2006), "Population Policies and Family Planning Programmes in India: A Review and Recommendations", Fifth Dr C. Chandrasekhar Memorial Lecture, International Institute for Population Sciences, Mumbai (February 3, 2006), IIPS Newsletter, October 2006, pp. 1-25.

Times of India (2006), "Cradle of Hunger: Child Malnutrition Rampant in Maharashtra and Elsewhere", Edit Page Article, April 19, p. 30.

Udupa, K.N. and Mukherji, Shekhar (1988), *Knowledge and Utilization of Primary Health Services by Rural Women of Varanasi District*, Indian Council of Medical Research (ICMR) Health Project, Institute of Medical Sciences, Banaras Hindu University, Varanasi, pp. 1-175.

UNICEF (2005), *The State of the World's Children, 2006,* UNICEF, United Nations, New York, December 14, 2005,

United Nations (1973), *Determinants and Consequences of Rapid Population Growth: New Findings,* New York, N.Y. pp. 4-9.

United Nations (1977), *Report of the Expert Group Meeting on Population Growth and Economic Development in Sub-national Areas,* Asian Studies No 40, UN-ESCAP, Bangkok, pp 17-18.

United Nations (1992), *World Population Monitoring, 1991*, U.N. Dept. of International Economic and Social Affairs, New York, N.Y., pp. 51-83.

United Nations (1993), *World Population Monitoring, 1992,* New York, N.Y.

United Nations Fund For Population Activities (UNFPA) (1994), *Programme of Action of International Conference on Population and Development (Cairo Conference)*, United Nations, New York.

United Nations (1997), *Human Development Report, 1997*, New York, N.Y.

United Nations (1998), *Human Development Report, 1998,* United Nations Development Programme (UNDP), United Nations, New York.

United Nations Development Programme (UNDP) (2003), *Human Development Report 2003*, UNDP, Oxford University Press, New Delhi.

United Nations Millennium Project (2005), *Investing in Development: A Practical Plan to Achieve the Millennium Development Goals,* United Nations Development Programmes, New York.

United Nations (2005), *Summary: Human Development Report 2005: International Cooperation at a Crossroads – Aid, Trade, and Security in an Unequal World*, UNDP, United Nations, 2005, pp. 19-26.

Vivekananda, Swami (1893), *Complete Works of Swami Vivekananda, Centenary Volumes, 1963, Volume I,* Udbodhan Karyalaya, Kolkata, p. 480, and various pages.

Vivekananda, Swami (1894), *Complete Works of Swami Vivekananda, Centenary Volumes, 1963, Volume II,* Udbodhan Karyalaya, Kolkata, pp 85-86, and various pages.

Vivekananda, Swami (1894), *Complete Works of Swami Vivekananda, Centenary Volumes, 1963, Volume III*, Udbodhan Karyalaya, Kolkata, p. 142, 224, 247, 318, 461, and various pages.

Vivekananda, Swami (1894), *Complete Works of Swami Vivekananda, Centenary Volumes, 1963, Volume IV*, Udbodhan Karyalaya, Kolkata, p. 246, 351, 367, 480, and various pages.

Vivekananda, Swami (1895), *Complete Works of Swami Vivekananda, Centenary Volumes, 1963, Volume V*, Udbodhan Karyalaya, Kolkata, pp. 17, 23, 51, 64, 23-24, 30, and various pages.

Vivekananda, Swami (1895), *Complete Works of Swami Vivekananda, Centenary Volumes, 1963, Volume VI*, Udbodhan Karyalaya, Kolkata, pp 61-62, 135, 264, 297, 384, and various pages.

Vivekananda, Swami (1895), *Complete Works of Swami Vivekananda, Centenary Volumes, 1963, Volume VII*, Udbodhan Karyalaya, Kolkata, p. 247, 447, and various pages.

Vivekananda, Swami (1896), *Complete Works of Swami Vivekananda, Centenary Volumes, 1963, Volume VIII*, Udbodhan Karyalaya, Kolkata, p. 150, 348, and various pages.

Wolpert Julian (1965), "Behavioural Aspects of the Decision to Migrate", Papers, Regional Science Association, Vol. 15, pp. 152-180.

Wood, Donald A. (1973) "Toward the Interpretations of Canonical Dimensions", *Multivariate Behavioural Research*, Vol. 7, No. 4, October 1973, pp. 477-482.

World Bank (1990), *World Development Report 1990: Poverty, World Development Indicators,* The World Bank, Washington D.C., pp. 56-89.

World Bank (1991), "Gender and Poverty in India", World Bank Working Paper, The World Bank, Washington D.C., pp. 21-35.

World Bank (1993), *World Development Report, 1993*, New York.

World Bank (1996), *India: Five Years of Stabilization and Reforms and the Challenges Ahead*, A World Bank Country Study, The World Bank, Washington D.C., pp. 77-98.

World Bank (1997), *World Development Report 1997: The State in a Changing World*, The World Bank, Washington D.C., pp. 111-130.

World Bank (2003), *World Development Report 2003, Sustainable Development in a Dynamic World: Transforming Institutions, Growth and Quality of Life*, The World Bank, Washington D.C., pp. 83-106.

World Bank (2003), "India's Sustaining Reforms, Reducing Poverty," *Development Policy Review*, July, The World Bank, Washington D.C., pp. 1-21, 23-45.

Zachariah, K.C., Rajan, Irudiya S., Sharma, P.S. et al. (1994), *Demographic Transition in Kerala in the 1980s,* Centre of Development Studies Monograph, Center for Development Studies, Thiruvananthapuram.

Index

Index